D0765738

Health Services Planning

Second Edition

Health Services Planning
Second Edition

Richard K. Thomas, Ph.D.

Kluwer Academic / Plenum Publishers
New York • Boston • London • Dordrecht • Moscow

ISBN 0-306-47804-8

© 2003 by Kluwer Academic/Plenum Publishers, New York
233 Spring Street, New York, New York 10013

http://www.kluweronline.com

10 9 8 7 6 5 4 3 2 1

A C.I.P. record for this book is available from the Library of Congress.

All rights reserved.

No part of this work may be reproduced, stored in a retrieval system, or transmitted in any form or
by any means, electronic, mechanical, photocopying, microfilming, recording, or otherwise, without
written permission from the Publisher, with the exception of any material supplied specifically for the
purpose of being entered and executed on a computer system, for exclusive use by the purchaser of
the work.

Permissions for books published in Europe: permissions@wkap.nl
Permissions for books published in the United States of America: permissions@wkap.com

Printed in the United States of America.

Preface to the Second Edition

When *Health Services Planning* was originally published in 1999, it was intended to fill a void that existed in the literature on the planning of health services. Its publication was also a response to developments in U.S. society in general and healthcare in particular that created an urgent need for the pursuit of at least some level of health planning. The 1990s had witnessed continued fragmentation of the public healthcare system and the introduction of new challenges such as the reemergence of long dormant communicable diseases. The growing number of uninsured individuals threatened to severely damage our ability to provide care. The closure of numerous hospitals and a large number of bankruptcies among healthcare organizations provided further evidence of the lack of planning for future exigencies.

Since that time the situation in the United States has further deteriorated in many ways, making the need for health planning even more urgent. Serious shortcomings in the public health arena have been identified and "safety net" hospitals have increasingly lost their ability to handle the overwhelming demand for their services. The Medicaid program is facing serious challenges and the ability of Medicare to sustain itself for the long run has been questioned. Add to this the threat of bioterrorism attacks and a public health data system that is of limited effectiveness and we have a situation that is ripe for disaster. Belatedly, federal and state agencies are attempting to "plan" for the possibility of a nuclear, biological, or chemical attack, but even here the efforts are uncoordinated and lacking in consistency nationwide.

Increasingly, the success stories spawned by the U.S. healthcare "system" are offset by reports of the inefficiencies and lack of effectiveness that continue to characterize it. Much of the confusion, wheel spinning, and missteps characterizing our healthcare system can be attributed to a lack of planning both systemwide and on the part of individual organizations. In an environment that is undergoing constant evolution and experiencing rapid change on many fronts, decision-makers require a framework for action. Without a plan in place, it is difficult if not impossible to make rational decisions.

Responsible parties in both the public and private sectors have come to realize that a systematic approach to the issues faced by healthcare is essential, and the 1990s witnessed a surge of interest in health services planning. As we enter the 21st century, the growing demand for community-based solutions to critical health problems has begun to create an environment supportive of public sector planning. Many daring individuals are even beginning to use the "p" word again. In the private sector, increasing competition, declining reimbursement, and a variety of other market forces are encouraging healthcare organizations to consider a planning-oriented response. The industry trend toward data-driven decision making is providing additional impetus for this movement. While there is still some resistance to "planning" per se, planning activities are emerging under the heading of "strategic initiatives," "business development," or some other moniker.

While planning may not be a panacea for all of the problems facing healthcare, it would certainly directly address issues related to cost, accessibility, and efficiency. Clearly, the less desirable characteristics of the system such as fragmentation, duplication, and lack of continuity can only be addressed within a planning framework.

This second edition of *Health Services Planning* retains the basic structure of the original. However, its contents have been systematically updated to reflect developments that have occurred in healthcare and health planning since the late 1990s. Some sections have been expanded and others contracted based on reader response to the first edition and developments in the field. The Additional Resources lists at the end of each chapter have been expanded to include relevant Web sites. Additional boxes have been added to provide more in the way of case studies.

If anything, the audience for a book such as this should be larger than for the first edition. The needs have become greater and the search for solutions more frantic. Health planning is increasingly seen as an issue not just for health professionals and government bureaucrats but also for people in many sectors of society who are affected by the deficiencies in the U.S. healthcare system. Hopefully, this revised work will provide the foundation for approaching health services planning for a wide range of concerned individuals.

The publication of this second edition of *Health Services Planning* reflects the input of a wide range of health professionals who, each in their own way, have contributed to the advancement of the field of health services planning. This includes those individuals in public sector environments who doggedly pursue to aims of health planning, often against overwhelming odds. It also includes those in healthcare organizations within the private healthcare sector who have pioneered the use of planning approaches in their particular domains. The experiences of individuals who are concerned over the state of the U.S. healthcare system and see planning as a means for addressing many of these concerns have provided useful material for this book. Their input in the form of anecdotes, suggestions, citations, and directions to resource materials have been invaluable.

I would particularly like to express appreciation to my friends and colleagues involved with the American Health Planning Association. The members of this organization have continued to carry the banner for health planning in the United States even when it hasn't been a popular cause to espouse. Their insistence on the importance of a planning approach for resolving the many issues facing healthcare in America has been inspiring. They have faithfully continued to preserve planning "lore" even when anti-planning interests appeared to hold sway.

Hopefully, this book will encourage a new generation of healthcare professionals to come to understand the important role that planning can play in creating a more efficient and more effective healthcare system. If this book can make some small contribution toward creating the type of healthcare system that Americans want and deserve, it will have been well worth the effort.

RICHARD K. THOMAS

Contents

I

Introduction to Health Services Planning

"Health services planning" is a term that is being used with increasing frequency today, reflecting the growing interest in the topic as we enter the 21st century. However, the term means different things to different people. In some cases it may refer to a vague notion of social engineering applied to healthcare. In others, it may refer to an activity as specific as the operation of a certificate-of-need process or the design of a health facility. A review of the planning literature reveals a variety of definitions in use, in fact, as well as cases in which the author does not even offer a definition. Indeed, there is little consensus among experts as to the definition of health planning and the concept is continuously being redefined as planning tries to "find itself" in the new millennium.

Health services planning has not been applied as extensively in the United States as it has in other developed countries. For that reason, it is appropriate to start from the beginning and present the basic concepts used in the field. The sections that follow in this chapter review the nature of planning in general and health services planning in particular. These sections are followed by a discussion of the issues surrounding health services planning in the contemporary healthcare environment.

WHAT IS PLANNING?

Let's begin with a basic definition of planning and work toward a more healthcare-specific version. A useful working definition would read as follows:

> *Planning is a process whereby a coordinated and comprehensive mechanism is developed for the efficient allocation of resources to meet a specific goal or goals.*

Regardless of the context, the various components of this definition can be applied. First, planning represents a process. In fact, the process may be viewed by some as more important than the outcome. Planning implies that attempts are made to coordinate the various aspects of the system being addressed. Further, planning activities are comprehensive in their approach in that they consider all relevant variables. Ultimately, the intent of the planning process is to achieve certain identified goals and to do this through the efficient allocation of available resources.

WHAT IS A PLAN?

Given this definition of planning, how, then, would a plan be defined? The plan is obviously the concrete product of the planning process, but this definition oversimplifies the significance of a plan. The printed product that results from the planning process should represent the formal codification of the plan. It provides the context in which planning should take place and should serve as a blueprint for reaching a specified goal or goals.

More importantly, the plan should serve as a context for decision making. Within the framework of the plan, administrators, planners, and business development staff should be able to systematically propose and implement any type of project. The plan provides the "criteria" for decision making by laying out the goals and objectives of the community or organization and specifying the point at which the community or the organization would like to be at some specified time in the future.

The planning process itself has substantial merit, even in the absence of a completed plan. In fact, it could be argued that a true plan is never completed. Completion implies the creation of a static document within the context of a dynamic environment. The plan should always be evolving and, in fact, it is virtually always the case that a plan is revised even before it is published. Similarly, it is seldom the case that certain objectives specified in the plan are not met either partially or fully prior to the plan being finalized.

Another reason for focusing on the process (planning) rather than the outcome (the plan) is because of the benefits that accrue from the process itself. The very act of going through the planning process forces a community or organization to examine who they are, what they are doing, and why they are doing it. Often, the by-products of the planning process are more important to the organization than the plan itself. This notion is summarized in a quote attributed to the British statesman Benjamin Disraeli who contended: "The plan is nothing; planning is everything."

WHAT IS HEALTH SERVICES PLANNING?

Having defined planning in a generic sense, how, then, should we define health services planning? Health services planning might be described as follows:

Health services planning is a process that appraises the overall health needs of a geographic area or population and determines how these needs can be met in the most effective manner through the allocation of existing and anticipated future resources.

As will be seen, this definition probably fits the notion of community-wide planning better than it does organization-level planning. Yet, the same concept applies to both. Ultimately, all planning comes down to identifying the needs of the target population (however defined) and then determining the best means for meeting those needs.

HOW IS HEALTH SERVICES PLANNING DIFFERENT?

Healthcare as an institution in U.S. society is unique in many ways. This uniqueness creates a special situation for the industry with regard to planning. Elasticity in the level of demand presents a challenge to health planners, and the fact that health services providers are often dealing with life-and-death situations adds an emotional dimension to the planning of health services not found in other arenas.

Healthcare is also set apart by the manner in which the industry is organized. The industry involves literally hundreds of thousands of essentially autonomous entities operating in a virtually uncoordinated manner. The various providers have limited incentives with regard to the coordination of efforts and are seldom constrained by any centralized agent of control. Most operate independently of most of the other organizations involved in the provision of care. Even within an organization such as a hospital, the number of separate "kingdoms" is astounding. Many of these internal departments actually work at cross-purposes with each other. Relationships within the organization are complex, and this alone creates a difficult planning environment.

Healthcare also is characterized by a wide variety of different customers and the nature of these customers varies from industry segment to industry segment. Patients represent only one group of customers, and an entity like a large hospital may have a dozen different customer groups with which to contend. Further, the various players in the industry have diverse objectives, some of which may be contrary to the objectives of other players.

The financial characteristics of healthcare also set it apart from other industries, with healthcare representing an exception to just about every "law" of economics. The role played by third-party payors is certainly unique, and the consequent indirectness characterizing decision-making confounds the planning process. The fact that the end-user may not make the consumption decision or pay for the service provided certainly creates a challenging context for health services planning.

Perhaps the most important factor that differentiates healthcare from other industries is the diversity of functions that often characterize healthcare providers. Not only do different entities perform different functions, but a single entity like a hospital will perform multiple functions simultaneously. For example, how does a church-sponsored hospital, for example, reconcile its mission of service and caring with the need to generate revenue above and beyond its expenses?

The obvious function of the health care system and its component organizations is to provide for the healthcare needs of the population. This is carried out most directly through patient care, and patient care is what comes to mind when we envision the healthcare system. However, there are thousands of healthcare organizations that are not involved in patient care. Even those who do provide care often serve a variety of functions. Many see themselves primarily as providing a community service; others see their role as essentially humanitarian. Some entities see themselves as contributing to the safety of the public, perhaps best exemplified by the various public health programs. Some organizations are clearly interested in the furtherance of certain religious perspectives, and others see themselves performing a social welfare role.

These examples do not include the economic functions that the healthcare system and its component organizations perform. Certainly the redistribution of resources and the creation of wealth and jobs are important. On the other hand, teaching and research are specifically designated functions of the healthcare system.

Beyond these overt functions of the system, there are "latent" functions identified by observers. The healthcare system serves in many ways as a mechanism of social control, defining the characteristics of individuals that are considered by society to be "normal" and "abnormal". In all societies, the healthcare system serves as an integrating mechanism for society, bringing the population together in response to illness and implicitly enforcing group values. The system also plays a role in explaining the "why" of sickness and death.

From any perspective, healthcare is not the typical industry. As an industry it has unique characteristics that make the direct application of planning techniques from other industries difficult. Even at the organization level, the variety of types of organizations creates a challenge for any health services planner.

THE POLITICAL NATURE OF PLANNING

Ideally, planning should be an objective process driven by technical considerations. In actual practice, though, planning inevitably involves "someone's" idea of the way things should be. Even when the plan represents group consensus, it is still a product of this group and not some other group. Thus, plans are never going to be completely objective in their formulation or implementation. They are likely to represent a compromise among vested interests in the community or "competing" forces within the particular organization. In fact, the broad participation that is currently encouraged at both the community and organizational planning levels assures that the process will be at least partially political.

One reason that planning inevitably has a political dimension is that plans are seldom formulated just for the sake of planning. Some *thing* virtually always serves to initiate the planning process. At the community level, it may be a crisis related to publicly funded care, a communicable disease epidemic, or runaway costs of care. At the organization level, it may be a crisis within the organization, changes in the external environment, the actions of competitors, or any number of other developments. The process may be driven by the interests of a particular group or even an individual with a specific agenda. Indeed, some proponents of planning may have a preconceived notion of what the organization should do and will attempt to use the planning process to reach *their* goals.

It should be remembered that *most* healthcare decisions are political. The decision of a hospital to offer a particular service or add new technology, the decision of a medical group to affiliate with Hospital A rather than Hospital B, and the decision to locate a clinic in an affluent suburb rather than the inner city are all made based on political, social and economic considerations rather than clinical ones. So it should be no surprise that the planning process is also political. Any health services plan is going to reflect the influence of the political, social and economic considerations that come into play in that particular healthcare environment, and the plan that results always reflects the environment that spawned it. The challenge for the planner is to balance the objective, technical dimension of planning with the realities of the context in which planning is taking place.

WHO NEEDS HEALTH PLANNING?

There are few healthcare organizations in today's environment that could not benefit from planning. In fact, virtually every organization is going to have to rely on planning to assure its continued viability in the future. The environment has become much too unstable and unpredictable to allow the capricious forces therein to control the destiny of a healthcare organization or health system. The industry maxim has become: Control or be controlled.

In the public sector, every community clearly needs to plan for its healthcare needs. Resources for the provision of health services are limited and are likely to become more limited for the foreseeable future. The cost involved in providing care continues to rise, and a growing army of uninsured Americans will continue to place a strain on the system. The continued maldistribution of services makes access to care a growing problem, and increasing demands for accountability contribute to a need for health services planning at the community level.

At the organization level, it is difficult to imagine any healthcare organization being able to position itself for the future without a plan in place. From the largest national hospital chain to the one-person clinician's office, every entity must be able to control its future to the extent it can. Multi-purpose organizations like hospitals must develop plans that allow them to adapt to the changing environment and coordinate the various and diverse components of their systems. Conglomerates that are the product of a merger of previously independent organizations face a particular challenge in meshing the organizational structures of disparate entities.

Health professionals such as physicians, therapists, and other clinicians also face the need to lay out a systematic road map for reaching the future. Any number of examples can be provided of practitioners who found themselves in one kind of a difficulty or another for failing to plan for various contingencies. Other institutional providers, such as nursing homes, home health agencies, and assisted living facilities, must similarly be able to chart a well thought out course.

Health insurance plans, including managed care plans, must be able to determine their future direction and implement a plan for reaching their goals. No success in the future is going to come through happenstance; every organization must take an active role in "inventing" its future. Health plans face the same challenge confronting healthcare providers; they must control their destinies or be controlled by an unpredictable environment.

PLANNING FOR WHOM?

The parties for whom the plan is being developed depend on the nature of the plan and the parties involved in the planning process. In community-wide planning, the plan ostensibly benefits the entire healthcare system and, by extension, all citizens of the community. In theory at least, the community health plan should represent the greatest good for the greatest number. The goals should be the provision of better access to care for all citizens, more efficient operation of the system, and more effective outcomes from the expenditure of public funds.

At the organization planning level, the objectives are much narrower. At this level, the self-interests of the organization are clearly the issue, and organization-level plans focus on the future needs of the organization (and by extension its customers) independent of the needs of the community. Inevitably, certain departments or individuals may benefit more than others, but, presumably, the intent of the plan is to enhance the effectiveness of the organization in reaching its corporate goals.

While community-wide planning and organization-level planning may appear to have mutually exclusive constituents, it is unrealistic to assume that the can be implemented totally independent of each other. Community-wide planning must take into consideration the needs of all entities involved in the provision of care, including for-profit healthcare organizations. Indeed, one of the constraints imposed on the federally mandated health planning of the 1960s and 70s was that plan development would not interfere with established practice patterns. On the other hand, no healthcare organization operating in a local context can afford to ignore the concerns of the local community and the health plans established for that community. Even today, certificate-of-need requirements and other regulations constrain the actions of private-sector healthcare organizations in some communities. Ultimately, community-wide plans must incorporate the perspectives of all players in the healthcare arena, and organization-level plans must accommodate themselves to the broader plans formulated for the community.

WHY IS HEALTH PLANNING NEEDED?

A number of reasons can be cited to justify the development of health services plans, although there is on-going debate over the appropriateness of some justifications for planning. Ultimately, it could be argued that planning is a virtue in its own right and that this should be enough reason in itself. The benefits derived from going through the planning process are multiple, even if no formal plan ever materializes. Yet this fact alone would seldom justify the initiation of the process.

Planning serves to engender coordination among the various components of a system or the subunits of an organization. Coordination is understandably required to implement a plan, but it is just as important to the planning process. Planning further serves to instill discipline into the operation of the system or organization. By drawing attention to the processes that are involved, planning serves as a force for efficiency.

The plan provides a powerful means for allocating resources. Indeed, the *raison d'etre* for planning could be argued to be the appropriate allocation of resources for future needs. There are always more demands for resources than there are available resources, and, in today's environment, there are certainly more opportunities than there are resources to exploit them. While the plan does not directly determine the manner in which resources are to be allocated, it does provide the framework within which decisions on resource allocation can be made.

Planning also serves the purpose of getting issues "out on the table" that would not otherwise be discussed. The process provides a venue for raising issues that might otherwise be ignored in the press of day-to-day operations. It allows the presentation of these issues in a context where they can be given thoughtful consideration and viewed within a framework in which other, perhaps competing, issues are being considered.

Another important function of the planning process is the setting of priorities, whether at the community or organization level. Priority setting is an inherent task within the planning process and one that impacts all other aspects of the organization. There are always too many worthy projects and too few resources to go around. Only within the context of a systematic plan is it possible to prioritize the various tasks that need to be performed.

Another function of planning, particularly in today's environment, is that of cost control. The knowledge base generated as a result of the planning process can become a tool for cost containment. The emphasis on coordination, efficiency, and accountability inherent in every plan provides the opportunity to introduce measures that are more cost-effective than existing practices.

The plan also serves as a mechanism for introducing accountability at both the community and organization levels. Indeed, this is one of the attributes that generates the most resistance to the planning process. Not only will the background research for the plan thoroughly examine existing community or organizational practices, but the implementation schedule adopted as part of the plan will clearly lay out the necessary tasks and assign responsibility. In this manner, it introduces a measure of accountability not otherwise present.

Another important function of the planning process relates to the collection of data. It could be argued that 80 percent of the planning process is devoted to the compilation of the necessary data and 20 percent is devoted to actual planning. More than a quarter century of planning experience suggests that the process of identifying sources of data, reviewing existing data on the community or the organization, and ultimately using these data as a foundation for planning activities provide an opportunity for both planners and managers to examine issues from a perspective not previously available. During the heyday of community-wide planning in the 1960s and 1970s, the data that were available to health professionals were better than they have ever been before or since. By the same token, the data generated through the organization planning process produces information that might not otherwise be available. This author has never participated in an organization planning process in which some of the information collected did not elicit surprise and/or grave concern from the organization's staff.

One final reason for planning, and one that perhaps overrides all of the others, is the need to establish a framework for decision making. In the final analysis, most healthcare decisions are made in a vacuum or at least under conditions involving less than optimal information. Because of this vacuum, it has been argued that hospital administrators are historically characterized by one of two modes of activity:

paralysis or impulsiveness. The number of "wrong" decisions made by healthcare organizations whether representing the community or their own self-interests are too numerous to recount. Without a plan for guidance, the chances of making an inappropriate decision multiply.

In many cases, the failure to make a decision is worse than a wrong decision. Many communities have failed to take appropriate action to address a looming crisis. Many organizations have lost market share or important referral relationships due to their failure to take decisive action. Paralysis results from not having a framework within which to make decisions or the criteria with which to evaluate the options. When confronted with a choice, decision makers must have a context within which to evaluate the situation. They must be able to determine how the proposed initiative fits into their overall plans and contributes to the specified goals and objectives of the community or the organization. A great opportunity is not really an opportunity if it does not contribute to the ultimate ends being pursued. The plan helps establish the criteria necessary for evaluating any such opportunity. These criteria may relate to the organization's mission, its revenue targets, the strategic initiatives that it is pursuing, or any number of other factors. What is critical is that criteria be in place so that timely and informed decisions can be made.

WHY THE RESISTANCE TO PLANNING?

The merits of planning for a function as important as the provision of health services should be obvious, and every other developed country has significant health planning capacity. Yet resistance to planning in general and to health services planning in particular reflects a prevailing—yet paradoxical—attitude within U.S. society. Americans may even be accused of "plan phobia". Even though we pride ourselves in our investments in research and development, the planning horizons for most U.S. corporations are typically the next quarter. Long-term benefits are typically sacrificed to bolster quarterly earnings. Although healthcare is not quite as shortsighted as other sectors of the economy, this neglect of planning is clearly present in healthcare.

Why, we have to ask ourselves, are we as a society so opposed to planning? One would think that, with the values that permeate American society, we would be obsessed with planning. As a society, we emphasize *control* of our environment, *prediction* of future developments, operational *efficiency*, and *coordination* of activities. It is difficult to see how any of these conditions can be achieved without planning. Americans also emphasize *activism* (or the taking of a proactive approach to the situation), and a *future orientation* that encourages them to make investments that will pay dividends in the future. If these values were not enough to encourage a planning mindset, we could all agree that, as a society, we are obsessed with the economic bottom line. If nothing else, this emphasis on *profitability* should mandate a strong planning orientation. How else can one assure control of the factors that are likely to affect long-term success? While other societies publish five- and ten-year plans for economic development, social programs, and other society-wide initiatives, no such federal planning activity takes place in the U.S. While foreign corporations are developing twenty-year plans, American corporations are obsessed with quarterly earnings.

Given the dominant traits of American society, how can we explain this phobia when it comes to planning? A number of explanations are offered for this resistance to planning. At the federal level (and down the governmental hierarchy to the community level) there is an almost irrational apprehension about the participation of government in the coordination of society's activities. The dominant philosophy in the economic system stems from a belief in the power of the "market" to drive institutions in the appropriate direction. Because of the influence of the economic system on U.S. society, this philosophy spills over into other areas including healthcare. Centralized planning is often equated with socialism and, at best, is thought to interfere with the operation of established patterns of service delivery. This perspective is reinforced by a widespread distrust of government on the part of the American people.

U.S. society is controlled for the most part by coalitions of special interest groups, and these groups greatly influence the operation of American institutions. Systematic attempts at planning run counter to the notion of "deal-making" that drives everything from national politics to corporate decision making to the development of health services. At the same time, the introduction of planning raises the specter of accountability for many groups that would rather toil in anonymity.

Nowhere is the lack of planning in the U.S. more obvious than in healthcare. In no other industry have the extant problems been so directly attributed to problems of coordination, communication, and cooperation. Virtually all of the problems that have dogged the healthcare industry—from fragmentation to duplication of services to ineffective data management—can be attributed to a failure to plan. Most important, the high cost of healthcare can also be attributed in great part to a lack of planning.

The healthcare industry is clearly characterized by some of the same apprehensions as U.S. society in general when it comes to planning. Certainly there is resistance to centralized coordination of activities that might be viewed as government "meddling". There is insistence that the market be left to drive the system, despite the general failure of this approach to appropriately direct the healthcare system in the past.

In healthcare, this concern over interference and accountability is magnified. In no other industry does one find so many autonomous entities with different agendas ostensibly attempting to contribute to a common goal. Within the hospital alone, there are many entities more concerned about their own welfare than they are about what should be the common goals of the organization.

Healthcare is also unique in that it is the only institution run essentially by "technicians." These technicians are clinicians—particularly the physicians who make most of the decisions—who argue that bureaucrats and administrators are not competent to make decisions and set policy for the healthcare system. Clinicians are "doers" who have little patience for drawn-out planning processes. Further, clinicians are inherently conservative in their approach; while ostensibly welcoming innovations in healthcare, they also resist any changes in practice patterns. This inherent conservatism works against the development of plans that carry the risk of upsetting the status quo.

One of the presumably beneficial functions of planning, the introduction of controls, has also been cited as a basis for resistance. The development of a plan implies the intention to control the future actions of members of the community or the organization. This not only applies to underlings who are expected to operationalize the plan (and perhaps radically change their day-to-day lives) but to top management as well. Corporate executives are, in effect, being directed by virtue of the plan to follow a particular course. Even if the plan offers very general guidelines for the future direction of the organization, management may see this as an infringement on their authority and a limitation on their ability to make mid-course adjustments in the operation of the organization.

Finally, there is the concern over the costs involved in the planning health services. This concern exists with regard to both community-wide and organization planning. The planning process is expensive in terms of both direct costs and indirect costs. Yet, at the same time, the costs of *not* planning have been found to be even greater when the implications for efficiency and effectiveness in the absence of planning are quantified.

WHAT A PLAN IS NOT

Whenever the issue of planning arises, the inevitable initial response is that "the last plan is gathering dust on the shelf." This reaction reflects a general failure to recognize what a plan is and is not. Even planners have not always appreciated this distinction, and it is understandable that many plans have remained unimplemented in the past.

A true plan should not be a static document. In fact, it should not be a document at all but the embodiment of a process. A plan is not a plan if it is not dynamic, evolving with the changing environment. Similarly, a true plan is not rigid but is extremely flexible. After all, the intent is not to anticipate and plan for every potential development, but to create a framework in which new developments can be addressed. A true plan is not a cookbook with step-by-step instructions for reaching a specified point in the future. It should embody the principles necessary for achieving the goals of the community or the organization.

Perhaps the best analogy compares planning to water safety. A plan should not be a life preserver to save a drowning swimmer but the swimming lessons that prepare the swimmer for any exigency. Thus, the plan does not provide the ultimate solution but offers the mechanism for finding the solution.

THE PLANNING TIME HORIZON

The question arises as to how far into the future one should peer when developing a plan. There is no one answer to this question, and for any type of plan it probably makes sense to think in terms of short-range, intermediate-range, and long-range planning. At a minimum, five years should be considered as the planning time frame. If a community health system is being planned, a twenty-year plan may be appropriate for systematically addressing the long-term development of the system, although from a pragmatic perspective that type of time horizon may not be practical in today's healthcare environment. Further, one is not likely to have adequate data for projecting more than five or ten years into the future.

In any case, a plan should be flexible enough to adapt to shifts in the environment, a factor that often encourages a shorter time horizon. However, the one- or two-year planning horizon typical of the industry is probably too short to adequately introduce the infrastructure changes necessary for advancing the state of the healthcare system. The issue of time horizons is discussed further in the respective chapters on community health planning and organization-level planning.

HEALTH SERVICE IN TODAY'S ENVIRONMENT

What is it about today's healthcare environment that is encouraging an interest in planning not witnessed for 20 years? Why is this happening at this point in time? There are numerous factors that could explain the growing urgency surrounding the planning of health services at all levels, but perhaps the most compelling reason is the increasing instability and lack of predictability pervading today's healthcare environment.

The primary impetus for planning can be summed up by reference to the paradigm shift that is occurring in U.S. healthcare. Most of the developments in recent years in healthcare can probably be attributed to the shift that has been occurring from an emphasis on "medical care" to a new emphasis on "healthcare". Medical care is narrowly defined and refers primarily to those functions that are under the influence of medical doctors. This paradigm reflects the underlying philosophy of care that evolved from germ theory at the beginning of this century. Medical care focuses on the clinical aspects of healthcare and neglects the non-medical aspects of sickness and health.

Healthcare refers to any activty that might be directly or indirectly related to preserving, maintaining, and/or enhancing health status. This concept includes not only the formal activities historically associated with the operation of the health-care system, but also such informal activities as preventive behavior, exercise, and diet. This paradigm shift has been boosted by the growing appreciation of the nonmedical aspects of healthcare and a new appreciation of the connection between lifestyle and health status. More than any other factor, however, has been the realization that mainstream American medicine built upon the old disease the-ory system was increasingly unsuited for the management of the new category of health problems that emerged during the last quarter of the 20th century. (This paradigm shift is discussed further in Chapter 3.)

In the final analysis, the historical lack of planning in healthcare itself pro-vides the best justification for future planning. When one considers the level of expenditures for health services and the fact that much of this is a result of inef-ficiencies in the operation of the system, it is hard to argue against a systematic approach to the challenges facing the industry. It could be argued that the United States spends enough money to provide "Cadillac" care to every man, woman, and child in the country, if the funds were appropriately managed and allocated. Yet, many citizens do without treatment or medication, millions of Americans do not have a personal physician, and the number of medically uninsured is estimated at over 40 million Americans.

By the same token, the importance of healthcare to our society—and our economy—would seem to make careful planning mandatory. To paraphrase a fa-miliar quote, "Healthcare is too important to be left to clinicians." While clinicians should not be excluded from the process, the planning perspective calls for a much wider view of the situation than has historically prevailed. When one considers the percentage of the population involved in the system and the cost of providing health services, the absence of a planning process seems totally unacceptable.

Healthcare is undergoing such rapid change that every new wave of reorga-nization leads to a different set of needs. The emergence of managed care alone spawned the need for a completely different set of planning agendas. Who would have thought that hospital administrators would ever say: "The only good bed is an empty bed"? Or that marketers would be asked to find the healthiest patients and not the sickest? Healthcare professionals in all types of organizations are faced with understanding an environment that is increasingly foreign to the industry.

As we enter the 21st century, most healthcare organizations are at a critical juncture. Their success depends increasingly upon their ability to adapt to a new environment. The situation calls for adopting a completely different mindset, a mindset in keeping with the anticipated industry developments of the new mil-lennium. Adapting to changes of this magnitude "on the fly" will not be a viable approach in the future. The rapidity of change and the significance of the decisions that must be made mandate a well-conceived framework for decision making in the form of community-wide and organizational-level plans.

There is an immediate need to reeducate healthcare professionals on the theories, methods and data used in health services planning, and this represents another reason for developing a planning agenda. Just as the hospital must be reengineered for the new environment, health professionals must be reeducated in order to continue to contribute to the planning process.

All of these factors make both the revitalization of health services planning and the timing of this book particularly appropriate. The problems extant in healthcare discussed in this chapter suggest a need for a new approach. The significance of decision making for any organization is much greater than in the past. It is one thing to be able to plan for the provision of health services in a stable, predictable environment. It is quite another matter to develop plans in the midst of an unstable, unpredictable environment. These activities raise the importance of planning within the healthcare organization several notches. The consequences of a wrong decision can be fatal for a healthcare organization. Both the demands being placed on the health services plan and the consequences of the actions of planners are reaching unprecedented levels.

The good news is that the capabilities for carrying out planning activities within healthcare have greatly improved. After a decade of missteps, some sound methodologies for health services planning have finally been established. Health-related data are becoming more readily available to support decision making by healthcare executives. Appropriate technology is increasingly available for application to the challenge of planning.

Since the initial publication of this book, the on-going deficiencies in the U.S. healthcare system have been punctuated by some dramatic events that have exposed the weaknesses of the system. These developments have created an environment that makes health services planning more important than ever before and the potential consequences of not planning greater than they have ever been.

2

An Overview of Health Planning

It is appropriate to start our discussion of health services planning by providing an overview of this function as carried out in the past and present. In Chapter 1 the nature of planning was discussed, and this chapter introduces the reader to various types of planning that might be considered under the general heading of health services planning. It summarizes the history of health services planning in the United States and provides an overview of its current status in this country.

For our purposes, health services planning will be divided into planning that takes place at the community level and planning at the organization level. This distinction between community-wide planning and organization-level planning will be maintained throughout the book. While the actual process of planning is quite similar, the objectives, the players, and the beneficiaries are quite different.

COMMUNITY-WIDE PLANNING

Community-wide planning involves the development of a health services plan that focuses on the total healthcare system that serves a designated geographic area. The starting point and the emphasis is the community and not the organizational players within that healthcare environment. This type of planning is called by a variety of names, most frequently comprehensive planning or system-level planning. The term "system-level" is confusing since it has come to be used in relation to large healthcare organizations that have structured themselves as "systems". Thus, the term "community-wide planning" will be used to refer to this type of planning activity.

A number of characteristics can be ascribed to community-wide planning. This form of planning is ostensibly comprehensive in its approach. The total system of care, defined in its broadest sense, should be considered in this process, with the "comprehensive health planning" initiatives of the 1960s and 1970s prototypical of this approach. At the same time, the total population is ostensibly the target of this process, and all citizens are the intended beneficiaries of the planning effort. To this end, the success of the community planning process is more often measured in terms of the overall health status of the community than in terms of individual health status or the impact of the process on specific healthcare organizations.

Community health plans tend to be relatively long range with regard to their time frame, typically involving a 5- to 10-year range. The more generalized the goal (e.g., raising the overall health status of the community), the greater the time required for plan implementation. This is not to say that short-term objectives are not addressed, but that changing the course of a community's healthcare system will take a considerable length of time.

Historically, community-wide planning has been sponsored by some branch of government. The planning initiatives of the 1960s and 1970s were initiated at the federal level and implemented through state and local governmental or quasi-governmental agencies. Community-wide planning is often thought of as "public sector" planning, although the impact of the planning activities often falls more directly on private sector organizations than on public entities. To a certain extent, community-wide planning does emphasize a "public health" approach to identifying problems within the community. These activities often include a regulatory component and may attempt to "control" utilization, costs and/or facilities development. Given the comprehensive nature of community-wide planning, it could be argued that only a government agency would be in a position to manage such a process. However, this has often created the uncomfortable situation whereby public ends are pursued by public agencies through attempts to control the behavior of private sector entities.

In the new community-wide planning environment that emerged during the 1990s, there was resistance to the type of "top-down" planning that characterized comprehensive health planning in the 1960s and 1970s. In fact, most current planning initiatives have originated at the local level rather than the state or federal levels. While governmental agencies may play a role, these new planning initiatives are not necessarily seen as governmental functions. Community groups and private sector healthcare organizations are being joined by business leaders in many communities to create a true public/private approach to resolving community-wide health problems.

The focus of community health planning has historically been on facilities and personnel, reflecting to a great extent the benchmarks traditionally utilized in assessing the status of the healthcare system. In the absence of more relevant status measures of the appropriateness of the system, health planners have determined the extent to which shortages or surpluses exist in terms of such tangible features of the system as hospital beds and physicians. Thus, the "health" of the system might be evaluated in terms of the number of hospital beds per 1,000 population or the physician-to-patient ratio.

Because of its comprehensive approach, community-wide planning often addresses topics or issues that would never be broached by most organizations involved in health planning for their own narrow purposes. These topics include public health, charity care, environmental concerns, and the non-medical factors that affect health status. Community-wide planning initiatives take into consideration the needs of the medically indigent and the extent to which the community's healthcare "safety net" operates effectively. Environmental pollution is often an issue in community-wide planning initiatives, but one that would seldom be addressed at the organization level of planning. Non-medical issues such as crime, housing, and domestic violence may be taken into consideration in developing a comprehensive understanding of the healthcare needs of the population.

Defining the "Community"

The "community" component of community-wide planning can be conceptualized at a number of different geographic levels. These levels generally correspond to a particular governmental or administrative level. Ideally, an integrated planning process involving all levels of government would be in place, as is the case in most European countries with centralized planning functions. This type of hierarchical structure is notably absent in the U.S. healthcare arena, however.

At the national level, health services planning is generally the responsibility of the central government. In most societies, in fact, health planning starts at the national level and is imposed downward through the healthcare system. In the United States, however, the ability of the central government to participate in health planning activities is seriously restricted. There are few powers granted to the federal government in this regard, leaving the central government much less involved in health planning activities than is the case in other industrialized nations.

A second level at which community-wide planning can occur is the regional level. In most centrally planned systems, regional planning encompasses designated geographic subunits of the national government. During the days of federally-sponsored comprehensive health planning in the United States, the entire nation was divided into planning regions. In the United States today, however, there are no formally designated administrative "regions", leaving no level of authority between the federal and state governments. However, certain "ad hoc" regions have been designated for which health services planning may occur. These would include regional authorities established to plan for the Appalachian and Mississippi Delta poverty areas. To the extent that health planners identify "unofficial" health services areas (e.g., the multi-county service area for a major medical center), the benefit of regional planning is recognized. Certain states maintain planning "regions" based on combinations of countries.

A third level at which planning can occur is the state level. In the United States and many other countries, the state or province has specified responsibilities (often including health services) and maintains a budget for carrying out these activities. In the United States, the state is essentially the next level of government below the national level. As a practical matter, much of the health planning that occurs in the United States today takes place at the state level.

The lowest level of government (and health services planning) in the United States is local government in the form of counties and municipalities. At this level, health planning authorities may be established to plan, regulate, and/or monitor the activities of the healthcare organizations within their jurisdiction. Cities may also establish health planning authorities, particularly if they contain large numbers of health facilities. Planning organizations at the local level typically have limited authority and often exist as volunary associations. There are a few exceptions where local health planning authorities have significant power, however.

Time Horizons

Health services plans may be distinguished in terms of their time horizons. They are typically categorized as short range, long range or intermediate range. A single plan, in fact, may include phases that relate to each of these time horizons. Short-range planning typically involves a time horizon of one to two years, while long-range planning typically covers five or more years. Intermediate-range planning, of course, falls in between.

Community-wide plans have typically been long-range by national planning standards, with a five-year horizon being common. For many, this appears to be a reasonable timeframe since it allows adequate time to bring about what are often significant changes but, at the same time, does not appear to alter existing practice patterns too rapidly. While planning activities should observe the five-year planning horizon, looking beyond five years in the current healthcare environment is considered risky by many observers.

With intermediate-range plans, typically extending less than five years into the future, the goals are understandably more modest. In community-wide planning, this may involve such activities as restructuring the local health authority board or establishing a community health information system. Radical changes in the healthcare delivery system, however, are not likely to be achieved in this timeframe.

Short-range planning is inconsistent with the community-wide planning concept. Little can be accomplished toward system-wide change in a one- or two-year planning timeframe. Some short-term activities that are supportive of longer-term goals may be implemented and not be seen as ends in their own right. The recruitment of a primary care physician for an underserved area or the establishment of a new healthcare clinic, for example, may be accomplished in this timeframe.

ORGANIZATION-LEVEL PLANNING

Organization-level planning refers to planning that occurs for and within a specific healthcare entity, and the majority of what could be considered health services planning today takes place within healthcare organizations and not at the community level. Although planning on the part of healthcare organizations has not been totally embraced, recent years have seen a surge in planning activity (although it may be referred to by some other term than "planning."). In fact, the scope of planning has expanded and the planning emphasis for healthcare organizations has become refocused.

Organization-level planning differs from community-wide planning in a number of important ways. Where community-wide planning is broad and comprehensive, organization-level planning is relatively narrow and focused. Where community-wide planning is intended to serve the needs of the total community, organization level planning is focused on the specific benefits to be derived by the organization involved in the planning. While community-wide planning seeks to encourage "system-wide" change, organization-level planning seeks to advance the goals of the individual organization independent of the community's delivery system.

While the goal of community-wide planning ideally is to improve the health status of the overall population, that of organization-level planning is to advance the interests of the organization. While community health planning has historically been a public function, with all that that implies, organization-level planning is usually restricted to private sector healthcare organizations. This last distinction has begun to blur as certain public organizations have started adopting corporate planning techniques and as public/private healthcare coalitions have emerged in certain communities.

Some of the new impetus for planning in healthcare has been generated by the rise of the for-profit national healthcare corporation. These entities are, for the most part, businesses first and healthcare organizations second. Among the business practices that these entities have brought to healthcare are strategic planning and business planning. The need to plan should be considered more urgent for private sector organizations in that their very survival has become increasingly dependent upon their ability to control their destinies.

Who Should Perform Organization-Level Planning?

From the largest national hospital chain to the one-person clinician's office, every healthcare organization must attemtp to control its future to the extent possible. Developing a plan does not assure that the future will be controlled, but it provides an advantage over those organizations that are operating without a plan. Clearly, multipurpose organizations like hospitals must develop plans that allow them to adapt to their changing environments and coordinate the various and diverse components of their systems. Other providers—physicians, therapists, and other clinicians—also face the need to lay out a systematic road map to the future. Other institutional providers, such as nursing homes, home health agencies, and assisted living facilities, must similarly be able to chart a well thought out course.

Health insurance plans, including managed care plans, must be able to determine their future direction and implement a plan for reaching their goals. No success in the future healthcare environment is likely to come through happenstance, and every healthcare organization must take an active role in "inventing" its own future.

Some for-profit corporations not involved in direct patient care have a longer history with various types of planning. Pharmaceutical companies and medical supply and equipment companies have historically operated more like entrepreneurs than healthcare organizations and have a long history of sound business operation. Medical laboratories and other support services also require planning input to determine the appropriate corporate direction.

Organizational Planning Levels

The most visible planning activities among healthcare organizations take place at the corporate level, with hospital-level planning being probably the representative example. In some cases, planning may be performed at the system level, involving perhaps several hospitals and other subsidiary components of the system. This might involve a national for-profit chain of hospitals or nursing homes, a home health organization with many subsidiary agencies, or a regional hospital network. However, planning at the health system level is particularly challenging due to the complexity and, often, geographical spread of the system components. At the same time, the need to merge various systems and corporate cultures mandates at least some level of planning at the system level.

At the facility level, planning is performed for a single facility and its associated services, even if the facility is part of a larger system. Historically, organization-level planning has centered on the hospital, at least among organizations involved in patient care. Clinics, specialty practices, nursing homes and residential treatment centers are other entities that might implement plans at this level.

At the subsidiary level, planning is performed for a unit that is a distinct subsidiary of a larger facility. For example, a hospital may own a home health agency and choose to plan for its development separately. In fact, licensure regulations may require that planning for the home health agency be carried out independent of hospital planning.

Planning can also occur at the division level within the organization, with the various divisions ideally combining to form a coherent organization-level plan. In a large organization, it may be difficult to carry out strategic planning for the entire organization without relying upon division-level plans. While these may ultimately be merged under the umbrella of the corporate structure within a large organization, much of the planning must occur at the divisional level.

Planning may also occur at the department level within the organization. Traditional organization-level planning that focused on budgets, facilities, and human resources generally occurred at this level. As the concept of strategic planning has become more accepted, departments are becoming more integrated into the enterprise-wide planning process.

Finally, planning may occur at the business unit level. This may involve a strategic business unit (SBU) or a product line. In this case, the planning activities may cut across some of the other levels (e.g., departments, divisions). The hospital service line has come to be seen by many as an appropriate unit for planning, since its success typically depends upon its ability to coordinate activities in a number of functional and specialty areas. The service line lends itself to the types of organizational planning that are becoming increasingly common, such as strategic planning, marketing planning, and business planning.

The nature of the planning process, the approach utilized, and the technical implementation of the plan are determined by the size, structure and culture of the organization. A national healthcare organization may be structured as a monolithic corporate entity with tight management controls throughout the organization. Or it may involve a number of loosely affiliated companies under a holding company umbrella. Certainly, private sector organizations are going to approach planning differently from public sector entities. Organizations involved in direct patient care are going to have a different perspective from those involved in support services. Organizations selling products will require a somewhat different approach from those providing services.

At different levels within the organization as well, different types of planning are likely to be emphasized. The higher the level, in general, the more likely the planning will be strategic in nature. The lower the level, the emphasis is more likely to be on operational planning.

Geographic Focus

The geographic focus for organization-level planning, as with community-wide planning, can reside at any level within the organization. Large medical supply companies may be international in their scope and carry out corporate planning at the global level. Even here, however, such organizations are likely to think in terms of national markets and, like domestic corporations focusing on the U.S. market, conduct planning at the national level.

While there are few strictly regional healthcare organizations in the United States, many national corporations divide their operations into regions and plan accordingly. Some large local systems may in effect constitute regional operations, and their planning activities may reflect this broader scope. Planning at the state level may occur in the case of organizations that are licensed to operate on a state basis or otherwise conduct business strictly within a particular state. Health insurance plans, including health maintenance organizations, are typically licensed by an agency of the specific state. This may mandate planning at the state level for these organizations.

Most healthcare providers are local in their orientation. In this context, "local" may refer to a single neighborhood or to a multicounty service area. It is at this level, however, at which the typical organization-level planner is likely to be working today. Thus, most of the organization-level planning that takes place today, on the part of healthcare providers, at least, focuses on the local level.

Functional Emphasis

Perhaps the best way to categorize the various types of organization-level planning is to think in terms of their functional emphasis. The functional emphasis focuses on the purpose the planning activity serves within the organization. Taking that approach, the following types of planning might be identified:

- ✓ *Strategic planning* involves matching organizational resources with organizational capabilities to position the organization to take advantage of opportunities in the market.
- ✓ *Marketing planning* involves a determination of the target for marketing activities and the appropriate "marketing mix" for achieving market-related goals.
- ✓ *Business planning* involves the coordination of resource allocation to achieve the business goals of the organization.
- ✓ *Financial planning* involves planning for the management of the organization's resources.
- ✓ *Facility planning* involves planning for the development, acquisition and management of the bricks-and-mortar of the the organization.
- ✓ *Technology planning* involves planning for the acquisition and management of equipment, computer resources and other technology-based assets.
- ✓ *Policy planning* involves high-level planning for the development of policies that will guide the direction of the organization in terms of mission, relationships, etc.
- ✓ *Program planning* involves planning for the development and management of the constellation of programs and services characterizing the organization.
- ✓ *Human resources planning* involves planning for the recruitment and management of personnel.
- ✓ *Operations planning* involves planning for the management of day-to-day instrumental activities of the organization.

Time Horizon

As with community-wide plans, organization-level plans may be distinguished in terms of their time horizons. They are typically categorized as short range, intermediate range or long range. A single plan, in fact, is likely to include phases that relate to each of these time horizons, although with organization-level planning, the time horizon will reflect the type of plan. Strategic planning by definition is longer range in its scope, while operations planning is much more restricted in terms of time horizon. Short-range planning typically involves a time horizon of one to two years, while long-range planning typically covers five or more years. Intermediate-range planning, of course, falls in between. As with community-wide planning, there is a reluctance to develop plans that extend more than five years into the future.

At the organization level, the rapidly changing nature of healthcare has, perhaps inappropriately, led to an emphasis on short-range planning. In addition, the entry into the field of publicly held national corporations who have to account to their shareholders every quarter has led to a more short-term orientation. As a result, long-range goals and even the organization's mission may be subservient to short-term concerns.

HEALTH PLANNING IN THE UNITED STATES: PAST AND PRESENT

Community-Wide Planning

History

The origin of health planning in the United States is often traced to the enactment of the Hill-Burton Act of 1946. This Act called for a national survey of hospital facilities and resulted in government funding for hundreds of hospitals. It was the first federal initiative of any magnitude directed toward healthcare, an arena that was not on the federal radar screen until the 1950s. While not a planning initiative per se, the implementation of the provisions of the legislation required the initiation of a number of planning-type activities (e.g., needs assessment, site selection, resource allocation).

Formal healthcare planning in the United States was established with the Comprehensive Health Planning Act of 1966. This planning initiative was in response to the discovery in the 1960s of large segments of the population that did not have access to mainstream healthcare, as well as to concerns over perceived inequities in the provision of services to different segments of the population. This act called for the establishment of a federally funded and coordinated planning initiative for assuring access to adequate healthcare for every American.

The program established state-wide and area-wide (i.e., sub-state) planning agencies for the implementation of the planning process. These agencies were charged with the development of state plans and were assigned responsibility for coordinating healthcare activities within the geographic areas under their jurisdiction. Planning agencies established guidelines for the development of facilities and programs.

The primary means of guiding the development of health services available to planning agencies was the review and evaluation of healthcare projects that were proposed by health care interests in the community. However, planning agencies could only make recommendations with regard to proposed projects and had limited power to affect change.

The Regional Medical Program (RMP) was another federal initiative established in the mid-1960s with responsibility for coordinating and promoting health services within identified health service areas. These programs were established nationwide and were charged with facilitating the diffusion of medical technology and other breakthroughs from major medical centers to surrounding areas. While planning was not a stated responsibility of these programs, a certain level of planning was required in order for the RMPs to successfully disseminate medical knowledge throughout their regions. The health focus of the Regional Medical Programs was categorical, addressing a small number of disease entities rather than the entire spectrum of health problems. In many parts of the country, RMPs coordinated their activities with existing health planning agencies (established under the health planning legislation of 1996). Even this collaboration was problematic since the two types of organizations often did not share the same boundaries.

Another landmark development of this period was the establishment of the Medicare and Medicaid programs. While neither Medicare nor Medicaid involved any substantial planning responsibilities, it has often been noted that operation of these two programs had a major impact on medical practice patterns and, in that sense, they served as a force for changing the nature of the healthcare system.

Planning activities were revitalized nationwide in 1974 with the enactment of the National Health Planning and Resources Development Act. This act was prompted by growing concern over the lack of uniformly effective methods of healthcare delivery, the maldistribution of healthcare facilities and personnel, and the increasing cost of care. With a better financial footing than the 1966 planning initiative, this act called for the creation of statewide health coordinating councils and the establishment of local health systems agencies.

To remedy the lack of authority characterizing earlier planning efforts, the new planning act featured the of the certificate-of-need process (CON) as a means of controlling the development of facilities and services. The CON process required any healthcare provider seeking to build additional facilities or add or change a service to demonstrate that the project was needed. The intent was to assure that any new project fit within the planning framework that had been developed at the state level. It was also intended to limit the duplication of services and equipment that was contributing to rising costs. (See Box 2-1 for a discussion of the certificate-of-need process.)

This "experiment" in health planning came to an end under the Reagan administration in the early 1980s. Despite some successes, comprehensive health planning had not created many political allies and essentially had few constituents. As a result, the demise of these programs represented the end of any formal federal planning initiatives. As we enter the 21st century, the federal government provides some limited support for health planning through initiatives like Healthy People 2010 and agencies like the Health Resources and Services Administration. Federally supported health planning initiatives are a distant memory.

BOX 2-1
The Certificate-of-Need Process

During the era of nationwide "comprehensive health planning" beginning in the mid-1960s and extending into the early 1980s, health planning agencies attempted to control the utilization of health services and ostensibly health-care costs through restrictions placed on the establishment and expansion of health services. The primary tool for implementing these restrictions was the certificate-of-need (CON) process. Eventually written into federal regulations, the CON process has been used (and abused) by various states as a means of controlling the building of facilities, the development of services, and the acquisition of expensive equipment on the part of healthcare providers.

The CON concept is relatively straightforward. It mandates that a certificate-of-need application be filed that justifies the proposed facility, equipment, or service based on certain criteria that reflect community needs. The underlying notion is that objective parties would review any proposal and either approve or disapprove its implementation. Under the aegis of comprehensive health planning, assessments were made at the local level and subsequently reviewed at the regional (sub-state) and state levels.

Under federally sponsored comprehensive health planning programs, uniform standards for the implementation of the CON process were enacted. Thus, each state followed similar guidelines and used similar criteria for reviewing applications. Each state was required to prepare a state health plan that adhered to federal standards. Further, each state was to establish local standards to supplement federal standards as a basis for evaluating the adequacy of a proposal. Thus, there were guidelines that specified the appropriate number of hospital beds or physicians per 1,000 residents or the catchment area appropriate for a particular piece of diagnostic equipment. The provisions of any proposed project were required to be consistent with the needs identified in the health plan and meet the criteria established to justify the service being proposed.

The initial implementation of CON legislation had little impact on the availability of facilities, services, and equipment. This was due primarily to the fact that health planning agencies had virtually no authority to enforce decisions made on CON applications. Healthcare organizations could, and often did, choose to ignore the ruling of the planning agency, and many cases

(continued)

can be cited in which facilities were built, services initiated or equipment purchased after the CON application was disapproved.

The health planning legislation enacted in the 1970s expanded the authority of health planning agencies and instituted disincentives that planning agencies could use to encourage compliance with CON rulings. One of these disincentives was the threat of withholding federal healthcare funds (e.g., Medicare reimbursement) from healthcare organizations that did not comply with CON rulings.

There has been considerable debate over the success of the CON process in controlling the supply of facilities, services, and equipment and over the ultimate contribution that this process has made to the quality of care and the cost of services. This is not to mention the controversy over the appropriateness of any type of formal controls on the activities of healthcare organizations. There is no consistent pattern with regard to the impact that CON legislation has in the states in which the process is in effect today. The process appears to have had a significant effect on the healthcare systems in some states and limited impact in others. To a great extent this reflects variations in the form of the CON programs take and in the manner in which they are implemented. After the elimination of federal funding for comprehensive health planning, the various states (and some local jurisdictions) adopted widely divergent guidelines for the CON process. Several states, in fact, eliminated the CON process altogether. Some of these, however, have since reinstituted some form of the CON review process. For most states, the process is under continual review, with periodic efforts initiated to change the process in one way or another.

Among the 36 states (and the District of Columbia) that had CON programs in place in 2001, the provisions of the programs vary widely (American Health Planning Association, 2002). Most states attempt to regulate capital expenditures, equipment acquisition, and the establishment of new services, although some regulate only one or two of these areas. Virtually all states that regulate capital expenditures have some minimum dollar threshold before a CON application is required. In many states, all hospital capital projects must be approved, but comparable projects proposed by a physician group may not require approval. The picture is further complicated by the fact that states vary with regard to the components of the system that are regulated. In some states, any new clinical service must be approved, while in others only home health or long-term care services, for example, require a CON application.

The preparation of a CON application is typically a complex process that requires expertise on a wide variety of subjects. The application must justify the need for the project based on the characteristics of the service area and existing practice patterns. The project must be demonstrated to be financially sound, and this often requires the involvement of expert business analysts. The project must meet all legal requirements (CON-mandated or otherwise), and physical plant components must be demonstrated to meet the guidelines set by the CON planning agency. Proponents typically have to demonstrate that they have community support for the project and that established utilization patterns will not be unduly disrupted. The project must adhere to the state health plan (if one exists) and to any guidelines in place related to minimum thresholds for services (e.g., a minimum of 20,000 residents to support a catherization laboratory). Because of the complexity of the CON application process, experts in the areas of market research, financial analysis, health law, architecture and engineering, and clnical areas, along with the standard complement of administrative types, are required for the successful development of a CON application.

A substantial application fee typically is required for the filing of a CON application and this in itself is a controversial issue. Some have argued that the filing fee itself constitutes a restraint on the free operation of the market in that it limits access to the process to those healthcare organizations that are already well established. In many states, the filing fee is used primarily to fund the operation of the CON agency.

There is no concensus as to the value of the certificate-of-need process as a tool in guiding the development of healthcare delivery systems. There are certainly arguments for and against this method of attempting to control the establishment of health services. The process itself continues to evolve, and modified versions of the CON process have been put in place in various states. Despite the reservations of some observers, it is likely that the CON process in some form will become increasingly important as the health planning movement becomes revitalized as the 21st century unfolds.

References: American Health Planning Association (2002). *National Directory of Health Planning, Policy and Regulatory Agencies.* Falls Church, VA: American Health Planning Association.

Current Status

Since the end of federally funded health planning initiatives in the early 1980s, virtually no health services planning has occurred at the national level. The planning apparatus, as limited as it was, suffered dismantlement under the Reagan administration. Today, there is no "home" in the federal structure for health planning. This is not to say that no planning-type activities occur, many do. However, their effect is felt very indirectly and these are not formally referred to as "planning" activities.

The absence of any formal health planning activities on the part of the federal government understates the influence that the federal government maintains over the direction that the healthcare system takes. While not considered true planning, the federal government is involved in a number of activities that implicitly influence healthcare policy and practice. The major influence is probably exerted through the control of funding. The federal government accounts for a major portion of the nation's healthcare expenditures and nearly 60 percent of the expenditures on direct patient care. These funds are expended primarily through the operation of the Medicare and Medicaid programs. It has been suggested, in fact, that the introduction of Medicare has had a greater influence on practice patterns within the U.S. healthcare system than any other single development.

A number of federal agencies are involved in programs that have planning-type components. The U.S. Public Health Service tracks the adequacy of primary care physicians and other clinicians and issues regular reports on health professional shortage areas. The PHS, in fact, is involved in programs such as the National Health Service Corps that seek to influence the distribution of primary care physicians into underserved areas. The Bureau of Health Professions, also within the Department of Health and Human Services, maintains databases on physicians and other medical personnel. Other agencies maintain inventories of health facilities and often evaluate the adequacy of such facilities for the communities they serve. The Center for Medicare and Medicaid Services (CMS) also maintains databases on a wide range of facility types. Another agency tracks enrollment in health maintenance organizations. While none of these activities constitute planning in a true sense, the operation of these programs influences the allocation of resources and the development of health-related policies at the national level.

The most visible planning-type activity sponsored by the federal government is probably the Healthy People 2010 initiative sponsored by the Office of Disease Prevention and Health Promotion within the Department of Health and Human Services. Originally formulated in the late 1980s, the HP2010 program involved the identification of areas of concern in healthcare that could benefit from the policy-making influence of the federal government. On-going research monitors areas of concern, and indicators have been developed to track the progress being made to address these issues. Goals and objectives have been developed for each category and benchmarks established to be reached by the year 2010. (See Box 2-2 for more detail on the Healthy People initiative.)

Further, by allocating funds—almost always with strings attached—for facilities development and health professions training, the federal government has influenced the number and location of hospitals and the characteristics of the physician pool. By influencing the use of medical education funds, for example, the federal government has attempted to redistribute physician personnel from specialty care to primary care. The funding of the nation's huge medical research industry has also been a major indirect contributor to the direction of the healthcare system. By setting funding priorities and allocating dollars accordingly, the federal government has dictated what is to be considered important for research purposes. The fact that prevention still is given a backseat to treatment and cure, for example, reflects the low priority placed on prevention within the federal research establishment.

Federal agencies also exert a planning-type influence through the regulatory powers held by the national government. These are felt in a variety of ways, from the operation of the Occupational Health and Safety Agency to the activities of the Food and Drug Administration to the regulations promulgated by the Centers for Medicare and Medicaid Services.

Planning activities at the regional level have never been well developed and limited venues exist today for introducing planning at that level. The only situations in which regional planning occurs in any sense is through the operation of regional authorities such as the Appalachian Regional Commission and the Mississippi Delta Regional Commission. While these are not healthcare initiatives per se, healthcare issues are often addressed. While such regional authorities may include funding for health-related activities, they generally have no authority for implementing healthcare initiatives.

Many states retained a health planning structure after the demise of federally-funded planning in the 1980s. Some continue to develop state health plans, with the level of effort, the scope, and the implications of the planning varying widely from state to state. Few state planning agencies have any significant authority to implement plans, with monitoring and oversight being essentially the limit of their influence.

One of the primary functions inherent in comprehensive health planning was the operation of the certificate-of-need process. Under the traditional health planning framework, any healthcare organization seeking to add or change a service or facility was required to certify that a need existed. This certification process was based on certain standards that were in place and on the priorities established within the particular state's health plan. The intent was to encourage the orderly development of facilities, equipment and services and, at the same time, limit duplication of services. As of 2001, 36 states and the District of Columbia continued to operate certificate-of-need programs, although at differing levels of intensity (American Health Planning Association, 2002).

BOX 2-2
Healthy People 2010

The Healthy People initiative sponsored by the federal government is perhaps the program that most closely resembles a national planning effort. The program is operated by the Office of Disease Prevention and Health Promotion within the U.S. Department of Health and Human Services. Inspired by a 1979 Surgeon General's report, the Healthy People initiative was established as a framework for improving the health status of the American population. While not a planning document in a technical sense, its intent is to encourage a second public health "revolution" that capitalizes on the significance of preventive health.

The Healthy People 2010 program was initiated in the 1990s as a successor to the Healthy People 2000 program established in 1990 as a comprehensive agenda for increasing years of healthy life, reducing disparities in health among different population groups, and improving access to preventive health services. For the federal government, the Healthy People 2010 provides a framework for measuring performance and serves as a strategic management tool. Success is measured by positive changes in health status, reduction in risk factors, and/or improved access to certain services.

In order to provide the foundation for the Healthy People initiative, extensive data collection activities were carried out related to 22 priority areas for 2000 and 28 priority areas for 2010. This effort involved the compilation of a great deal of information on these topics that can be used as background for the establishment of program objectives. Continuous monitoring is undertaken in order to track the progress being made in reaching Healthy People 2010 objectives.

For each of the 28 priority areas a series of objectives was established, resulting in a total of 467 objectives. For the priority area of "Maternal and Infant Health", for example, the objectives include the following:

1. Reduce the infant mortality rate to no more than 4.5 deaths per 1,000 live births by the year 2010.
2. Reduce the fetal death rate to no more than 4.1 deaths per 1,000 live births by the year 2010.
3. Reduce the maternal mortality rate to no more than 3.3 deaths per 100,000 live births by the year 2010.

Most of the objectives also spawn subobjectives that are even more specific. For example, the objective of reducing the infant mortality rate is accompanied by subobjectives that address the infant mortality rates for specific subpopulations (e.g., African Americans, Hispanics). In fact, a major difference between the HP2000 and HP2010 initiatives is the latter's greater emphasis on disparities in health status among various population groups. Since the inception of the Healthy People initiative, improved data collection has made more precise peformance measurement possible.

While the Healthy People 2010 program provides a framework for planning, there is no formal implementation plan for reaching its objectives. Further, the program has no authority to mandate activities that would contribute to its stated objectives. Some indirect influence is exerted, however, through the selective channeling of federal research funds. Applicants for federal grant money, for example, must demonstrate that the projects being proposed are consistent with Healthy People 2010 objectives.

The priority areas for the Healthy People 2010 initiative include the following:

1. Access to quality health services
2. Arthritis, osteoporosis, and chronic back conditions
3. Cancer
4. Chronic kidney disease
5. Diabetes
6. Disability and secondary conditions
7. Educational and community -based programs
8. Environmental health
9. Family planning
10. Food safety
11. Health communications
12. Heart disease and stroke
13. HIV
14. Immunization and infectious diseases
15. Injury/violence prevention
16. Maternal, infant, and child health
17. Medical product safety
18. Mental health and mental disorders
19. Nutrition and overweight
20. Occupational safety and health
21. Oral health
22. Physical activity and fitness
23. Public health infrastructure
24. Respiratory disease
25. Sexually transmitted diseases
26. Substance abuse
27. Tobacco use
28. Vision and hearing

Additional information on HealthyPeople 2010 can be obtained from the Office of Disease Prevention and Health Promotion in Washington, DC, or from the HealthyPeople Web site at www.healthypeople.gov.

States exert some of the same indirect influences on the healthcare system that the federal government does. Healthcare is a major item in all state budgets, with the Medicaid program typically representing a major line item. Public health expenditures are also likely to be a significant budget item, and the allocation of funds for direct patient care (e.g., for mental health services) may be substantial. The control of funding for the Medicaid program alone has no doubt done much to influence practice patterns.

State agencies are responsible for most licensing and regulation of health facilities and personnel. Hospitals, nursing homes, home health agencies and many other facilities and programs must meet state requirements for licensure and abide by state-initiated regulations. Many types of health professionals must maintain state-issued licenses in order to practice. While these are seldom considered planning activities, they exert an indirect influence on the practice patterns found within a state. Attempts by various state licensing agencies to exclude foreign-trained physicians from licensure, for example, represent an indirect planning activity related to healthcare personnel.

State agencies have considerable public health responsibilities, including the monitoring of environmental conditions and other threats to the health of the populace. While the operation of these programs does not constitute true planning, their presence does influence the approach taken to the management of numerous health issues. Increasingly, public health agencies are being required to think strategically and to develop at least some semblance of a strategic plan.

At the local (city or county) level, the extent of planning activities varies widely. Most communities do not maintain formal planning organizations today. However, in a few communities well-established planning authorities may exert inordinate influence. For the most part, planning activities at this level are voluntary on the part of the participants, and local planning agencies typically have limited funds and few regulatory powers.

Numerous national initiatives, particularly on the part of major foundations, have encouraged grassroots planning activities at the local level. The Local Initiative Funding Program (Robert Wood Johnson Foundation) and the Coalition for Healthier Cities and Communities are two examples. The National Association of County and City Health Officials (NACCHO) also plays an active role in encouraging local health planning activities through its Turning Point Program. NACCHO has also been instrumental in the development of the Mobilizing for Action through Planning and Partnerships (MAPP). These organizations have provided seed money and technical support for the development of public/private consortia designed to establish a planning process, however, informal, at the community level.

Local health authorities formally established for the management of the public health system or some other "public" health function may, through their normal operations, constitute an indirect force for health planning. They influence which services are reserved for the public sector and thereby have an impact on private sector practice patterns. If, for example, the county hospital board establishes a neonatal intensive care unit in the public hospital, this may preclude the need for such services in the private sector.

Local health departments may be large and influential organizations, particularly in major cities. Examples include the Los Angeles health department with a three billion dollar budget, the New York health authority with its system of public hospitals, and the City of Chicago health department with 1,600 employees. The policies and subsequent actions of such agencies no doubt have implications for the direction taken by the local healthcare system.

The 1990s witnessed renewed interest in community-wide health planning and this revival has extended to the 21st century. After a decade-long absence, the-term "planning" began to reappear in the healthcare literature during the mid-90s. The topic of planning is becoming more frequently listed in professional association programs, and there is growing public discourse surrounding the issue of health planning.

A number of factors have no doubt contributed to this reemergence of interest. At a theoretical level, the paradigm shift from a medical care emphasis to a healthcare emphasis calls for a different approach to the management of health and illness, an approach more sympathetic to systematic planning. At a more practical level, the recognition that the problems surrounding healthcare are not going to go away and the fact that many of these problems can be traced to a lack of planning are contributing to this revitalization. The attention drawn to community-based healthcare initiatives by the Clinton administration as it struggled with healthcare reform in the early 1990s probably was another contributing factor.

While full-scale planning activities are still uncommon, a number of planning-like activities can be seen. Attempts at developing community health information management systems (CHMIS) in a number of communities reflect the felt need to coordinate patient information. Other data generation and dissemination efforts further reflect this trend toward a more systematic approach to the management of the healthcare delivery system. The growing interest in "population-based" healthcare–on the part of both public and private sector healthcare organizations– further reflects this emerging planning orientation.

Regardless of the form that this new planning takes, it is undoubtedly going to be a lot different from the traditional approach embodied by the comprehensive health planning initiatives of the 1960s and 1970s. The healthcare world has changed dramatically and the planning approach must be revised to reflect this. Unprecedented resources are available to put into the planning effort, and there appears to be an opportunity to establish a community-wide planning framework that can be successful in this new environment. (A detailed discussion of the future of health services planning is included in Chapter 13.)

Organization-Level Planning

Under the "expansionist model" that drove healthcare from the end of World War II to the 1980s, planning focused almost exclusively on facilities and capital expenditures and on operations. Organization-level planning, in fact, was very much operations oriented throughout the 1970s. Since the concern was with day-to-day activities, a short-range focus on budgets, facilities and programs dominated organization-level planning. Hospitals were the healthcare provider organizations most actively involved in planning. They were also the most internally focused ones and unlikely to think in terms of external factors.

The 1970s became a period of "institutional planning" which, although incorporating more "modern" planning techniques, continued to focus on bricks-and-mortar issues. In the 1980s "operational planning" was emphasized, with a focus on day-to-day operations, budgets, facilities management, and certificate-of-need activities.

By the mid-1980s the external environment began to exert its influence, and the world began to change for healthcare providers. Hospitals for the first time were faced with competition, deregulation, reduced reimbursement, and decreased utilization. In short, hospitals and other healthcare organizations were forced to start thinking strategically. The shift from a product orientation to a service orientation occurred during this period, and healthcare organizations became market oriented and consumer driven. These developments facilitated the shift from an operations orientation to a strategic orientation. The wave of mergers and acquisitions that characterized the 1990s served to encourage organization-level planning on the one hand, while making it an even greater challenge on the other.

By the 1990s the planning concept had been widely accepted by healthcare organizations, if not totally incorporated into their cultures. Prompted by the industry-wide paradigm shift from medical care to healthcare, healthcare organizations began moving away from the more traditional types of facilities, budgeting and operations planning toward strategic, marketing and business planning.

RELATIONSHIP BETWEEN COMMUNITY-WIDE AND ORGANIZATION-LEVEL PLANNING

Historically, there has been little relationship between planning at the community level and organization-level planning. The two types of planning have involved different entities and have been triggered by different factors in the environment. Realistically, community-wide planning has never been as comprehensive as it theoretically should be, and significant fragmentation has always existed even in the face of aggressive community-wide planning. Until the 1980s organization-level planning was not concerned with the external environment, and no connection was seen between the internally-oriented planning of the organization and the community-wide planning carried out by government agencies. The only interface typically occurred when a private sector healthcare organization had to pose its project proposal within the context of an existing health plan.

Today, there appears to be considerable convergence between the two types of planning. The reemerging community health planning movement appears to be adopting some of the techniques from organization-level planning and proponents of the new community health planning are encouraging the participation of private sector providers. The impetus for some of these community health planning movements has come from business leaders, and the emergence of new planning initiatives that include both public and private entities is encouraging.

Healthcare organizations, on the other hand, have come to realize that planning in isolation is not truly planning. Many organizations are beginning to take a population-based approach that, by definition, causes them to include a much wider range of community entities in their planning activities. Examples of joint efforts to develop community health information systems and the appearance of public/private initiatives aimed at community health issues suggest that a certain level of convergance is occurring. In addition, providers with tax-exempt status are increasingly being pressured to coordinate their initiatives with community-wide initiatives that are underway. (These issues are discussed further in Chapter 13.)

HEALTH PLANNING IN OTHER COUNTRIES

One other perspective that is worthwhile pursing in our introductory discussion of health services planning is the comparative perspective. How does health planning in the United States—particularly community-wide planning—compare to the health planning activities of other countries?

The United States is exceptional among comparable industrialized countries in its lack of health planning. Most European countries, along with Canada and Japan, have centralized healthcare systems characterized by strong planning components. In fact, most of these countries have a long history of government involvement in the planning of health services. Unlike the U.S., private sector healthcare is severely limited or unknown in these societies.

Health planning in most industrialized countries is integrated into broader social and economic planning functions. Health is seldom seen as an independent issue but as one very much wrapped up with socioeconomic considerations. For these reasons, health planning in such societies tends to be very comprehensive in its approach. Top-down planning is the rule, with policies set in many cases at the upper administrative levels and passed down to lower levels of the organization.

Even among developing countries, there is growing emphasis on system-wide health planning. While many aspects of the U.S. healthcare system are admired, the U.S. is unlikely to serve as a model for countries seeking to initiate health planning at the national level. Other countries must be looked to for examples of national planning efforts.

References

American Health Planning Association (2002). *National Directory of Health Planning, Policy and Regulatory Agencies*. Ninth edition. Falls Church, VA: American Health Planning Association.

Additional Resources

Benjamin, A. E., & Downs, G. W. (1982). Evaluating the National Health Planning and Resources Development Act: learning from experience? *Journal of Health Politics and Law*, 7(3), 707–722.

Coalition for Healthier Cities and Communities, Boulder, CO. Web site: http://www.healthycommunities.org.

Eagar, Kathy (2002). *Health Planning*. St. Leonards, NSW, Australia: Allen and Unwin.

Green, Andrew (1999). *An Introduction to Health Planning in Developing Countries* (2nd ed.). London: Oxford.

Health Policy and Planning (periodical). London: Oxford University Press.

Institute of Medicine (1993). *Access to Healthcare in America*. Washington, DC: National Academy Press.

Landrum, L. B. (n.d.). *Health planning is alive and well*. Retrieved February 1, 2003, from http://www.ahpanet.org/policy.html.

Marcyznski-Music, K. K. (1994). *Healthcare Solutions: Designing Community-Based Systems That Work*. San Francisco, CA: Jossey-Bass.

National Association of County and City Health Officials, Washington, DC. Web site: http://www.naccho.org.

Reeves, Philip N., and Russell C. Coile, Jr. (1989). *Introduction to Health Planning*. Arlington, VA: Information Resources Press.

Reinke, William A. (editor) (1997). *Health Planning for Effective Management*. London: Oxford.

Rohrer, James E. (1996). *Planning for Community-Oriented Health Systems*. Washington, DC: American Public Health Association.

Robert Wood Johnson Foundation, Princeton, NJ. Web site: http://www.rwjf.org.

Steen, John W. (n.d.). *Certificate of Need: A Review*. Web site: http://www.ahpanet.org/articles.html

U.S. Department of Health and Human Services, Office of Disease Prevention and Health Promotion. Healthy People 2010 Web site: www.healthypeople.gov.

3

The Social and Health Systems Context for Health Services Planning

Any planning activity requires a complete understanding of the context in which planning is taking place. It is impossible to understand a healthcare system without an appreciation for the environment in which it exists. For effective planning to occur, planners must first fully understand the nature of the existing system for which they are planning, including the background on how the system evolved to the point it has.

By the same token, effective planning cannot occur without an indepth comprehension of the population that the plan is meant to serve. The social, political and economic characteristics of the target population must be thoroughly understood, along with the lifestyles, attitudes and other traits that characterize the population.

While it is not possible to describe all of the social and health systems dimensions that are important for framing a health plan, the important issues are hopefully addressed in the sections that follow. This chapter also reviews the development of the U.S. healthcare during the second half of the 20th century within the context of the social, demographic and healthcare developments that affected it.

THE SOCIOCULTURAL CONTEXT

The healthcare system of any society can only be understood within the socio-cultural context of that society. Similarly, the approach to planning (indeed, even the fact that a planning initiative exists) reflects the structure and the value system of the particular society. No two healthcare delivery systems are exactly alike, with the differences primarily a function of the contexts within which they exist. Thus, the social structure of a society, along with its cultural values, serves to define the healthcare system. The form and function of the healthcare system reflect the form and function of the society in which it resides (Parsons, 1951).

Every society has certain functions that must be performed if that society is to survive. These functions include reproduction of new society members, social-ization of them, distribution of resources, maintenance of internal order, provision for defense, accommodation of the supernatural, and, importantly for our pur-poses, providing for the health and well-being of its population. Societal structures (referred to as "institutions") are established to meet these needs. In every society some form of family evolves to manage reproduction, some form of educational system to deal with socialization, some form of economic system to deal with the allocation of resources, and so forth. A service system of some type evolves to deal with the health and welfare of the population.

The form that a particular institution takes varies from society to society. A society's cultural history, its environment, and its relationship with other soci-eties all contribute to the shaping of its various institutions. These are numerous forms that can be taken by the family, the political institution, and the economic institution, with the particular form being uniquely tailored to the situation of that society. Similarly, there are a variety of forms the healthcare institution can take.

Considering the types of health systems that exist among the world's soci-eties, one might speak in terms of "traditional" healthcare systems (e.g., shaman-ism among American Indians), more complex traditional systems such as holistic Asian systems (e.g., Aryuvedic healthcare), capitalistic systems (e.g., the for-profit healthcare in the United States), socialized systems (e.g., the National Health Service in Great Britain), and Communistic systems such as those that once ex-isted in the what was then the Soviet Union and can be found today perhaps only in Cuba.

No one system of healthcare delivery is intrinsically better or worse than any other; each has evolved in response to particular social, cultural, and environmental considerations, and each is uniquely suited to its particular society. If the system is not suited to the society, it must transform itself in response to societal needs or disappear.

The importance of any institution varies from society to society. Historical and environmental factors, as well as the particular society's value system, influence the importance of the respective institutions. Traditional societies emphasize the family and religious institutions, and the economic and healthcare institutions may be poorly developed. Modern industrial societies tend to place more emphasis on the economic and educational institutions, while the family and religious institutions tend to be relatively neglected. In recent decades, the healthcare institution has become increasingly important in industrial societies as well. This has been particularly the case in the United States.

It is only in modern industrial society that healthcare has developed as a distinct institution. For most of human history, society's provision for the healthcare needs of the population has occurred within the framework of the family or the religious institution. Traditional societies typically lack the scientific underpinnings for the development of formal healthcare systems. An absence of emphasis on rationality and a dependence on the supernatural as an explanatory factor in the existence of health, illness and death typically preclude the development of a healthcare system set apart from other institutions. As societies have become more complex, healthcare systems have come increasingly distinct and separate from other institutions of society and even from the social service system.

The Cultural Framework

The restructuring of U.S. institutions during the 20th century was accompanied by a cultural revolution resulting in extensive value reorientation within American society. The values associated with traditional societies that emphasized kinship, community, authority, and primary relationships became overshadowed by the values of modern industrialized societies, such as secularism, urbanism, and self-actualization.

The "modern" values that emerged within the U.S. after World War II supported the development of a healthcare system that was to become the epitome of modern "Western" medicine. The values that emerged in the twentieth century and still serve to color the nature of American society today placed emphasis on economic success, educational achievement, and scientific and technological advancement. These values supported the ascendancy of healthcare as a dominant institution during the last half of that century.

Implicit throughout the evolution of American healthcare has been the importance of economic success, and the U.S. system emerged as the only for-profit healthcare system in the world. Today, the profit-motive remains strong as for-profit national chains have absorbed much of the nation's health services delivery capacity. The free enterprise aspect of healthcare is linked to other American values such as freedom of choice and individualism.

Other values became important as American culture evolved in the 20th century. For example, change became recognized as a value in its own right. At the same time an activist orientation emerged that called for a proactive approach to all issues, including healthcare. The aggressive approach taken by Americans in the face of health problems reflects this activist orientation.

The conceptualization of "health" as a value in U.S. society represented a major development in the emergence of the healthcare institution. Prior to World War II, health was not perceived as a distinct value but was vaguely tied in with other notions of well-being. Public opinion polls prior to World War II did not identify personal health as an issue for the U.S. populace, nor was healthcare delivery considered a societal concern. By the 1960s, however, personal health had climbed to the top of the public opinion polls as an issue and the adequate provision of health services became an important issue in the mind of the American public.

Once health became established as a value, it was a short step to establishing a formal healthcare system as the institutional means for achieving that value. An environment was created that encouraged the emergence of a powerful institution that supported many contemporary American values. Some of them, like the value placed on human life, were considered immutable. The emerging scientific, technological and research communities contributed to the growth of the industry. Support from the economic, political, and educational institutions assured the ascendancy of this new institutional form.

Societal Trends

The 20th century witnessed a growing dependence on formal institutions of all types in the United States, and this created a favorable environment for the emergence of a healthcare institution. The political and educational systems, for example, came to be seen as responsible for functions performed informally in earlier times. Healthcare, however, provides possibly the best example of this emergent dependence on formal solutions, since it is an institution whose very development was a result of this transformation. Our great-grandparents would have considered formal healthcare as a last resort in the face of sickness and disability. Few of them ever entered a hospital, and not many more regularly utilized physicians. Today the healthcare system is seen as the first line of resistance, not only for clear-cut medical problems, but also for a broad range of psychological, social, interpersonal, and spiritual problems.

The transformation of American society in the 20th century clearly affected the provision of healthcare, as the traditional managers of sickness and death—the family and the church—gave way to more formal responses to health problems. The health of the population became in part the responsibility of the economic, educational, and political systems and, eventually, of a fully developed and powerful healthcare system. Traditional, informal responses to health problems gave way to complex, institutional responses. "High touch" home remedies could not compete in an environment that valued high-tech (and subsequently high status) responses to health problems.

Demographic Trends

Today, perhaps more than at any time in the past, demographic trends are shaping the demand for health services, both at the national and local level. By looking at specific demographic attributes of the U.S. population and their present and future trends, analysts can predict both the level and types of health services that will be utilized at various distant time periods. These demographic trends are important in that they contributed to the composition of the U.S. population; this, in turn, has influenced the morbidity profile of the population. The healthcare system that emerges should ultimately represent a response to the morbidity characteristics of the population. Indeed, the demographic transformation of the American population in the 20th century might be considered a major, if not the major, determinant of the needs to be addressed by the healthcare system.

This is the case due to another transformation that demographic trends spawned. The changing demographic characteristics triggered the "epidemiologic transition" that took place in the United States in the second half of the 20th century. As the mortality rate for the American population declined during the that century and life expectancy increased, a significant change occurred in the morbidity and mortality profile of the population (Omran, 1971).

Throughout recorded history, acute health conditions had constituted the major health threat and the leading causes of death. Communicable, infectious and parasitic conditions, accidents, complications of childbirth, and other acute conditions were a constant companion to human beings. At the beginning of the 20th century, the leading causes of death were such conditions as tuberculosis, influenza, and other communicable diseases.

During the second half of the 20th century, the changing demographic profile prompted a shift away from acute conditions to chronic conditions as the predominant health problems. Improved living conditions, better nutrition and higher standards of living, accompanied by advances in medical science, reduced or eliminated the burden of disease from acute conditions. This void was filled, however, by the emergence of chronic conditions as the leading health problems and leading causes of death. The older population that resulted from these developments was now plagued by hypertension, arthritis, and diabetes, as well as numerous conditions that reflected the lifestyles that emerged within the American population in the second half of that century. (See Box 3-1 for additional detail on the epidemiologic transition.)

This section cannot begin to address all of the demographic trends now underway nor all of the related issues addressed by health demographers. Therefore, it focuses on the key demographic trends and their likely implications for health services planning.

The Changing Age Structure

The first, and perhaps most important, demographic trend in the United States is the population's changing age distribution. The aging of America has obviously been one of the most publicized demographic trends in history. The implications of this trend for health services demand have been well-documented, with age arguably the single most important predictor of the demand for health services.

BOX 3-1
The Epidemiologic Transition

Perhaps the most significant trend affecting healthcare during the 20th century was the shift from acute conditions as the dominant type of health problem to chronic conditions. Referred to as the "epidemiologic transition", this development had major implications for the healthcare delivery system and, indeed, for our perceptions of the very nature of health and illness. Acute conditions such as infectious and communicable diseases and accidents have been the leading health problems and causes of death throughout human history. Until well into the 20th century in the United States, yellow fever, whooping cough, influenza, and tuberculosis were leading causes of death. Acute conditions such as these are characterized by rapid onset, rapid and predictable progression, and some ultimate disposition (i.e., either recovery or death). Further, most acute conditions can be attributed to some disease organism within the affected party's environment.

The predominance of acute conditions led scientists to develop the germ theory of disease causation. This in turn led to the development of the medical model approach to addressing health problems. The medical model assumes that the causes of virtually all conditions can be isolated in the form of microorganisms or otherwise reduced to physical or biochemical causes. If these etiological factors can be counteracted, then a cure can be achieved. This approach became the foundation of 20th century Western medicine and continues to be a dominant paradigm in healthcare today.

By the middle of the 20th century, acute conditions began to be displaced by chronic conditions as the primary type of health problem. Chronic conditions tend to be gradual in their onset, of long or infinite duration, and often cumulative in their effect. Chronic conditions are less likely to be caused by factors external to the individual (although some causes are clearly exogenous) and are more likely to arise from within the victim and reflect social and psychological influences. Thus, chronic conditions are more frequently linked to lifestyle, environmental factors, and even the psychological state of the affected party. The chronic conditions that have become increasingly common include arthritis, hypertension, and diabetes. Although

The "internal" restructuring of the age distribution of the population has particular significance for the demand for health services. Population growth within the older age cohorts (age 55 and over), particularly among the oldest-old (age 85 and over), is faster than that for the younger cohorts. The total population increased

sometimes resulting in death (although almost indirectly), chronic conditions seldom contribute directly to mortality but are more likely to interfere with the affected party's quality of life and/or result in disability. Unlike acute conditions, chronic conditions can seldom be cured and often become life-long afflictions for those so affected.

Two important interdependent factors have contributed to the epidemiologic transition. The first is the impact of medical science on acute conditions. During the 20th century the United States witnessed the eradication of most of the major killers from earlier times and a general reduction in the burden of disease on society. Once individuals were spared the premature deaths often caused by acute conditions, they were able to live long enough for chronic conditions to take their toll.

The second factor contributing to the epidemiologic transition was the better living conditions and higher socioeconomic status that came to characterize Americans during the 20th century. A safer environment, better nutrition and other factors contributed to a healthier and more long-lived population. Americans were able to survive to much older ages on the average. While acute conditions are no respecter of age, they often have their greatest impact on the youngest age cohorts. Chronic conditions, on the other hand, are much more common among older populations. As the U.S. population has continued to age, the older cohorts have grown in significance while the younger cohorts have declined. As older persons have come to account for a larger proportion of the population, chronic conditions have become more common.

With chronic conditions dominating the morbidity profile, a growing mismatch has developed between the dominant approach of the healthcare system and the healthcare needs of the population. The medical model was developed to address acute conditions and is much less salient with regard to the management of chronic conditions. Although the healthcare delivery system is adapting to the epidemiologic transition, it still has a long way to go to successfully address the needs of a population characterized primarily by chronic conditions.

Reference: A. R. Omran (1971). "The Epidemiologic Transition: A Theory of the Epidemiology of Population Change," *Milbank Memorial Fund Quarterly* 49:515ff.

by 13 percent between 1990 and 2000, while the population 85 and over increased by over 36 percent. The movement of the baby boomers into the "middle ages" will make the 45–65 age group the largest age cohort in the first decade of the 21st century. Several younger cohorts (i.e., those 25–34) experienced a net loss of population during that decade. A continued "shortage" of younger working age individuals (i.e., those 25–40) will persist throughout the first decade of the 21st century, until the baby boom echo cohort enters this age group toward the end of that decade (U.S. Census Bureau, 2003).

The factor above with the most implications for future healthcare demand is the movement of the huge baby boom cohort into the "middle ages". The first of some 77 million baby boomers turned 50 during the 1990s. This is a cohort that grew up in affluence and comfort, and they are used to having things, including their health, in working order. When they have to contend with the onset of chronic disease and the natural deterioration that comes with aging, the healthcare system will be significantly impacted.

An automatic accompaniment to the aging of America has been the feminization of its population. The changing age distribution has important implications for the population's male/female ratio. Generally speaking, the older the population, the greater the "excess" of females. Except for the very youngest ages, females outnumber males in every age cohort. Among seniors, females outnumber males two to one, and, at the oldest ages, there may be four times as many women as men. This results in an older ages structure for women and, in 2000, the median age for women was 38.0 years compared to 36.5 years for men. Further, 23.2 percent of the female population was 55 or over, compared to 18.9 percent of the male population. In 2000, the "excess" of females over males in the population amounted to over five million in the United States.

Racial and Ethnic Diversity

Another demographic trend that characterizes American society as it enters the 21st century is its increasing racial and ethnic diversity. America has once again become a nation of immigrants, with the numbers of newcomers from foreign lands during the 1990s equaling historic highs, and long-established ethnic and racial minorities are growing at faster rates than are native-born whites. As a result, the visibility of non-Hispanic whites in the U.S. population is decreasing (U.S. Census Bureau, 2003).

The cumulative effect of the trends of the past several years has been a diminishing of the relative size of the white population (especially the non-Hispanic white population) and the growing significance of the black, Asian and Hispanic components of the U.S. population. The 2000 census revealed an America that was 75.1 percent white, 12.5 percent black, 3.7 percent Asian-American and Pacific Islander, and less than one percent American Indian/Alaskan Native (based on reporting of a single race). The remainder fell into the "other" racial category or reported two or more races.

The figure for the white population includes most Hispanics and they accounted for 12.5 percent of the total population (not factoring in the undercount of Hispanics). Thus, non-Hispanic whites accounted for approximately 63 percent of the U.S. population in 2000. This compares to 71 percent in 1980 and

67 percent in 1990. Since most of the anticipated population growth during the next two decades will be a function of immigration, the proportion of non-Hispanic whites within the population will continue to decline.

A great deal of variation in age exists among the racial and ethnic groups, a factor that allows demographers to make relatively accurate projections of the future racial and ethnic composition of the population. The Anglo (non-Hispanic white) population has by far the oldest age structure and the Hispanic population the youngest, with a difference of over ten years in median age in 2000 (38.6 versus 28.1 years). The median age for the black population is 30.2 years and for the Asian population 32.7 years. The differential in age distribution is expected to continue into the foreseeable future, as illustrated by the relative proportions of children recorded for the various racial and ethnic groups. A telling statistic is the fact that, in 2000, minorities accounted for over 46 percent of the children under 5, but account for only 37 percent of the total population.

Given the fact that the U.S. healthcare system has historically been geared to the needs of the mainstream white population, the trend toward greater racial and ethnic diversity can not help but have major implications for the nature of the system. Any planning activities must take into consideration the changing characteristics of the population and the demands that these changes will make for the system.

Changing Household and Family Structure

Another demographic development characterizing U.S. society is its changing household and family structure. This trend is no surprise to demographers, although it has seldom been linked to health issues. For decades, the family has been undergoing change. First it was high divorce rates; then it was less people marrying (and those who did marry married at a later age); then it was less people having children (and those that did have children had fewer of them and at a later age).

In 2000, the census reported that 54.4 percent of the U.S. population over 15 was married, a very low figure by historical standards. Some 27.1 percent had never married, 11.9 percent were separated or divorced, and 6.6 percent were widowed (U.S. Census Bureau, 2003). These figures are all high by historical standards. Given that health status and health behavior differs considerably among the various marital statuses, the current and future array of statuses should be a concern for the health planner.

These changes in marital status have had major implications for the U.S. household structure. It has meant that what is popularly considered the "typical" American family (with two parents and x number of children) has become a rarity, accounting for only 24 percent of the households in 2000. Today, married couple (without children) households have become the most common household form, but this type of household accounts for less than 28 percent of total households. "Non-traditional" households have become the norm, and an unprecedented proportion of households are one-person households.

As with marital status, the changing household structure has important implications for both health status and health behavior. The demands placed on the healthcare system by two-parent families, single-parent families, and elderly people living alone vary widely and require different responses on the part of the healthcare system. The continued diversification of U.S. household types for the foreseeable future will require commensurate modifications in the healthcare delivery system.

Consumer Attitudes

Although patterns of consumer attitudes in U.S. society tend to be complex, it is clear that a new orientation is occurring with regard to healthcare. For the most part, today's consumer is much more knowledgeable about the healthcare system, much more open to innovative approaches, and much more intent on playing an active role in the diagnostic, therapeutic and health maintenance processes.

These new attitudes are concentrated among the under-50 population and among certain demographically distinct groups. The movement toward gaining control of one's health has been spearheaded by the baby boom cohort that is now beginning to face the chronic conditions associated with "middle age". This is the population that has been responsible for the success of health maintenance organizations, urgent care centers and birthing centers. This is the group that has been influential in limiting the discretion and control of physicians and hospitals. This cohort has also provided the impetus for the rise of "alternative therapy" as a competitor for mainstream allopathic medicine.

The approach to healthcare favored by the baby boom population is more patient centered than the traditional approach and is more likely to emphasize the non-medical aspects of healthcare. In general, baby boomers are less trusting of professionals and institutions and are control oriented to the point of stubbornness. This group is more self-reliant than previous post-WWII generations and places greater value on self care and home care. It is both outcomes oriented and cost sensitive. It is a generation that prides itself in getting results and extracting value for its expenditures. While this cohort began influencing the healthcare system by "voting with its feet" during the 1980s, its members are increasingly in the positions of power that allow them to influence the reshaping the healthcare landscape.

To a certain extent, these new attitudes toward healthcare reflect the rise of consumerism related to all segments of society. *Consumers* (as opposed to *patients*) expect to receive adequate information, demand to participate in healthcare decisions that directly affect them, and expect the healthcare they receive to be of the highest possible quality. Consumers want to receive their healthcare close to their homes, with minimal interruption to their family life and work schedules. They also want to maximize the value that they receive for their healthcare expenditures. Thus, addressing the needs of consumers requires a different approach from addressing the needs of patients.

THE TRANSFORMATION OF THE U.S. HEALTHCARE SYSTEM

It is not appropriate to speak of a modern healthcare system in the United States until after World War II. Prior to that time, healthcare as an institution was poorly developed and accounted for a negligible proportion of societal resources. It remained an institutional non-entity until the period following World War II when it began a rapid rise to become a major U.S. institution.

There are two aspects of any healthcare system to be considered: (1) the disease theory system and (2) the health services delivery system. The disease theory system involves the underlying philosophies and assumptions that support the system. It represents the explanatory framework that addresses the nature of sickness and disease and serves as the foundation for the health services delivery system. Just as scientific medicine rooted in germ theory provides the underpinning for modern American healthcare, a religious belief system based on the influence of the supernatural provided the disease theory system for many traditional healthcare systems.

The delivery system involves the actual provision of healthcare. This is the component with which the general public is most familiar. Unless some type of crisis or public debate develops, participants in the delivery system are not likely to give much consideration to the underlying disease theory system. Nevertheless, changes in the nature of the disease theory system will have major implications for the health services delivery system and the thrust of any health planning.

The development of the healthcare system following World War II can be divided into six stages, roughly equating with the five decades of the last half of the 20th century and the first decade of the 21st. Each of these stages will be briefly discussed in turn.

The 1950s: The Emergence of "Modern" Medicine

As American society entered a new period of growth and prosperity following the end of World War II, the modern U.S. healthcare system began to take shape. The economic growth of the period resulted in increased demand for a wide range of goods and services, including healthcare. "Health" was coming to be recognized as a value in its own right, and considerable resources were expended on a fledging healthcare system that had lain dormant during the war.

The 1950s witnessed the first significant involvement of the federal government in healthcare, as the Hill-Burton Act resulted in the construction of hundreds of hospitals to meet pent up postwar demand. Health insurance was becoming common and, spurred by the influence of trade unions, healthcare benefits became a major issue at the bargaining table.

World War II had also served as a giant "laboratory" for pioneering a wide range of medical and surgical procedures. Trauma surgery was essentially unknown prior to the war, and trauma and burn treatment capabilities were now available to apply in a civilian context. New drug therapies were being introduced, and formal health services were coming to be seen as a solution for an increasing number of problems.

The 1960s: The Golden Age of American Medicine

During the 1960s the healthcare institution in the United States experienced unprecedented expansion in personnel and facilities. The hospital emerged as the center of the system, and the physician—much maligned in earlier decades—came to occupy the pivotal role in the treatment of disease. Physician salaries and the prestige associated with their positions grew exponentially (Starr, 1982).

Private insurance became widespread, offered primarily through employer-sponsored plans. The Medicare and Medicaid programs were introduced and these initiatives expanded access to healthcare (at government expense) to the elderly and poor, respectively.

New therapeutic techniques were being developed, accompanied by growth in the variety of technologies and support personnel required. New conditions (e.g., alcoholism, hyperactivity) were identified as appropriate for medical treatment, causing an increasing proportion of the population to come under "medical management". Complete consumer trust existed in the healthcare system in general and in hospitals and physicians in particular.

Some murmurs of dissent were heard due to the lack of access for certain segments of the population. Even here, there was virtually no criticism of the disease theory system that underlay the delivery system. It was felt that the infrastructure was sound and that tinkering with the delivery system was all that was required.

The 1970s: Questioning the System

Entering the 1970s the healthcare system appeared to be continuing along a track of expansion and growth. New techniques continued to be introduced, and there appeared to be no limit to the application of biomedical technology. Even more new conditions were identified, and increasing numbers of citizens were brought under medical management financed through private insurance and government-subsidized plans. The hospital was entrenched as the focal point of the system, and the physician continued to control more than 80 percent of the expenditures on health services.

During this decade a number of issues began to be raised concerning the healthcare system and its operation. Issues of access and equity that were first voiced in the 1960s reached a point where they could no longer be ignored. Large segments of the population appeared to be excluded from mainstream medicine. Further, the effectiveness of the system in dealing with the overall health status of the population was brought into question. Standard health status indicators suggested that the U.S. population was lagging behind many other countries in improving health status.

While many issues were raised during the 1970s, the increasing cost of care garnered the most attention. Clearly, the United States had the world's most expensive healthcare system. The costs were high and they were increasing much faster than those in other sectors of the economy. While it was once assumed that resources for the provision of healthcare were infinite, it came to be realized that there was a limit on what could be spent to provide health services. Coupled with questions about access and effectiveness, the escalating cost of care caused widespread alarm.

During this period the underlying foundation of the healthcare system was questioned for the first time. Earlier criticism had been directed at the operation of the system, and it had been assumed that the disease theory system was appropriate. Hence, a "band-aid" approach had been advocated rather than major surgery. As the 1970s ended, more and more voices were being raised concerning the underlying assumptions of the system.

The 1980s: The Great Transformation

The 1980s will no doubt be seen by historians as a watershed for U.S. healthcare. The numerous issues that had been emerging over the previous two decades came to a head as the 1980s began. By the end of the decade, American healthcare had become almost unrecognizable to veteran health professionals. Virtually every aspect of the system had undergone transformation, and a new paradigm began to emerge as the basis for the disease theory system (Strauss and Corbin, 1988).

The escalating—and seemingly uncontrollable—costs associated with healthcare prompted the Medicare administration to introduce the prospective payment system. Other insurers soon followed suit with a variety of cost-containment methods. Employers, who were footing much of the bill for increasing healthcare costs, began to take a more active role in the management of their plans.

The decade also witnessed the introduction of new financial arrangements and organizational structures. Experiments abounded in an attempt to find ways to more effectively and efficiently provide health services. The major consequence of these activities was the introduction of managed care as an approach to controlling the utilization of services and, ultimately, the cost borne by insurers. The managed care concept called for incentives on the part of all parties for more appropriate use of the system.

This transformation resulted in considerable shifts in both power and risk within the system. The power that resided in hospital administrators and physicians was blamed for much of the excess costs and inefficiency in the system. Third-party payors, employers and consumers began to attempt to share in this power. Large groups of purchasers emerged that began to negotiate for lower costs in exchange for their "wholesale" business. Insurers, who had historically borne most of the financial risk involved in the financing of health services, began shifting some of this risk to providers and consumers.

Developments outside of healthcare were also having significant influence. Chief among these was the changing nature of the American population. The acute conditions that had dominated the healthcare scene since the inception of modern medicine were being supplanted by the chronic conditions characteristic of an older population. The respiratory conditions, parasitic diseases, and playground injuries of earlier decades were being replaced in the physician's waiting room by arthritis, hypertension, and diabetes. The mismatch between the capabilities of the healthcare system, and the needs of the patients it was designed to serve became so severe that a disease theory system began to emerge.

The 1990s: The Shifting Paradigm

Although change occurs unevenly throughout a system as complex as American healthcare, many are arguing that by the late 1990s a true paradigm shift was occurring. Simply put, this involved a shift from an emphasis on "medical care" to one on "healthcare". *Medical care* is narrowly defined in terms of the formal services provided by the healthcare system and refers primarily to those activities that are under the control of medical doctors. This concept focuses on the clinical or treatment aspects of care and excludes the non-medical aspects of healthcare. *Healthcare* refers to any function that might be directly or indirectly related to preserving, maintaining, and/or enhancing health status. This concept includes not only formal activities (such as visiting a health professional) but also such informal activities as preventive care (e.g., brushing teeth), exercise, proper diet, and other health maintenance activities.

Since the 1970s there has been a movement of activities and emphasis away from medical care toward healthcare. The importance of the non-medical aspects of care has become increasingly appreciated. The growing awareness of the connection between health status and lifestyle and the realization that medical care is limited in its ability to control the disorders of modern society have prompted a move away from a strictly medical model of health and illness to one that incorporates more of a social and psychological perspective (Engel 1977).

Demographic factors have played no small role in this process. Unquestionably, the influence of the large baby boom cohort has been felt with regard to these issues. This population more than any other has led the movement toward a value reorientation as it relates to healthcare. It has been this cohort that has emphasized convenience, value, responsiveness, patient participation, accountability, and other attributes not traditionally found in the U.S. system of healthcare delivery. It has also been the cohort that has been instrumental in the emergence of urgent care centers, freestanding surgery facilities, and health maintenance organizations as standard features of the system.

Despite this changing orientation, an imbalance remained in the system with regard to the allocation of resources to its various components. Treatment still commands the lion's share of the healthcare dollar, and most research is still focused on developing cures rather than preventive measures. The hospital remains the focal point of the system, and the physician continues to be its primary gatekeeper. Nevertheless, each of these underpinnings of medical care was substantially weakened during the 1980s, with a definitive shift toward a healthcare-oriented paradigm evident during the 1990s. (See Box 3.2 for a discussion of this paradigm shift.)

At the close of the 20th century, the healthcare institution continued to be beset by many problems. It could be argued that the system was too expensive (particularly in view of its inability to effectively address contemporary health problems and raise the overall health status of the population) and that large segments of the population were excluded from mainstream medicine. The fact that "administrative costs" account for an estimated 23 percent of the U.S. healthcare dollar (compared to less than 10 percent in socialized systems) suggests that there are considerable inefficiencies in the system. (For a review of the status of the United States healthcare system at the end of the 20th century, see Wilensky and Newhouse, 1999.)

2000–2010: New Millennium Healthcare

As the 21st century begins, U.S. healthcare appears to be entering yet another phase, one that reflects both late 20th-century developments and newly emerging trends. The further entrenchment of the healthcare paradigm appears to be occurring, as the medical model continues to lose its salience. This trend is driven in part by the resurgence of consumerism that is being witnessed and the emergence of a consumer-choice market. At the same time, financial exigencies and consumer demand are encouraging more holistic, less intensive approaches to care.

The new millennium is witnessing continued disparities in healthcare, exacerbated by the growing number of uninsured individuals and a depressed economy that turns healthcare into a "luxury" for many Americans. Disparities exist in health status among various racial and ethnic groups and among those of differing socioeconomic status. Disparities exist in the use of health services and even in the types of treatment that are provided individuals in different social categories.

The first decade of the twenty-first century is also witnessing a further reaction to managed care. Capitated reimbursement arrangements are becoming less common, the gatekeeper concept is being abandoned, and consumer choice is being reintroduced into the market. Baby boomers are increasingly driving the market, shaping patterns of utilization and creating a demand for new services. At the same time, the growing population of elderly Americans is creating a demand for senior services far greater than anything ever experienced in the past.

BOX 3-2
From Medical Care to Healthcare

Most observers of the healthcare scene argue that the overarching development in healthcare of the late 20th century was the paradigm shift from an emphasis on medical care to an emphasis on healthcare. Although the two terms are often used interchangeably, there are major differences characterizing the two concepts, differences that have major implications for health planning.

Medical care is narrowly defined in terms of the formal services provided by the healthcare system. It refers primarily to those functions of the system that are under the influence of medical doctors. This concept focuses on the clinical aspects of care—i.e., diagnosis and treatment—and excludes consideration of the nonmedical aspects of care. *Healthcare* is more broadly defined and refers to any activity that directly or indirectly contributes to preserving, maintaining, and/or enhancing health status. Healthcare includes not only formal health-seeking activities (e.g., visiting a health professional), but also involvement in oral hygiene, exercise and healthy eating h habits.

Since the beginning of the 20th century, the dominant paradigm in Western medical science has been the medical model of disease. Built on the germ theory formulated late in the 19th century, the medical model provides an appropriate framework within which to address and respond to the acute health conditions prevalent well into the 20th century. Since the 1970s, however, there has been a steady movement of activities and emphases away from medical care and toward healthcare. Despite the ever-increasing sophistication of medical technology, the importance of the nonmedical aspects of care has become increasingly appreciated. The growing awareness of the connection between health status and lifestyle and the realization that medical care is limited in its ability to cure the disorders of modern society have prompted a move away from a strictly medical model of health and illness to one that incorporates more of a social and psychological perspective.

A number of factors have contributed directly or indirectly to this shift in orientation. Clearly, the "epidemiologic transition," through which acute

---

Information technology is becoming an increasingly important driving force. The new healthcare calls for effective information management and data analysis. The demands of the Health Insurance Portability and Accountability Act (HIPAA) are bringing information technology issues to the forefront. This is being accompanied by the rise of e-health, perhaps the most significant development in

conditions have been displaced by chronic disorders, has played a major role. As acute conditions waned in importance and chronic and degenerative conditions came to be predominant, the medical model began to lose some of its salience. Once the cause of most health conditions ceased to be microorganisms within the environment and became aspects of lifestyle, a new model of health and illness was required. The chronic conditions that had come to account for the majority of health problems did not respond well to the treatment-and-cure approach of the medical model. Chronic conditions could not be cured but had to be "managed" over a lifetime, and this called for a quite different approach.

Independent of this trend has been the growing dissatisfaction of patients with the operation of the healthcare system. Further, the runaway costs of the system have led observers of all persuasions to question the wisdom of pursuing the one-size-fits-all approach to solving health problems traditional in medical care.

Demographic change has played a significant role in this paradigm shift as well, with the influence of the large baby boom cohort being a major factor. This population, more than any other group in U.S. society, has led the movement toward the changing emphasis in healthcare. This cohort emphasizes convenience, value, responsiveness, patient participation, and other attributes not traditionally incorporated into the medical model. This cohort has been instrumental in the emergence of urgent care centers, innovative outpatient facilities, and HMOs as standard features of the healthcare system.

The transition from medical care to healthcare has affected everything from the standard definitions of health and illness to the manner in which healthcare is delivered. Health status is now defined as a continuous process rather than in terms of a specific episode of care. The causes of ill-health are now sought in the environment and the social context of the individual as often as they are sought under the microscope. The importance of the nonmedical component of therapy has come to be recognized and fathers are now allowed to participate in childbirth and families are encouraged to participate in the treatment of cancer patients. Perhaps the most significant indicator of the paradigm shift is the fact that the term "patient" itself is increasingly being replaced with terms like "client", "consumer", and even "customer."

healthcare in several years. The use of the Internet in the distribution of health information, the servicing of patients and plan enrollees, and the distribution of healthcare products promises to significantly change relationships within the healthcare arena.

References

Engle, George (1977). "The Need for A New Medical Model: A Challenge for Biomedicine," *Science* 196: 129–135.

Omran, A. R. (1971). "The Epidemiologic Transition: A Theory of the Epidemiology of Population Change," *Milbank Memorial Fund Quarterly* 49:515ff.

Parsons, Talcott (1951). *The Social System*. New York: Free Press.

Starr, Paul C. (1982). *The Social Transformation of American Medicine: The Rise of a Sovereign Profession and the Making of a Vast Industry*. New York: Basic Books.

Strauss, A., and J.M. Corbin (1988). *Shaping a New Health Care System*. San Francisco: Jossey-Bass.

Wilensky, G.R., and J.P. Newhouse (1999). "Medicine: What's Right, What's Wrong, What's Next?", *Health Affairs*, 18:92–106.

United States Census Bureau (2003). "American FactFinder", accessed at URL: http://factfinder.census.gov/servlet/BasicFactsServlet.

Additional Resources

Pol, Louis G., and Richard K. Thomas (2001). *The Demography of Health and Healthcare*. (2nd edition). New York: Plenum.

4

Health Services Demand and Utilization

INTRODUCTION

The demand for health services ultimately drives all healthcare planning activities. In fact, the demand for services is the *raison d'etre* for any healthcare organization. Most decisions on whether or not to offer a service will be predicated upon presumed levels of demand. Once a service is offered, virtually all decisions related to the continued provision of that service will be a function of the level of demand. For this reason, health planners spend a great deal of their time and effort trying to determine current and future levels of demand for total health services or for the specific services offered by the organization involved in the planning process.

The issue of demand carries us back to the question of who (or what) are we planning for. In the case of community-wide planning, the demand for the widest range of services possible must be taken into consideration. For planning to be truly comprehensive, the demand for virtually every type of service must be determined, ranging from consumer education programs to chronic disease management to trauma care.

At the organization level, the focus is considerably narrower. The emphasis will be on the demand for the services currently offered by the organization or for services that are being considered for offering. If the organization is multipurpose like a hospital, the planner will need to consider a relatively wide range of services (although not as comprehensive as that considered by the community health planner). On the other hand, a local home health agency serving exclusively Medicare patients will be concerned with a fairly narrow range of services.

The factors influencing the level of demand for health services have become increasingly complex, and past utilization patterns are seldom predictive of future utilization. The significant demographic, socioeconomic and psychographic transformation that the U.S. population has been undergoing has served to "naturally" modify the level of demand. At the same time, managed care arrangements and other developments in healthcare "artificially" influence the level of the demand for health services. These developments have made the task of projecting demand for health services an increasingly challenging task at a time when the ability to do so is critical to the survival of most organizations.

DEFINING "DEMAND"

"Demand" is an imprecise concept as applied to health service's and the term is often used interchangeably with other terms. In fact, there is technically no one definition of demand in common usage. The concept is sufficiently vague and is used in so many different ways that it is difficult to provide an operational definition.

Part of the confusion in terms of defining (and measuring) health services demand stems from a lack of agreement as to *who* the customer for health services is. Typically the services demanded by the end-user, usually the patient, are the primary consideration. However, other customer groups such as physicians, health plans, and employers may play a part in determining demand. For health plans, the customer may actually be the benefits manager for an employer-sponsored plan. For medical supply or equipment companies it may be retail distributors.

Perhaps the best way to approach the demand concept is by examining its component parts. From a planning perspective, demand can be conceptualized as the ultimate result of the combined effect of: 1) healthcare needs; 2) healthcare wants; 3) recommended standards for healthcare; and 4) actual utilization patterns (Berkowitz et al, 1997).

Healthcare Needs

Healthcare needs can be defined in terms of the overall health status of a population or more specifically in terms of the number of conditions that require medical treatment found within that population. The health conditions included here are those that an objective evaluation–e.g., a physical examination–would uncover within the population. These might be thought of as the *absolute* needs that exist in "nature" without the influence of any other factors. All things being equal, the absolute level of need should not vary much from population to population. These epidemiologically based needs that a team of health professionals would identify in a "sweep" through a community could be considered to represent the "true" prevalence of illness within the population.

A population with certain characteristics can be expected to experience a specified level of various health conditions based on these characteristics. However, these absolute needs, at least in contemporary societies, do not translate directly into demand. In fact, the mismatch between these baseline needs and the ultimate utilization of services is substantial. There are many conditions that go untreated (indeed, even undiagnosed) for various reasons. There are many other conditions for which treatment is obtained that would not be identified among the absolute needs of the population. For example, no team of epidemiologists assessing the healthcare needs of a community is likely to identify the sagging facial skin as a health problem. Yet, tens of thousands of facelifts are performed in the United States every year by medical doctors. The existence of a clinically confirmed need, then, is not a prerequisite for the presence of demand for a service.

Healthcare Wants

Health care wants can be conceptualized as the wishes or desires for health services on the part of a population. Unlike needs, wants would not necessarily be uncovered by a sweep of public health investigators through the community. Wants are shaped less by the absolute needs of the population than by the variety of factors that influence the consumption of other goods and services besides healthcare. In fact, many of the health services consumed are considered medically unnecessary or elective. These reflect the operation of wants rather than needs. Examples of these services include tummy tucks and laser eye surgery for nearsightedness. The U.S. healthcare system has adapted itself to the existence of wants as well as needs, and important components of the system cater to those desiring elective services.

The extent to which health care wants are a consideration in the planning process depends on the type of planning being performed. Community-wide planning ideally should emphasize the baseline needs of the population, although, realistically, the wants of the population must be taken into consideration if the approach is to be truly comprehensive. At the organizational level, the type of organization and the services it offers will dictate whether needs or wants are the main consideration. Certainly an AIDS clinic deals with basic needs, and there are few elective procedures relevant to the treatment of patients with AIDS. On the other hand, a plastic surgeon specializing in body sculpting is likely to focus on the want-driven demand generated by those motivated by vanity. At the same time, if this plastic surgeon also maintains a reconstructive surgery practice for trauma victims, both wants and needs may be a consideration in planning.

Recommended Standards for Healthcare

The third dimension involves recommended standards for the provision of healthcare. As healthcare professionals have become more attuned to prevention and health maintenance, the number of recommended procedures has increased. This component involves primarily diagnostic procedures or disease management procedures that are recommended for patients with certain symptoms or who are at risk for certain health problems.

The medical community has developed standards that call for diagnostic tests at a certain frequency, the performance of certain medical procedures at specified times, and the implementation of various treatment plans on the part of certain patients. A wide range of diagnostic procedures are now indicated for certain age groups and other population segments at risk of various health conditions. For example, an annual mammogram is recommended for all women over 50, regular prostate exams for all men over 40, and regular cholesterol exams for individuals at risk of certain conditions.

As Americans have become increasingly health conscious, a growing number of standards have been put into place. For example, a few years ago cholesterol tests were limited to patients actively under medical management. Today, cholesterol tests are recommended for everyone at specific intervals, along with pap smears and breast exams for women, prostate exams for men, and a growing number of other diagnostic and screening procedures.

Health Services Utilization

The fourth dimension involves the actual utilization of health services. The utilization level is frequently used as a proxy measure for demand, in that utilization rates can be calculated for virtually any type of health service or product. More data are available related to health services utilization than for the other dimensions of demand, primarily because utilization data are routinely collected for administrative purposes whenever a health service is provided. Utilization rates indicate the level of activity within the healthcare system, as opposed to theoretical demand.

Because of the perceived relationship between demand and utilization, analysts may sometimes work backward from utilization levels and use them as a proxy for demand. However, utilization does not equal demand and, depending on the circumstances, the level of demand may exceed actual utilization or, conversely, utilization levels may exceed reasonable demand for services. For example, there may be less utilization than expected because of limited access to health services. On the other hand, some services may be overutilized for various reasons (e.g., insurance coverage, physician practice patterns) unrelated to the level of demand.

FACTORS INFLUENCING DEMAND

The factors that combine to influence the level of demand today are multiple and their interactions are complex. Knowledge of the cultural background, lifestyle patterns, and financing arrangements of a population may be a better predictor of the type and level of services that will be utilized than knowledge of the actual level of morbidity characterizing a population. The section below describes some of the factors influencing the level of demand.

Population Characteristics

A variety of population characteristics influence the demand for health services. These can be categorized in terms of their effect on health status and/or health behavior. While a detailed discussion is not possible in this context, the correlation between population characteristics and health status and health behavior are summarized below. (See Pol and Thomas [2000] for a detailed review of the relationship between demographic characteristics and both health status and health behavior.)

At first blush one would think that the state of the population in terms of *biological factors* would play a significant role in health behavior. Although health problems may be thought of as essentially biological problems, the correlation between the morbidity profile of a population and its healthcare utilization is not nearly that direct. While biological characteristics may predispose the individual to various health problems, other factors may eventually determine the type and amount of health services utilized. Biological factors are comparable to the healthcare "needs" described above and may or may not translate into utilization.

Psychological factors correlated with health services demand include personality types and attitudinal traits, as well as the emotional responses evoked by health problems. Clearly, fear, vanity, and pride come into play in the use of health services. The relationship between these factors and health behavior can become exceedingly complex as can be seen in the case of the hypochondriac or in cases where fear pushes one person to seek treatment but prevents another from visiting the physician. In the contemporary U.S. healthcare environment, fear, pride and vanity play a large role in the demand for many elective procedures (e.g., cosmetic surgery, stomach resection). Because of the individualized nature of psychological traits, it is difficult to directly correlate them with health services utilization. In any case, there is limited useful data available on psychological characteristics available to planners.

A number of *demographic characteristics* influence utilization. *Age* is probably the single best predictor of health services utilization. Age is related not only to levels of service utilization but to the type of services utilized and the circumstances under which they are received. This is true whether the indicator is for inpatient care, tests and procedures performed, or virtually and other measure of utilization. Different conditions are associated with each age cohort, resulting in demands for differing types of services.

The *sex* of the consumer is another factor influencing utilization rates. In the U.S., females are more involved in the healthcare system than men and are heavier users of health services in general. They tend to visit physicians more often, take more prescription drugs, and, in general, use other facilities and personnel more often. Women are also more aware of the health services that are available and quicker to turn to health professionals when symptoms occur.

Racial and ethnic characteristics influence the demand for health services, with the most clear-cut differences identified between African-Americans and non-Hispanic whites. Certain Asian populations and many ethnic groups also display distinctive utilization patterns. While differences in utilization may be traced to differences in the types of health problems experienced by these populations, many of the differences reflect variations in lifestyle patterns and cultural preferences. Different perceptions of and expectations for the healthcare system are also likely to exist among various racial and ethnic populations.

Marital status is related not only to levels of demand but to the type of services utilized and the circumstances under which they are received. Different levels of morbidity are associated with each marital status category, resulting in demands for differing levels and types of services. These factors, along with the lifestyles associated with various marital statuses, probably have more impact on utilization than do actual differentials in morbidity.

The *income level* of a population is probably one of the best predicators of the utilization of health services. The distribution of health problems within the population is highly income specific. There is a correlation between income level and the amount of health services utilized, as well as with the types of services utilized and the circumstances under which they are received as well. This is true whether the indicator is for inpatient care, outpatient care, tests and procedures performed, or virtually any other measure of utilization.

The relationship between *educational level* and utilization resembles that for income. The distribution of health problems within the population is to a certain extent associated with educational status, and the educational level of the population is probably one of the better predictors of the demand for health services. Education is related to both the type and level of health services utilization.

There is a relatively direct and positive relationship between *occupational and industrial characteristics* of a population and health services utilization. The type of occupation, as well as occupational status, has been correlated with the utilization of health services. Different levels of morbidity are associated with each occupational status category, resulting in a demand for different levels and types of services.

Associations between *religious affiliation and degree of religiosity* and health behavior are probably the most idiosyncratic of any of the demographically related associations. These relationships have been exposed to limited research so that clear patterns are difficult to discern. Further, in the United States, religious affiliation and participation tend to be associated with so many other variables that is difficult to isolate the influence of these variables per se. Nevertheless, there is evidence that health status, and the subsequent use of services, is correlated with measures of religiosity and this may be an important factor in some communities.

Lifestyle and psychographic factors have important implications for health-care wants, needs, and behavior. The propensity to utilize health services may be more highly correlated with lifestyle characteristics than it is with other variables. A specific constellation of health behavior can be associated with each lifestyle category, making lifestyle an important predictor of health behavior. To a certain extent, lifestyles override, or at least refine, differences based on demographic traits.

Technological Factors

The healthcare technology available to a society has a significant influence on the consumption of health services, since the services that can be made available will be a function of the technology to which the system has access. In the United States, the technological advances of the past few years have routinized many procedures considered impossible in the past and played a major role in changing the setting in which healthcare is provided. During the last two decades of the 20th century, surgery was transformed from a predominantly inpatient activity to a predominantly outpatient endeavor.

Advances in technology usually lead to higher levels of utilization of the services that are supported by the new technology. Indeed, some operations like laser eye surgery could never have been performed without certain technological advances. Thus, the availability of certain types of technology on the part of a provider is a controlling factor with regard to the services that can be performed.

Further, technological advances have been responsible for major changes in the practice of medicine and, thus, in utilization patterns. Technological advances have facilitated major changes in surgical techniques and supported the emergence of home health care as a major component of the industry. In fact, the short recovery time now possible with less invasive surgical techniques has served to reduce the average length of hospital stay and boost the growth of the home healthcare industry.

The impact of technology has been particularly felt in the area of diagnostic testing in recent years. The variety of tests that can be performed has increased dramatically. Examples include advanced diagnostic imaging and home testing procedures.

Structural Factors

One final consideration in the examination of demand involves the *structural factors* that encourage or discourage the use of health services. Chief among these are the financial arrangements that exist for paying for care. One indicator of the likely level of demand is the type and extent of health insurance coverage for individuals and families. The availability of insurance has been identified as one of the best predictors of the demand for services. When insurers introduce copayments and/or higher deductibles into their insurance plans, the use of health services often declines in response. When reimbursement for a service is offered, the use of that service tends to increase.

Changing reimbursement arrangements also exert an influence on practice patterns. Hospitals face restrictions on the services they can provide, introduced by health plans that are trying to control claims, while changing reimbursement patterns and regulatory pressures are forcing physicians to change their practice patterns as well. It has been suggested, in fact, that reimbursement provisions under the Medicare program over the past 15 years have done more to influence practice patterns of U.S. healthcare providers than the combined effect of technological developments during the same time period.

The emergence of managed care as a dominant organizational structure within healthcare has also had an impact on utilization patterns. In fact, the very concept of managed care emphasizes the ability of health plans to control the utilization of services on the part of their enrollees. For example, health plans are increasingly encouraging their members to obtain certain services, while at the same time discouraging them from obtaining others. Many health plans are now moving toward the concept of "demand management" in which they attempt to control utilization before the fact by managing the level of demand among enrollees.

The second structural consideration has to do with the availability of services in the form of facilities and personnel. Until recent cost-containment measures were instituted, it was apparent that the level of health services utilization was to a great extent a function of the facilities and health professionals available. It was remarkable to observe that, if a community built a new hospital or recruited additional physicians, it suddenly found the demand for hospital care and physician services escalating. Situations can be observed in which the demand for services is not being met because of a lack of facilities or personnel. In others an oversupply of

---

BOX 4-1
The Dartmouth Atlas of Healthcare

The analysis of healthcare service areas has been hampered historically by a lack of data on realistically defined medical catchment areas. The development of accurate boundaries for market areas often required extensive primary research and, if a large number of markets were involved, this process could be extremely tedious and time consuming. In addition, health planners often did not have access to the data necessary for delineating appropriate service area boundaries.

Health planners can benefit from work completed by the Dartmouth University Medical School with funding from the Robert Wood Johnson Foundation. Researchers at the Center for Evaluative Clinical Sciences used Medicare utilization data to divide the United States into clearly identifiable hospital service areas. For the 1999 release (the most recent), Medicare data for 1996 was allocated to 306 hospital referral areas and 3,436 hospital service areas. The results of this project have been published in *The Dartmouth Atlas of Healthcare in the United States* and made available on line at www.dartmouthatlas.org.

The core publication is the first widely available reference to detail and compare the dramatic differences in healthcare resources, utilization,

facilities and/or personnel may result in the overutilization of health services—i.e., at a level that exceeds reasonable demand.

To the extent that a maldistribution of health facilities and personnel persists in the United States, there are going to be chronic problems with regard to access. Even in urban areas with ample community resources, some of the resources may not be truly accessible to all segments of the population. Until access can be factored out as a variable, it will continue to influence the level of health services utilization.

Research over the past two decades has revealed a surprising variation in the patterns of practice of physicians and, to a lesser extent, hospitals. Far from being an exact science, medicine involves frequent value judgments on the part of physicians and other practitioners. While there are individual differences among physicians within the same market area in terms of the volume and types of services provided to similar patients, there are even more striking variations from market to market (The Center for Evaluative Clinical Sciences, 1999). Local practice patterns significantly influence the level of service utilization, creating differences of several magnitudes between market areas in some instances. (See Box 4-1 for a description of the Dartmouth Atlas of Health Care that illustrates variations in practice patterns across the nation.)

and expenditures at the national, regional and local hospital market areas across the nation. Regional supplements have been produced along with state-specific products for a few states. Reports on categorical diseases (e.g., cardiology) are beginning to be produced.

Unlike traditional approaches to service area delineation that follow political boundaries, the Dartmouth study examined sub-county referral patterns in order to establish more realistic services areas. The Dartmouth Atlas offers many revealing insights into the state of our healthcare delivery system, particularly the large variations found from community to community in the utilization rate for health services. The authors have concluded that, indeed, geography is destiny when it comes to the use of health services.

The Atlas allows the analyst to focus on a carefully defined hospital service area and access a wide variety of statistics specific to that service area. Or the analyst may wish to compare a variety of service areas in different parts of the country on the basis of certain characteristics. Information is available at the service area level on hospital resources, expenditures, utilization and outcomes. Data are also available on Medicare expenditures, the distribution of physicians and performance rates for common procedures.

Reference: Center for Evaluative Clinical Sciences (1999). *The Dartmouth Atlas of Health Care*. Hanover, NH: Center for Evaluative Clinical Sciences.

THE ELASTICITY OF HEALTH SERVICES DEMAND

The recorded level of health services utilization reflects a combination of the needs, wants, and recommended standards of the population, as well as the impact of the structural factors noted above. While each category of "demand" represents a different type of challenge for health services planners, the real challenge is to be able to determine what combination of these factors is relevant for a particular situation. The determination of demand is clearly a multifaceted process that involves a number of different dimensions. While it may be appropriate, depending on the situation, to use either need, want, recommended standards, or utilization as a proxy for demand, ultimately some type of blended concept must be developed that more precisely specifies effective demand.

A surprising fact to many is that the demand for most health services is relatively elastic. Although economists once considered medical care to be the one service for which demand was truely inelastic, this is not a contemporary perspective. The assumption had been that, if an individual was sick, the individual would consume health services, *and*, if an individual received health services, he must be sick. This assumption only applies, however, to rare life-threatening situations for which treatment will almost invariably be received regardless of any other characteristics of the patient or the healthcare system. For every episode requiring life-saving efforts, there are thousands of healthcare consumption situations, many involving individuals who are not technically sick. The ultimate level of health services utilized rises and falls in response to a wide range of factors.

MEASURING HEALTH SERVICES UTILIZATION

The indicators that are commonly used to measure health services utilization are discussed in the sections that follow. Each of the key utilization indicators is discussed in turn, although the various aspects of these indicators cannot be discussed in detail in the limited space available here and not all possible indicators are included. (See Box 4-2 for an overview of coding systems employed to measure utilization.)

Hospital admissions is one of the most frequently used indicators of health services utilization, since the hospital represents the focal point for treatment in the system. The terms "admissions" and "discharges" are used to refer to episodes of inpatient hospital utilization. The hospital admissions rate serves as a proxy for a variety of other indicators, since hospital admissions are correlated with tests conducted, surgeries performed, and allocation of other resources. Since hospital care is both labor and capital intensive, one admission carries a great deal of weight in terms of significance in overall health care expenditures. Admissions may be measured for the entire community or for the particular facility or may be decomposed into components of utilization. This could involve the calculation of admission rates by clinical specialty, demographic attribute, geographic origin, payor category, and so on.

BOX 4-2
Coding Systems in Healthcare

The health services planner is likely to be overwhelmed by the variety of coding schemes that are utilized in the U.S. healthcare system. Unfortunately, a number of different systems are in use, and it is impossible to understand the functioning of the system without a working knowledge of the manner in which conditions and procedures are classified and recorded. The classification systems briefly described below are commonly used; however, more information than can be provided here will ultimately be required to gain an understanding of these various systems.

International Classification of Diseases

The most widely recognized and used disease classification system is the *International Classification of Diseases*, now in its tenth edition (abbreviated ICD-10). The ICD system is the official classification scheme developed by the World Health Organization (WHO), the healthcare arm of the United Nations. In the United States a version of the ICD system is used that reflects the modifications necessary in keeping with current medical practice in American hospitals. The ICD-9 version is slowing being replaced in the U.S. by ICD-10.

The ICD system is designed for the classification of morbidity and mortality information and for the indexing of diseases and procedures that occur within hospital settings and certain other healthcare settings. The present classification system includes two components: diagnoses and procedures. Two different sets of codes are assigned to the respective components and the codes are detailed enough that very fine distinctions can be made among different diagnoses and procedures. (A different system is used for recording procedures in physicians' offices and other outpatient settings.)

Originally, the ICD system was designed to facilitate communication concerning diseases worldwide, to provide a basis for statistical recording-keeping and epidemiological studies, and to facilitate research into the quality of healthcare. However, additional functions have evolved in which the system is used as a coding scheme for facilitating payment for health services, evaluating utilization patterns, and studying the appropriateness of healthcare costs. While the epidemiologist may find this system invaluable for studying the distribution and spread of disease, its primary use within the U.S. healthcare system has come to be related to financial management (i.e., as a coding system for patient billing).

The disease classification component is composed of 17 disease and injury categories, along with two "supplementary" classifications. Within each

(continued)

of these major categories, specific conditions are listed in detail. A three-digit number is assigned to the various major subdivisions within each of the 17 categories. These three-digit numbers are extended another digit to indicate a subcategory within the larger category (in order to add clinical detail or isolate terms for clinical accuracy). A fifth digit is sometimes added to specify any factors further associated with that particular diagnosis. For example, with the ICD-9 version Hodgkin's disease, a form of malignant neoplasm or cancer, is coded 201. A particular type of Hodgkin's disease, Hodgkin's sarcoma, is coded 201.2. If the Hodgkin's sarcoma affects the lymph nodes of the neck, it is coded 201.21.

The supplementary classifications are a concession to the fact that many non-medical factors are involved in the onset of disease, responses to disease, and the use of services. These additional categories attempt to identify causes of disease or injury states that are external to the biophysical system.

Procedure categories were introduced for the first time with the ICD-9 version. The procedure component is divided into 16 categories. Of these, 15 are keyed to specific body systems (e.g., nervous system, digestive system), and one involves diagnostic procedures and residual therapeutic procedures. A two-digit scheme is used, with a code being carried out to two decimal places when necessary to provide more detail. The system was designed to accommodate usage to both hospital and ambulatory care settings.

Much like the disease-coding scheme, the procedure-classification system is heavily used for financial management and the determination of patterns of utilization, although it retains its uses for epidemiological studies.

Current Procedural Terminology

While the ICD classification system focuses on procedures performed under the auspices of a hospital or clinic, the Current Procedural Terminology (CPT) system relates exclusively to procedures and services performed by physicians. Physician-provided procedures and services are divided into five categories: medicine, anesthesiology, surgery, radiology, and pathology and laboratory services. In its fourth edition (CPT-4), this system identifies each procedure and service with a five-digit code number. This method attempts to facilitate accurate, specific, and uniform coding for physician offices.

Examples of coded procedures include surgical operations, office visits, and x-ray readings. The most accurate descriptor is determined form the CPT guidebook by the provider and that code is assigned. In addition to the identifying code, the five-digit number allows for modifiers to be appended. Modifiers may indicate situations in which an adjunctive service was performed. The manual also contains some useful information on accepted definitions for levels of care and extensiveness of consultation. Some 7,000 variations of procedures and services are catalogued.

Another set of codes has been developed to supplement the CPT codes. The Common Procedure Coding System (HCPCS) was developed by the Health Care Financing Administration before its name was changed to Centers for Medicare and Medicaid Services. HCPCS involves a listing of services provided by physicians and other providers that are not covered under the CPT coding scheme. These include certain physician services along with nonphysician services such as ambulance, physical therapy, and durable medical equipment.

Diagnosis Related Groups

Spiraling healthcare costs during the 1980s launched an era of cost containment. Efforts aimed at slowing healthcare expenditures have been initiated primarily by the federal government in response to the financial demands placed on the Medicare program, the Medicaid program, and other federally supported healthcare initiatives. The most significant step in this regard has been the introduction of prospective payment as the basis for reimbursement for health services rendered under the Medicare program. Hospitals, physicians, and certain other providers of healthcare are informed at the beginning of the financial accounting period the amount that the federal government will pay for inpatient services for a particular category of patient.

The prospective payment system (PPS) limits the amount of reimbursement for services provided to each category of patient based on rates determined by the Centers for Medicare and Medicaid Services (CMS), the federal agency that administers the Medicare program.

The basis for prospective payment is the *diagnosis related group* (DRG). Using the patient's primary diagnosis as the starting point, CMS has developed a mechanism for grouping all hospital patients into over 500 DRGs. The idea is to link payment to the consumption of resources, with the assumption that a patient's diagnosis should be the best predictor of resource utilization. The primary diagnosis is modified by such factors as other coexisting diagnoses, the presence of complications, the patient's age, and the usual length of hospital stay in order to derive the 500+ diagnostic categories.

For many purposes—e.g., general reporting, statistical analysis, planning—DRGs represent too fine a distinction among conditions. For these purposes, DRGs have been grouped into 23 major diagnostic categories (MDCs). These MDCs are based primarily on the different body systems.

(continued)

DRGs are categorized as either medical DRGs or surgical DRGs. In the calculation of reimbursement for services, each DRG is given a weight. The weight is the major factor in a complicated formula for determining the rate of reimbursement for each hospital participating in the Medicare program.

Although introduced for use in federal healthcare programs, the DRG system was quickly adopted by other health plans as a basis for reimbursement. This system has become the standard classification system in use for hospitalized patients in the U.S. and has been adopted by other countries around the world.

Ambulatory Payment Classification

As the prospective payment system based on DRGs was being implemented to control the cost of inpatient care for Medicare, much of the medical treatment was being shifted to an outpatient or ambulatory setting. Any cost savings realized by the Medicare program on the inpatient side were being eroded by growing expenditures for ambulatory services. This situation prompted the development of a system similar to DRGs for the outpatient environment referred to as the *Ambulatory Payment Classification* (APC).

As with DRGs, APCs focus on the facility component of healthcare costs and not on physician charges. The intent of CMS is to contain outpatient facility costs, introduce some controls over outpatient services utilization, and create a prospective system that works similar to DRGs. The

Patient days refers to the number of hospital days generated by a particular population and is usually calculated in terms of the number of patient days generated per 1,000 residents. This indicator refines hospital admissions as an indicator by reflecting the total utilization of resources, since measuring patient days serves to adjust for variations in length of stay for various conditions. Like admission rates, patient days may be calculated by diagnosis, type of hospital, patient origin, and payer category. Changes in reimbursement procedures, in fact, have made the patient day more of a standard unit for the measurement of resource utilization than the hospital admission.

Another indicator used to measure hospital utilization is the *average length of stay*. This is typically reported in terms of the average number of days patients remain in the facility during a specified time period. This indicator provides a good measure of resource utilization as well. In fact, Medicare and many health care plans reimburse hospitals on a per diem rate.

There are several *other facility indicators* that might also be mentioned. While not all of them carry the significance of hospital admissions, each is important in

basis for the fee is the patient visit rather than the entire episode as in the case of DRGs. An APC-specific diagnosis code has been developed and CPT codes continue to be used to classify procedures and ancillary services. Introduced in August of 2000, APC codes are now being widely used in outpatient facilities.

Diagnostic and Statistical Manual of Mental Disorders

The definitive reference on the classification of mental disorders is the *Diagnostic and Statistical Manual of Mental Disorders* (fourth edition), commonly referred to as DSM-IV. Published by the American Psychiatric Association, the DSM remains the last word in mental disease classification, despite long-standing criticism of the classification scheme. Its 17 major categories of mental illness and over 450 identified mental conditions are considered exhaustive.

The DSM classification system is derived in part from the ICD system discussed earlier. It is essentially structured in the same manner, using a five-digit code. The fourth digit indicates the variety of the particular disorder under discussion, and the fifth digit refers to any special consideration related to the case. The nature of the fifth-digit modifier varies depending on the disorder under consideration. Unlike the other classification systems discussed, the DSM system contains rather detailed descriptions of the disorders categorized therein and serves as a useful reference in this regard.

its own way. Utilization rates may be calculated for nursing homes, hospital emergency rooms, hospital outpatient departments, urgent-care centers, surgery centers, and freestanding diagnostic centers, among others.

Perhaps one of the most useful indicators of health services utilization is the volume of physician encounters. This is typically measured in terms of *physician office visits* although telephone contact and physician visits to hospitalized patients are sometimes considered. The physician is the "gatekeeper" for most types of health services, and physician utilization is a more direct measure of utilization levels than hospital admissions, since virtually everyone uses a physician's services at some time. Physician utilization rates are often broken down by specialty, since the utilization of the different specialties varies dramatically.

There are *other types of personnel* for whom utilization rates might be calculated. Most of these, like physicians and dentists, are independent practitioners who practice without the supervision of other medical personnel. Examples include optometrists, podiatrists, chiropractors, nurse practitioners, and physician's assistants, as well as various mental health counselors and therapists. Other health care personnel, who generally cannot operate independently but for whom utilization rates might be calculated, include home health nurses and various technical personnel. Physical therapists and speech therapists are other categories of healthcare personnel for whom utilization rates might be developed if, for example, the analyst was involved in planning for rehabilitation services.

As the importance of home healthcare has grown in recent years, the volume of *home health visits* has taken on more importance. The range of services provided has been expanded and a much broader segment of the patient population is considered appropriate for home care. Home care utilization is typically measured in terms of visits by various types of personnel. Thus, a population might be considered to have a certain number of home nurse visits or home physical therapist visits as indicators of utilization. Alternatively, the number of residences (i.e., the rate per 1,000) receiving home care might be calculated.

Another indicator of the use of health services that is sometimes used is the level of *drug utilization*. Although patient care providers typically have limited use for information on drug utilization, analysts representing other entities such as pharmaceutical companies do. These analyses typically focus on the consumption of prescription drugs, since these (rather than over-the-counter medicine) are thought to more closely reflect actual utilization of the formal healthcare system. While the level of drug prescribing can be determined from physician and pharmacist records, rates of consumption for nonprescription drugs must be determined more indirectly.

Rates of prescription drug utilization are typically calculated in terms of the number of prescriptions within a given year per 1,000 population. Alternatively, the average number of prescriptions written annually per person may be calculated. Occasionally, the level of drug consumption might be estimated based on the quantities of pharmaceuticals prescribed.

The indicators of utilization considered the most salient will depend on the level of planning that is taking place and the type of plan. In the case of community-wide planning, the planner will probably be interested in most of the indicators discussed above, due to the comprehensive nature of this type of planning. At the organization level, the type of utilization indicators of interest depends on the nature of the organization and the type of plan that is being implemented.

ESTIMATING THE DEMAND FOR HEALTH SERVICES

Knowledge about the current level of demand for health services, however measured, is important for the planning process. Even more important, however, is the anticipated future level of demand characterizing the population under study. A variety of techniques have been developed for projecting future demand, and three of these are discuss below.

Traditional Utilization Projections

The simplest and most straightforward approach to projecting the utilization of health services involves straight-line projections that extend historical trends. For example, it was common in the past to review several years' experience with hospital admissions and then extrapolate this trend into the future. This approach was very intuitive in that, if the trend had been upward, it continued to rise. On the other hand, if a downward trend had been recorded, the assumption was that historical patterns would persist in the future.

Few market analysts would utilize this approach in today's healthcare environment. Developments external to the healthcare arena have such an impact on the demand for services and ultimate patterns of utilization that the past no longer serves as a guide to the future when it comes to the utilization of health services. This situation has forced a much more sophisticated approach to the projection of utilization.

Population-Based Models

The most powerful factor in terms of predicting health services utilization is the size of the population. A change in the number of people served tends to have greater impact in terms of changes in utilization expected in the future than virtually any other factor. Because of the importance of population size and because population projections are likely to be both readily available and fairly reliable, population-based projections have become the most common predictive technique used in forecasting health services use.

The simplest approach involves multiplying the projected population by known utilization rates. Thus, population-based models involve two components: 1) appropriate population estimates and projections; and 2) accurate utilization rates. Population estimates and projections are available from a variety of sources and for various levels of geography.

While some benefit can be derived from basing the demand estimates on the total population, the analysis typically examines utilization in terms of age and sex. Changes in age distribution occur frequently, and these changes can have a major effect on utilization. Utilization patterns for males and females vary significantly, and these must be taken into consideration. The easiest way to express the effect of age is to employ sex- and age-specific use rates. As more data have become available, the population may also be examined in terms of race and income. In some cases, it may be possible to decompose the population in terms of payor category.

Thus, utilization rates may be expressed in terms of hospital admissions or physician visits per 1,000 residents per year, patient days per 1,000 residents per year, live births per 1,000 females age 15 to 44 per year, and so forth. These rates can be adjusted to account for regional differences when appropriate. The utilization rates of interest can be applied to different age/sex categories and adjusted for other attributes to the extent they are available.

While population-based demand projection models in all of their permutations offer an intuitively appealing approach to the issue, there are limitations to their usefulness. On the one hand, the mobility of the population in contemporary America introduces an element of uncertainty into the projection process. The cohort affect certainly plays a role in determining differential utilization patterns, and it is no longer safe to contend, for example, that the utilization patterns of 65-year-olds today will be the same as for 65-year-olds twenty years ago. Thus, applying an age-specific rate to today's elderly that is based on past experience may be risky.

Utilization rates themselves are given to change. All things being equal in terms of population characteristics, there are numerous factors that influence utilization rates. Many of these have already been discussed and they include the availability of services, financing arrangements, and the level of managed care penetration. Who could have predicted, for example, the decline in hospital admissions that resulted from the introduction of the Medicare prospective payment system and the emergence of managed care? The influence of developments of this type make the prediction of future levels of utilization a challenge.

Econometric Models

Econometric models include a variety of different techniques for projecting future phenomena in complex situations. In their simplest form, econometric models represent a type of time series analysis. In effect, they attempt to statistically improve on the projection model discussed above that extrapolates past trends into the future.

Econometric models use equations that project utilization as a function of the interplay of various independent variables. With a complex phenomenon like the utilization of health services, it makes sense to consider forecasting based on multiple factors rather than a single one. The more the factors involved in predicting future utilization, the greater the probability of an accurate projection. Econometric prediction addresses such factors in a series of mathematical expressions. The equation that is ultimately used is the one that best "fits the curve" in terms of historic demand. However, for this complex form of econometrics to work, projections are needed for numerous independent variables in the equation.

Many analysts have attempted to apply econometric models to the prediction of health services demand. In today's environment, however, econometric models have limited utility because of the unpredictability and instability in the healthcare environment.

References

Berkowitz, Eric N., Pol, Louis G., and Richard K. Thomas (1997). *Healthcare Market Research*. Burr Ridge, IL: Irwin Professional Publishing.

Center for Evaluative Clinical Sciences (1999). *The Dartmouth Atlas of Health Care*. Hanover, NH: Center for Evaluative Clinical Sciences.

Pol, Louis G., and Richard K. Thomas (2000). *The Demography of Health and Health Care*. New York: Plenum.

Additional Resources

American Medical Association (CPT Codes). Website at URL: www.ama-assn.org.

American Psychiatric Association (Diagnostic and Statistical Manual). Website at URL: www.psych.org/clin_ res/dsm/dsmintro813ø1.cfm.

Center for Medicare and Medicaid Services (Diagnosis Related Groups, Healthcare Common Procedures Coding System, Ambulatory Payment Classification). Website at URL: www.cms.gov.

5

The Planning Process

INTRODUCTION

Health planning involves a series of steps that move the process from the first organizational meeting to a finalized plan (and beyond). While the planning process has become increasingly standardized, there is no *one* process that fits all situations. While the variations that exist share common traits, each takes a slightly different approach. The process for community-wide planning is somewhat different from that for organization-level planning, and each type of organizational plan calls for variations in the planning process.

Despite these differences, all planning processes include certain components, and the sections that follow offer a "generic" outline of this process. The extent to which this process varies for different levels of planning and different types of plans will be noted in the discussion.

THE PLANNING MODEL

The model diagrammed below (Figure 5-1) presents a general framework for the planning process. It applies to virtually any type of planning and is charming in its simplicity. There are two types of factors that influence the current status of the community's health system or the healthcare organization: internal factors and external factors. Combined, these determine the current situation of the community

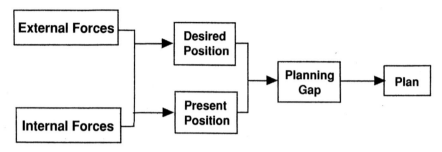

Figure 5-1. The Planning Model.

or the organization. Once the desired situation has been specified, the difference between the existing situation and the desired situation (the "planning gap") can be determined. Once identified, the planning gap becomes the target for subsequent planning activities. Although the discussion that follows suggests a much more complicated process, ultimately health services planning comes down to the ability to identify gaps and address them.

STEPS IN THE PLANNING PROCESS

Planning for Planning

A great deal of preparation is involved in the planning process, thus "planning for planning" consumes much of the early effort. The first step in any planning process involves identifying the mandate under which the planners are to operate. The planning process may be initiated, for example, in response to a felt need within the community, a health problem that is not being adequately addressed, or a crisis faced by an organization. It may also be driven by some political motivation or some immediate financial consideration. The "why" of the planning process is likely to color all subsequent activities and should be addressed early in the process.

Much of the early planning activity is organizational in nature. It involves identifying the key stakeholders, decision makers, and resource persons that must be taken into consideration. At the community level, identifying these players and soliciting participation is as much a political process as it is a technical process. While there is no foolproof combination of team members that assures success, certain categories of participants must be included whether the planning is taking place at the community level or the organization level. These include representatives of the various stakeholders, key decision makers, opinion leaders, and representatives of various substantive areas. It is important that the planning process be inclusive, involving people who have significant influence in the community (for example, elected officials), as well as the people who are most likely to be affected by the plan (such as residents of low-income neighborhoods.)

In order to plan for the total community, participants should include represen-tatives of both private sector providers and public health agencies, both physical medicine and mental health interests, and acute, chronic and long-term care ser-vices. To be truly community based, representatives of "marginal" clinical groups such as chiropractors, podiatrists, psychologists, and alternative therapists should be included.

At the organization level, the selection of key participants is equally important. In fact, it is much easier for one inappropriately chosen participant to torpedo the planning effort with an organization than it is at the community level due to the more "public" nature of the latter. The selection of participants is particularly ticklish within the organization, in that the process may have problematic outcomes for some of those chosen to participate.

At the organization level, the internal participants in the planning process should be drawn from a wide range of functional areas, starting with management. Certainly the staff of the marketing department should play a key role and, if there is a research department, the efforts of the two should be combined. Depending on the issues, finance, human resources, or other key departments, including clinical departments, may play a role. Moreover, it is hard to imagine an efficient planning process being carried out today without the full cooperation of the information systems department.

The planning process itself needs to be outlined at this stage. The format for the process, the objectives of the process (not the plan at this point), and such practical issues as the frequency of planning team meetings should be considered. Importantly, the purpose of these meetings–e.g., work sessions, progress reporting, decision making–must be determined. (Figure 5-2 depicts the steps in the planning process as described below.)

Stating Assumptions

One of the critical steps at the outset (and actually at any juncture in the plan-ning process) is the stating of assumptions. "Assumptions" are the understandings that drive the planning process, and, if they are not specified early in the process, the planning team may find itself well down the road holding conflicting notions of what the process is really about. Assumptions might be made concerning the macro-environment (e.g., depressed economic conditions expected for the near term), the regulatory environment (e.g., stricter CON regulations are anticipated), or the micro-environment (e.g., Competitor X will continue increasing its mar-ket share). Assumptions can also relate to demographic trends, reimbursement practices, internal resource availability, and any number of other aspects of the healthcare system.

From a community-wide planning perspective, an assumption might be made, on the one hand, that any plan that disturbs existing practice patterns will not be acceptable. Obviously, such an assumption places serious constraints on the process. On the other hand, an assumption may be made that, for this planning

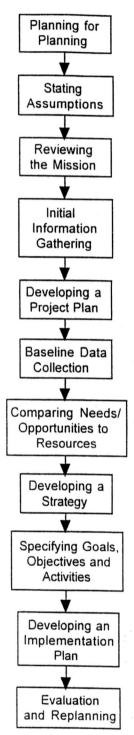

Figure 5-2. The Planning Process.

initiative, "nothing is sacred", thereby giving the planners, theoretically at least, a free hand to consider any options. These assumptions might be thought of as the "facts of life" with which the planners are going to have to live.

Assumptions should be made by organization-level planners about the market that is being considered. These would include assumptions related to the nature of the market (and its population), the political climate, the position of other providers, and so forth. At the organization level, assumptions might also be made concerning the internal environment. These may relate to financial status, personnel capabilities, existing contracts, and the like. For example, the assumption that virtually no financial resources are available internally for plan implementation is an important constraining factor.

Assumptions should also be stated with regard to the scope of the planning process. While it is hoped that the process at the community level will be comprehensive, this cannot be assumed. There may be reasons that certain aspects of the system are not taken into consideration in this process. For example, it has not made sense in the past to include local military facilities in the planning process, since they involve distinct services that cater to a discrete population, with neither services nor population overlapping with the community. The scope of the process is clearly an area of potential controversy, and assumptions regarding the scope should be agreed upon as early in the process as possible.

Some assumptions can–and should–be stated at the outset of the planning process. Others will be developed as information is collected and more indepth knowledge is gained concerning the community, its healthcare needs, and its resources. The same will be true in the planning process for an organization. Although assumptions will undoubtedly be refined as the planning process continues, it is important to begin with at least general assumptions identified.

Reviewing the Mission

In any planning initiative, the mission(s) of the entities involved should be considered. If no planning process is currently in place at the community level, a mission statement should be developed early in the process. If a planning process is already established, the mission driving that process needs to be revisited. In those rare cases in which a single agency is charged with the development of the community-wide plan, the mission statement of that agency should be reviewed. The mission established for community-wide planning will inevitably be broad and idealistic and should guide the goal-setting process.

At the organization level, the mission statement of the organization should be examined early in the planning process. It is important to reach consensus on the mission, since the thrust of subsequent planning will be guided by the mission statement. In a rapidly changing environment, it may be found that the activities of the organization may no longer match its mission statement, or that the nature of the organization's current activities may call for a revised mission statement. Until some level of consensus on mission is reached, it is not likely that much effective planning will take place within the organization.

Initial Information Gathering

No planning process should ever begin "cold". A lack of knowledge displayed in the first organizational meeting is likely to forever sour any possible progress. As much before-the-fact knowledge as possible should be obtained from any available source. For community-wide planners, this may involve a "literature review" of materials that have been prepared on the local healthcare system. Newspaper articles that describe various aspects of the system may be available, and many communities produce health-related publications. Increasingly, community report cards are being developed by various organizations, and this information may help inform the process.

Healthcare organizations within the community typically publish documents that describe the organization and its operation. Some of these, like policy and procedure manuals, may have been developed for internal use. Others, like marketing material, are for public consumption. Publicly-held companies and organizations that are tax exempt must both file reports on their status. The document review should include any previous plans that have been developed and any research projects or consultant studies that have been conducted. While these reports are likely to have limitations, they can provide at least a partial view of certain aspects of the system.

This review should be accompanied by interviews with knowledgeable individuals within the community, both inside and outside of the medical establishment. For community-wide planning, the scope should be as wide as possible. There are always going to be varying "versions" of the healthcare story, with the assessment of the system changing with one's perspective. At a minimum, one should be familiar with the perspectives of the key institutional players, major decision makers and opinion leaders, and political influentials.

This initial information gathering process should also reveal something about the history of the current system. While planning is futuristic in its outlook, the future of any community health system is likely to be inextricably intertwined with its past. Current relationships take the form they do because of historical developments, and past experiences and relationships will color any future developments.

This point is equally valid at the organization level. The organization's "life history" will be instructive in developing a plan for its future. The corporate culture will exert a strong influence on the planning process, and this culture typically can only be understood in the light of its historical development. For this reason, a historical review of the organization is an essential component of most internal audits.

During initial information gathering, the major issues that are driving the process should be identified. While these issues will be continuously clarified during the planning process, the initial identification of issues provides a starting point for further research. While the issues at the community level are likely to be much broader than those for the organization, they have the same effect in terms of the planning process. They may or may not be the issues that are ultimately addressed, but the fact that someone considers them issues must be taken into account.

This background research should identify the decision-making process for the community healthcare system, at least to the extent it can be isolated. How are decisions made with regard to the expenditure of public healthcare funds? What healthcare organizations are influential politically? Who has the grassroots support of the community?

At the organization level, the identification of decision makers is even more important. The ultimate success of the planning process will have as much to do with internal relationships as it does with external factors. Initial information gathering should determine who plays what roles and how the relative clout of the respective parties is likely to impact the planning process.

As part of this process, any potential barriers to the planning initiative should be identified. Certain barriers are likely to become obvious during this early stage of inquiry, and individuals or organizations that are clearly resistant to the planning process are likely to surface. Any immutable patterns of behavior on the part of members of the medical community should be identified. While some barriers can be surmounted, others might not be. These understandings become a part of the assumptions that drive the process.

The Project Plan

Early in the process of planning for planning, a project plan should be developed. The project plan systematically depicts the various steps in the planning process and specifies the sequence to be followed. The project plan also indicates the relationships that exist between the various tasks and, importantly, the extent to which the completion of some tasks is a prerequisite for the accomplishment of others.

Project planning tools like Gantt charts facilitate plan development. Project management tools such as the program evaluation review technique (PERT) and the critical path method (CPM) offer useful aids for estimating the resources needed for the project and clarifying the planning and control process. PERT involves dividing the total research project into its smallest component activities, determining the sequence in which these activities must be performed, attaching a time estimate for each activity, and presenting them in the form of a flow chart that allows a visual inspection of the overall process. The time estimates allow planners to determine the "critical path" through the chart. These tools can be readily accessed today using computer software packages. (See Figure 5-3 for a simplified depiction of a Gantt chart.)

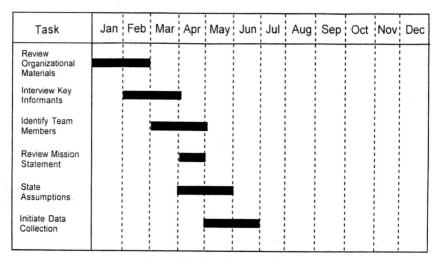

Figure 5-3. Sample Gantt Chart.

Environmental Assessment

The first step in the formal data collection process involves an environmental assessment, regardless of whether the planner focuses on a community or an organization. Also referred to as a situational analysis, this assessment typically begins at the macro-level of analysis. This would ordinarily involve analysis at the national level, although, for some organizations with multinational operations, it could take place at the international level. The macro-level analysis should be followed by analysis at the regional level if appropriate. The environmental assessment at the state level is particularly important, given the role that states play in the regulation of healthcare. Finally, the assessment should address the micro-level or the local environment. Ultimately, most healthcare organizations operate locally, and the local environment should be carefully analyzed within the context of national and state developments. The topics to be covered are identified below, with more detail provided in Chapters 6 and 7.

As a starting point in the environmental assessment, broad *societal trends* should be analyzed and their implications for the local environment considered. Among those to be considered are demographic trends, economic developments, lifestyle trends, and even shifts in attitudes. The same type of analysis should be applied to *healthcare industry trends* to identify any developments that are likely to affect the community or the organization. These could include trends in reimbursement (discussed below), changing organizational structures within the delivery system, and the introduction of new treatment modalities.

Regulatory, political and legal developments should be reviewed for their implications for the community or the organization. At the federal and state levels, a number of regulatory functions exist, while states have primary responsibility for licensing health facilities and personnel. The potential impact of regulatory, political, and legal developments at all levels of government should be considered.

Developments in the area of *technology* can exert a major influence on the course of the healthcare system. Technology here is considered in the broadest possible light, covering medical and surgical treatment modalities, pharmaceuticals, biomedical equipment, and information management. Most observers have been surprised at the impact of the Internet on healthcare, and other technology trends that are likely to impact the system or the organization should be identified.

Reimbursement arrangements related to the provision of care are a major factor to be considered in the analysis of a healthcare system. The reimbursement provisions promulgated by Medicare have a substantial impact on practice patterns, and the influence of managed care on the healthcare system cannot be ignored. Anticipated changes in reimbursement can become the single most important considerations in some planning contexts.

This review of the social, political, economic and technological trends affecting the environment provides a starting point for subsequent background research and a context within which additional knowledge can be framed. These trends should be initially analyzed at the macro-level and subsequently "stepped down" to the geographic level appropriate for the community or organization in question.

Baseline Data Collection

The environmental assessment provides the backdrop for the collection of baseline data on the community or the organization. This process identifies the who, what, when, where and how of the community and its healthcare system or, in the case of organization-level planning, the current position of the organization vis-à-vis the market. These data provide the basis for comparative analyses and are the yardstick by which the success of the planning process will be measured.

In compiling baseline data for planning purposes, certain steps in the process should be followed. Whether the situation is being analyzed in terms of demographic characteristics, health status, or health resource availability, the same sequence should be followed. For every component analyzed, the planner should identify, inventory or quantify, profile, and assess. These steps are discussed in turn:

Identify. The first step always involves the identification of the factors on which data are to be collected. For example, the demographic traits, health status indicators, and categories of resources that are to be studied should be specified. This process should be as comprehensive as possible, realizing, however, that additional variables may be identified as the process unfolds.

Inventory/Quantify. Once the relevant factors have been identified, they must be inventoried. An "inventory" of demographic characteristics can involve a range of population characteristics. Similarly, an inventory of health status characteristics could involve the quantification of various indicators. An inventory of services or facilities may involve a straightforward count of relevant units. For example, if inpatient capacity was identified as a factor to be considered, the hospital bed inventory would be quantified.

Profile. Once the inventories are complete and the various measures have been quantified, it is possible to profile the community or the organization in terms of the relevant variables. This profile represents a composite "snap shot" of the community as it currently is constituted or the current status of the organization. The profile will typically involve comparisons to other settings or existing benchmarks. No judgment is made at this point, but a state-of-the-community or state-of-the-organization picture is generated.

Assess. The final step in the process involves an assessment of the conditions that have been identified. Once the community has been profiled in terms of demographic characteristics, for example, it is possible to interpret this information within the context of the planning process. Once the profile of the organization has been established in terms of utilization rates, it is possible to give meaning to these statistics. Questions such as the following can then be addressed. What are the implications of continued population redistribution for health services demands? What are the implications of the continued aging of the population? How does the overall health status of the community compare to that of other communities? Is the physician-to-population ratio favorable or unfavorable? What does the decrease in cardiology volume mean? The answers to these and similar questions will provide a starting point for subsequent planning activities.

Profiling the Community

With community-wide planning, the delineation of the "community" will usually be obvious. It will typically coincide with the geographic unit that comes under the jurisdiction of the government entity that is involved in planning. Thus, if the state of Mississippi is initiating a community-wide planning process, the State would be considered the "community". If the Jackson County planning authority is sponsoring the initiative, Jackson County is likely to constitute the community.

There may be situations in which the boundaries of the community are not clearly defined. For example, a regional planning authority may be established to address the needs of an area that cuts across state lines and involves a number of counties. The delineation of the boundaries of the community in this case requires a different approach. Techniques developed for determining the service area for a specific healthcare organization might be used in these cases. (These techniques are discussed in Chapter 7.)

As part of this community profiling process, the regional setting should be taken into consideration, and different regions of the country have their own cultural patterns. The *community type* should also be a consideration when collecting baseline data. Whether the dominant community type within the planning area is urban, suburban or rural will have important implications for both health status and health behavior. The community assessment process should also consider local *environmental factors* to the extent that they impact health status.

In the case of organization-level planning, the service area might be conceptualized as its "market", and the market for the organization may coincide with the service area for community planning purposes. On the other hand, the market area boundaries for an organization may extend beyond the jurisdiction of the planning agency or, in other cases, may be more restrictive than the area covered in community planning. Or, the market for the organization may not be tied to geography but represent a subgroup of the total community, as in the case of a cosmetic surgery practice that caters only to older, upscale individuals who can afford this vanity service.

Profiling the Organization

At the organization level, the collection of baseline data begins with the organization itself. Healthcare organizations routinely generate a large amount of data as a by-product of their normal operations. Many types of data can typically be extracted from internal records, including patient characteristics, utilization trends, and sources of revenue.

Systematic acquisition of internal data typically involves the performance of an *internal audit*. The internal audit involves a number of components. An audit examines the organization's *structure*, its *processes*, its *customers*, and its *resources*. The components included and the emphases placed on them will depend on the nature of the planning engagement. (The planning audit is more fully discussed in Chapter 7.)

The audit process involves the identification of the separate units within the organization, and these are subsequently described and assessed. A hospital, for example, will have a number of departments that must be considered. A specialty group practice may include both diagnostic and therapeutic components or feature a number of service lines to be considered. The current status of each organizational component should be reviewed, along with past trends and expected future developments.

The following list illustrates aspects of the organization that might be addressed by means of an internal audit:

- Services and products offered
- Nature, number and characteristics of customers
- Utilization patterns for services and products
- Sales volumes for services and products
- Staffing levels and personnel characteristics
- Internal management processes

- Financial characteristics
- Pricing structure
- Marketing arrangements
- Locations of service outlets
- Referral relationships

At the end of this process, the planner should be able to answer the questions raised at the outset: Who we are? What we are doing to whom? Where we are doing it? How are we doing it? And, ultimately, how well we are doing it?

Profiling the Population

The characteristics of the population residing in the community or the organization's market area are typically determined through an *external audit* that expands on the environmental assessment. Many of the same types of data will be collected for both the community and organization planning levels. The main categories of data that should be collected on the community's population include: demographic data, sociocultural data, psychographic or lifestyle data, and data on insurance coverage and consumer attitudes. (Details of these characteristics are provided in Chapters 6 and 7.)

In assessing the health status of a population, community-wide planners frequently make use of some type of health status index that serves to quantify the needs of the community and its sub-communities. The current health status of the community will be an important determinant of the level of demand for health services and serves as the baseline against which the effectiveness of planning can be measured. The emphasis, of course, will be on those dimensions that are relevant to the needs of the community or the organization. These would include fertility characteristics, morbidity characteristics and mortality characteristics. (The health status of the population can be determined following the steps outlined in Chapters 6 and 7.)

Planners are particularly concerned with the patterns of health behavior that characterize a population. Health behavior can be defined as any action aimed at restoring, preserving, and/or enhancing health status. Formal health behavior is defined in terms of such indicators of utilization as physician visits, hospital admissions, and drug prescriptions. Health behavior also includes informal actions on the part of individuals that are designed to prevent health problems and maintain, enhance or promote health. Historically, the emphasis in the analysis of health behavior has been on the formal services provided by healthcare practitioners, although increasing attention is being paid to informal health behavior.

While community health planners will be interested in the broad range of health behavior, organization-based planners focus on those indicators of health behavior that are most relevant for their operations. Hospitals, for example, are likely to require information on many of the indicators of interest to community planners. Organizations offering more limited services will focus on the specific indicators of utilization relevant to their needs.

The information developed through the external audit provides the basis for estimating the demand for health services characterizing the target population. The identified level of need can subsequently be compared to the community resources described below in order to determine the planning gap.

Community Resources Inventory

The other side of the coin from the need assessment is the resource inventory. The healthcare resources available to the community must be identified and ultimately matched to the needs identified for the target population. These resources include health facilities and equipment, healthcare programs and services, health personnel, financing options and existing networks and relationships at a minimum. (These indicators are addressed in more detail in Chapters 6 and 7.)

The list of factors to be considered in the community-wide planning process may appear overwhelming, but this is the level of comprehensiveness that is required in order to develop an adequate picture of the community under study. All of these components are important in one way or another, and almost any one of them could have a substantial impact on the system.

At the organization level, the resource inventory will inevitably be much more focused than that for community-wide planning. The emphasis will be on those facilities, programs, personnel and other resources that are relevant to the organization in question. Ultimately, the resources that are inventoried will reflect the type of organization, the nature of its services, and the type of planning being conducted.

Assessing Health Status and Healthcare Resources

It is essential, once the community's needs and resources have been identified and inventoried, that they be evaluated. A number of approaches can be utilized in this regard, although all ultimately involve some type of comparative analysis. The assessment of an indicator of health status, for example, could involve a comparison with that same indicator at a previous point in time, a comparison with the indicator for a comparable community, a comparison with the state or national average, or a comparison with some standard that has been established. In fact, an indicator should probably be assessed from all of these perspectives.

At this point, various analytical techniques might be utilized, such as a gap analysis or SWOT analysis. These techniques are useful in determining the state of the community or the state of the organization prior to proceeding with the planning process. These analytical techniques are discussed in more detail in subsequent chapters.

Summarizing the Preliminary Analysis

Enough information should now be available to present a summary statement of the analysis up to this point. This may involve a state-of-the-community report for community-wide planning or a state-of-the-organization report for organization-level planning. This report should include a comprehensive description of the community or organizational environment, a status report on the internal situation (in the case of an organization), and a report describing the overall status of the community or market area.

This status report should include the strengths, weaknesses, opportunities and threats identified during the analysis. It should also include an "issues statement" based on the results of the analysis to this point. The issues statement will help clarify the process and narrow the focus of the planning team. This is also a point at which the mission statement and the original assumptions should be revisited.

This report presents an opportunity to frankly describe the state of the community's health system or the state of the organization and serves as the launching point for subsequent plan development. This is a critical point in the planning process, in that it presents the baseline data against which any progress will be measured. It also assures that everyone involved in the process is on the same page, agreeing with the stated assumptions and the understandings generated by the process up to this point.

Considering Strategies

This is a point at which the choice of strategy might be considered (although some planners would place this step later in the process). While strategies are typically associated with organization-level planning, they should not be ignored when community-level planning is being conducted. The strategy refers to the generalized approach that is to be taken in response to the challenges identified.

With community-level planning, this may mean choosing between a public health approach, a free market approach, an educational model of development, or a public/private consortium approach, to name a few. Any one of these could be thought of as a strategy and serve as the framework for subsequent planning. Any strategy developed for community-wide planning should meet several criteria. It should provide overall direction for the initiative, fit the available resources, minimize resistance, reach the appropriate targeted groups, and, ultimately, advance the vision of the community.

At the organization level, the choice of strategy is critical. The strategy sets the tone for subsequent planning activities and, in effect, sets the parameters within which the planners must operate. Examples of strategies that might be adopted by organization-level planners include a market dominance strategy, a niche strategy, a flanking strategy, or a coalition strategy, to name a few. (Specific strategies are discussed in more detail in Chapter 8).

The research undertaken to this point should have generated enough information on the planning environment and the issues to be addressed to allow for at least a general strategy to be identified. While the precise strategic approach to be taken may not be specified at this point, at least the options can be narrowed. This will serve to focus subsequent planning activities by eliminating strategies that are considered unproductive. Under a community-wide planning scenario, for example, it may be determined that changing the lifestyle patterns of the population represents a more realistic path to reaching planning objectives than does the control of facilities construction. Clearly, that planning approach will be quite different than if facility regulation was the focus. Similarly, if a hospital determines, based on available data, that it cannot compete head on with the major player in the market area, its adoption of a "second fiddle" or "flanking" strategy will channel planning in a different direction than if a more confrontational approach was chosen.

Inventing the Future

The final consideration at this juncture is the development of a scenario that depicts where the community or organization would like to be at some specified point in the future. Time-horizons of five, ten, and fifteen years might be considered. A scenario should be developed that describes the range of services that are envisioned, the patterns of referral and utilization, the health status of the community, and so forth for specified points in the future. At the organization level, the scenario should describe the organization as envisioned in terms of future characteristics such as size, personnel composition, service complement, position in the market, stance relative to competitors, volume of services, locations, payor mix, and any other characteristic that is considered important.

The desired future position represents the target that the planning process is intended to achieve. Of course, the visionary should be tempered by the feasible and the ideal by the practical. One approach, in fact, might be to develop a best case/worst case/probable case set of scenarios.

DEVELOPING THE PLAN

The effort up to this point provides the foundation for the actual development of the plan. If the initial work is properly carried out, the planning process should flow smoothly, at least from a technical perspective.

Setting the Goal(s)

Goals are generalized statements about an ideal state for the community or organization that will serve as the target for future development. The goal specifies the desired form of the community healthcare system or, alternatively, the future characteristics of the organization. The goal represents the generalized accomplishments that the planners would like to achieve. Goals establish the tone for the rest of the planning process, since all subsequent components are derived from them. The goal or goals that are established should reflect the information that was provided in the summary report based on initial information gathering. As in other planning activities, the goal should meet certain criteria before it is accepted, including compatibility with the stated mission.

Goals tend to be idealistic, and this is particularly true in the community-wide planning context. At the community level, the goal may call for "establishing an effective and efficient delivery system that serves the needs of the entire community". At the organization level, on the other hand, the goal will be more specific to the mission of the organization and may, for example, call for "positioning ABC orthopedic group as the premier sports medicine program in the region".

The number of goals to be established depends on the complexity and size of the organization, the nature of the issues at hand, and the type of planning being undertaken. If the focus is narrow, a single goal may be appropriate. On the other hand, the complexity of many healthcare organizations mandates the establishment of multiple goals. Goals ultimately may be established specific to particular issues or units within the organization.

Specifying Objectives

Objectives refer to the specific targets to be reached in support of goal attainment. To many these represent the "tactics" that support the plan's strategies. Objectives should be developed in response to the major opportunities or problems identified and should represent potential solutions (or at least part of the solution) for these issues.

While goals are general statements, objectives should be very specific and stated in clear and concise terms. Any concepts referenced in an objective must be operationalizable and measurable. Objectives must also be time bound, with clear deadlines established for their accomplishment. Finally, they must be amenable to evaluation. This characteristic is particularly critical since the success of the process will be measured by the extent to which objectives have been met. This is a critical point in the planning process since the baseline traits to be used for evaluation must be measurable.

Objectives are stated in such terms as: The rate of teen pregnancy in the community will be reduced from 15 percent to 10 percent by the end of 2005 (in support of the goal of improving the reproductive health of the community). Or, the hospital's orthopedic practice will recruit a sports medicine specialist within the next twelve months (in support of the stated goal of expanding the organization's orthopedic service lines).

Several objectives may be specified for each goal. Four or five would not be uncommon, although many more than that becomes unwieldy (especially if more than one goal is being considered). Multiple objectives are common since it is likely that action will be required on a number of different fronts in order to attain a specified goal. The objectives should be reviewed by any appropriate parties and possibly by some outside the organization such as experts on the local healthcare system.

It may be useful to organize planning team members into working committees for each specific objective. These work groups should deal with the various substantive issues that must be addressed (e.g., reproductive health, chronic disease). This approach serves to coordinate and focus efforts so the work group will have the greatest possible impact. At the community level, appropriate "support" organizations should be brought in to assist with plan implementation and to provide exposure to "best practices" related to their areas of expertise.

Any barriers to accomplishing the stated objectives of the system or the organization should be identified and assessed. The extent to which these barriers can be overcome must be determined. A specialty practice, for example, may have felt that its market share could be greatly enhanced by assigning half of its physicians to the other local hospital. However, upon further reflection, it was determined that its primary competitor who was entrenched at the other facility would create such a furor that any advantage would be compromised. In the case of insurmountable barriers, an objective may simply have to be eliminated.

Prioritizing Objectives

The planning process typically generates a number of equally important objectives. In many cases it may not be feasible to pursue all of the objectives that have been identified. Even if staff, money and other resources are not an issue, it may not be possible to address all of them within a reasonable timeframe or to pursue all objectives simultaneously. As a result, the prioritization of objectives becomes an important step in the process.

There is no one foolproof procedure for prioritizing objectives and the approach to prioritization is likely to vary with the situation. Whatever approach is used, consensus should be developed on the prioritization process before it is time to implement it.

There are a number of questions that might be asked to help determine the order of priority for the pursuit of objectives. While these probably relate more directly to organization-level planning than to community-wide planning, most of them can be adapted to either situation. Representative questions include:

- What are the most urgent issues, issues that could lead to dire consequences if they are not resolved?
- What are the pivotal issues, issues that contribute most directly to the mission and goal?
- Which objectives must be addressed as a prerequisite for achieving other objectives?

- What objectives will provide the greatest return for the planning "investment"?
- Which objectives can be achieved quicker, easier and less expensively than others?
- Which objectives will result in the most visible or most tangible results?
- Which objectives will have the most lasting impact and/or can maintain themselves over time?
- Are objectives with short-term benefits more important than those with long-term benefits?
- Which objectives face the least barriers?
- What is the level of risk characterizing the options and to what extent is risk an issue?
- Which objectives will involve multiple benefits if they are achieved?
- Which objectives are critical to filling important gaps in services or addressing organizational weaknesses?
- To what extent is there likely to be a negative response to the achieving of an objective?

The challenge is to identify on the front end the criteria that are most important. It may even be necessary to utilize different sets of criteria within a single planning initiative due to the nature of the project. The application of these priorities is likely to result in the elimination of some objectives that may not be workable, although they may have seemed like a good idea when they were first proposed.

One other consideration at this point is the possibility of unanticipated consequences resulting from the meeting of any of the objectives. Although it may appear tedious, it is important to specify the likely consequences of carrying out each objective. This should involve a determination of both intended and unintended consequences. Too often the positive aspects of the situation are examined in isolation from the negative consequences that may result from the pursuit of the objective.

Specifying Actions

The next step in the planning process is a critical one, in that this is where the planning team specifies the actions to be carried out. For each of the objectives that have been identified (and survived the various "cuts"), a set of actions must be specified. This process essentially breaks the procedure for meeting objectives down into manageable steps. It is one thing to indicate what actions should be taken, it is another to specify *how* they are to be carried out. For this reason, an implementation approach must be developed that lays out the required tasks.

A number of action steps are likely to be required for each objective. Just as several objectives must be met in order to attain a single goal, numerous actions must be performed to achieve an objective. These actions take a wide range of forms, from the most mundane of support activities to highly complex tasks. Many of these actions imply a certain sequence and this is a point at which the original project plan might be further refined to specify the sequencing of the action steps.

IMPLEMENTING THE PLAN

Planning is ultimately only an exercise, albeit a meaningful one. The payoff comes in the implementation of the plan. The planning process creates a road map which the community or the organization must use to get where it wants to go. It is at the implementation stage, however, that the process often breaks down. The oft-repeated maxim that "the last plan is still sitting on the shelf" generally reflects a failure in implementation rather than any flaw in the plan itself.

The transition from planning to implementation is difficult under the best of circumstances. It involves a hand-off from the planning team to the management team. Implementation must occur at several different levels and within different sectors of the community or divisions of the organization. For this reason, the implementation of the plan requires a level of coordination that few organizations and certainly few communities have in place.

To a certain extent, planning is talk, but implementation is action. Very little about the system or the organization has to be changed during the planning process (although some change inevitably occurs as a by-product). However, the implementation plan is likely to require significant change within the community or the organization. These changes are likely to affect management processes, information systems, and the corporate culture, in addition to more mundane work routines.

Implementation is particularly a challenge for planners at the community level. There is not likely to be an obvious organization to take charge of the implementation process. The planning process typically represents a coalition of various community organizations, with no one organization capable of managing implementation (even if all others agreed that they should do it). Further, there is likely to be no organization in a position to coordinate the various parties, both public and private, that must be included in the process. Within an organization, the ability to assign responsibility for plan implementation certainly exists, although there will always be difficulties in carving out staff time from existing responsibilities. This challenge is made greater for working managers, unless the activities generated by the plan already fall under the responsibilities of the manager.

Steps in Implementation

In order to approach plan implementation systematically, the planning team should develop both a detailed project plan and an implementation matrix. An implementation matrix can be developed using a spreadsheet and should lay out who is to

Activity	Responsible Party	Other Relevant Parties	Start Date	Deadline for Completion	Resource Requirements	Prerequisites	Comments
Task 1							
Task 2							
Task 3							
Task 4							
Task 5							
Task 6							
Task 7							
Task 8							
Task 9							
Task 10							

Figure 5-4. Sample Implementation Matrix.

do what and when they are to do it. The matrix should list every action called for by the plan, breaking each action down into tasks, if appropriate. For each action or task the responsible party should be identified, along with any secondary parties that should be involved in this activity. The matrix should indicate resource requirements (in terms of staff time, money and other requirements). The start and end dates for this activity should be identified. Any prerequisites for accomplishing this task should be identified at the outset and factored into the project plan. Finally, benchmarks should be established that allow the planning team to determine when the activity has been completed. (Figure 5-4 presents an example of an implementation matrix.)

The nature of the progress indicators used will be determined by the type of plan. In many cases, *operational* benchmarks will be important. These may relate to utilization levels, facility development, or staffing changes, as well as others. *Clinical* standards may be established in many cases as well. These may focus on outcomes such as a reduction in the hospital mortality rate or improvement in surgical outcomes. *Financial* benchmarks are likely to be included in many plans. The success of planning activities will often be measured in terms of such factors as revenue, profit, or return on investment.

Requirements for Implementation

The resource requirements from the implementation matrix should be combined to determine total project resource requirements. This will determine the extent to which the project will require *operating funds* and *capital investment*, including any *facilities and equipment* requirements. In addition, the *human resource* requirements should be determined, and *information system* requirements specified. Any changes in *governance or management* will need to be outlined, along with anticipated *marketing* needs. Once the individual resource requirements has been specified, the total resource requirements of the project will be identified for the first time.

The prerequisites for plan implementation noted above ultimately must involve the budgetary process. In fact, the failure of many planning initiatives can be attributed to the inability to translate plans into budgets. This represents a challenge for any organization, and the shorter the time frame the greater the challenge. The budgetary process might be considered antithetical to the strategic planning process in that it reflects a refinement of current budgetary requirements rather than a proactive consideration of future organizational needs. For this reason, the planning process must include those parties in the organization who are likely to influence the budgetary process.

The implementation requirements must be addressed in relation to available funds and any other fiscal constraints. The fact that financial resources will almost always be limited means that adjustments may be required in the implementation plan. This may mean that activities have to be delayed, modified or eliminated altogether. This is one of the reasons that objectives should be prioritized during the formulation of the plan.

Means of Implementation

Implementation of the plan at the community level will involve a wide variety of community organizations, and this creates an inevitable management challenge for community-wide health planning efforts. In some cases, it may be possible to use the authority vested in the planning entity to enforce changes through regulatory efforts. In most cases, however, the changes must be voluntary so the process focuses on more of education, persuasion and coordination than on control. At the organization level, the means used to implement the plan will of necessity transcend various departments and units.

The implementation process is likely to employ both direct means and indirect means. The direct means of implementation have been addressed to a certain extent through the development of the implementation matrix and the identification of resource requirements. *Budgeting activities* that provide for the allocation of resources are typically utilized to directly facilitate plan. Direct methods may also include changes in *policies and procedures* to allow various activities to occur. In the case of community-wide planning, direct means may involve the enactment of regulations that affect the actions of healthcare organizations. Ultimately, the organization-level plan may require changes in the *organizational structure* and/or *management processes*. The extent to which these direct means of implementation are utilized depend, of course, on the type of organization and the type of plan.

Indirect means of plan implementation might also utilized. These are indirect in the sense that they support plan implementation rather than being directly involved in task performance. At the organization level these methods might include making changes in *physical facilities* that allow certain activities to occur. Various forms of *communication* might be utilized to support implementation. Certain *symbolic actions* might be taken that provide psychological support for the operationalization of the plan.

Perhaps the most extensive of the indirect means deals with the community mindset or the *corporate culture* of the organization. At the community level, the emphasis may be on creating an environment that encourages healthy lifestyles and behavior patterns. In many cases, the corporate culture will have to be modified in order for plan implementation to occur at the corporate level. If a planning mindset does not already exist, this will have to be incorporated into the culture. If the culture emphasizes strict organizational divisions, a new way of thinking may have to be introduced in order to implement the plan across divisional lines.

"PRODUCTS" GENERATED BY THE PLANNING PROCESS

The most tangible "product" derived from the planning process is the planning document that is inevitably generated. This is where the process is "put to paper" in a document that summarizes the background information, lays out the vision developed through the process, and describes how this vision will be attained. This document should also include an implementation plan that will specify the steps that must be followed to turn the plan into action.

The process should also generate a database of information on the community and/or the organization that can be utilized to support future planning activities and even unrelated projects. In some cases, the plan may be long forgotten, but its legacy of a comprehensive database on the community or the organization may live on. In fact, the creation of such a resource should be an explicit objective of any planning process. A database can be updated, expanded and otherwise developed over time to not only support this project but to support future initiatives of various types.

Less tangible products include a new perspective on the nature of the system or the organization, the identification of available resources (perhaps heretofore unknown), a new understanding of the players in the community or within the organization, and so forth.

An even more important intangible product is the establishment of a process for planning that, hopefully, will persist after the end of the discrete project. Remember, "the plan is nothing, but planning is everything". If a planning mindset has been inculcated, the process will take on a life of its own. Planning should become established as an inherent part of the operation rather than an episodic event. This mindset should be developed to the point that decision makers stop and think about "the plan" before they make any important decision.

THE EVALUATION PLAN

The notion of evaluating the planning project should be top of mind on the first day of the process and the means for evaluation should be built into the process itself. Evaluation is necessary to determine the success of the process. This is important to those involved in the process, as well as to any parties that may be assessing the value of the planning initiative. For example, grantmakers and funders will usually want to know how many people were reached and served by the initiative, as well as whether the initiative had the community-level impact it was intended to have. Community groups may want to use evaluation results to guide them in decisions about their programs, and where they should put their efforts. Researchers will most likely be interested in proving whether any improvements in community health were caused by your programs or initiatives.

Evaluation techniques focus to two types of analysis: process (or formative) analysis and outcome (or summative) analysis. The former evaluates systems, procedures, communication processes, and other factors that contribute to the efficient operation of a program. Outcome evaluation focuses more on end results or what is ultimately accomplished. Process evaluation essentially measures efficiency, while outcome evaluation measures effectiveness (Adams and Schvaneveldt, 1991).

Process evaluation and outcome evaluation may overlap in various stages of the analysis. For example, it is not enough to report that regular planning meetings are being held. The process evaluation should measure the extent to which the meetings are achieving the results that they are intended to. Both types of evaluation have a role to play in the project. Using the project plan as a guide, the process can be monitored and regular progress reports presented.

Evaluation should involve on-going monitoring of the planning process, including benchmarks and/or milestones for assessment along the way. This will require the clarification of the objectives and goals of your initiative. According to the Community Tool Box (developed by the University of Kansas), the following issues should be addressed during the evaluation process:

- ✓ *Planning and implementation issues*: How well was the program or initiative planned out, and how well was that plan put into practice?
- ✓ *Assessing attainment of objectives*: How well has the program or initiative met its stated objectives?
- ✓ *Impact on participants*: How much and what kind of a difference has the program or initiative made for its targets of change?
- ✓ *Impact on the community*: How much and what kind of a difference has the program or initiative made on the community as a whole?

Data collection and benchmarking are extremely important to understand progress and community improvements, and documenting the process of community or organizational change is a task that should occur on a regular basis. Community-wide planners should submit updates to the public and organization-level planners to the key parties involved in the organization.

Once the questions to be answered through the evaluation have been identified, the next step is to decide which methods will best address those questions. Some of the methods to be utilized include: a monitoring and feedback system; member surveys about the initiative; goal attainment report; behavioral surveys; interviews with key participants; and, for community-wide planning, community-level indicators of impact.

Although evaluation techniques are often praised for their bottom-line objectivity, they are also useful in healthcare where it is not possible to place a dollar value on everything. Thus, cost-effectiveness analysis can take into consideration the intangible aspects of the service delivery process in its evaluation. Thus, strict cost/benefit analyses are likely to be less suitable for use in healthcare than in most other industries.

REVISION AND REPLANNING

As noted earlier, it is unlikely that a health plan will be completed without being modified in one way or another. This type of "on the fly" revision is inevitable in a rapidly changing environment. At the end of the planning period, it is important to reassess the internal characteristics of the organization and the state of the external environment. Questions should be raised such as: What developments have subsequently occurred that will affect the plan or the implementation of its provisions? What actions have been taken supportive of the plan that were not anticipated? Have there been developments that affect resource requirements? Have actions on the part of competitors affected the "strategic balance"?

Ideally, each component of the planning process should be revisited with these concerns in mind. The assumptions should be reviewed along with the mission statement. The baseline data should be updated to account for the time lapse since the planning process was initiated. The emphasis here will, of course, depend on the type of plan.

The strategy chosen should be reviewed to determine if it is still the best approach in view of possible changes in the environment. For example, has the collaborative strategy selected failed due to unanticipated competition on the part of "collaborators"? The goals and objectives should be revisited to assure that they are still appropriate in the light of any changes in either the internal or external environment.

Realistically, the planning process is likely to require a substantial shift in mindset for most healthcare organizations. For continuous revision and replanning to occur, the organization must truly become a "planning organization". This level of commitment will require that planning become an inherent part of the culture. If this can be accomplished, the above activities should easily follow.

References

Adams, G. R., and J. D. Schvaneveldt (1991). *Understanding Research Methods*. New York: Longman.

Additional Resources

American Health Planning Association. Health planning tools at URL: www.ahpanet.org.
Fawcett, S. B., Harris, K. J., Paine-Andrews, A., Richter, K. P., Lewis, R. K., Francisco, V., Arbaje, A., Davis, A., Cheng, H. in collaboration with Johnston, J. (1995). Reducing risk for chronic disease: an action planning guide for community-based initiatives. Lawrence, KS: Work Group on Health Promotion and Community Development, University of Kansas.
National Association of County and City Health Officials, *Mobilizing for Action Through Planning and Partnerships*. Web-based planning guide at URL: http://ctb.lsi.ukans.edu.
Public Health Foundation (1999). *Healthy People 2010 Toolkit: A Field Guide to Health Planning*. Washington, DC: Public Health Foundation.
University of Kansas, *Community Toolbox*. Web-based planning guide. URL: http://ctb.lsi.ukans.edu.

6

The Community Assessment Process

INTRODUCTION

The community assessment component is a critical part of the community-wide planning process. Without this assessment as a foundation for the planning process, any planning would be "shooting in the dark". Not only would planners lack a general understanding of the environment, but the uniqueness of the community could not be appreciated.

This chapter presents a general framework for conducting a community assessment. It lays out the steps involved in performing the assessment preparatory to carrying out the planning process. The outline presented is relatively generic, and the planner should realize that this framework may need to be adapted to the situation of the particular community.

The first step in the community assessment process involves the development of a general picture of the community and its healthcare system. This process will include a review of pertinent background materials and interviews with key participants in the community health system. The intent is to develop enough background on the community to thoughtfully craft the remainder of the plan.

A "literature review" should be conducted, including any materials that have been prepared on the local healthcare system. Newspaper articles may have been published that describe various aspects of the system, and many communities produce health-related publications. This review of print materials should include any previous plans that have been developed and any research projects or consultant studies that have been conducted. University researchers are likely to have conducted studies on the local healthcare system, and government agencies often compile reports on various aspects of the system. Health facilities may have submitted certificate-of-need applications or other reports to governmental agencies, and these are often a matter of public record.

A second component of this stage of information gathering involves interviews with knowledgeable individuals within the community, both inside and out of the medical establishment. Those interviewed should include anyone currently involved in planning activities in the community, representatives of the major private sector healthcare organizations, public health leaders, and representatives of the physician community. Major decision makers, opinion leaders, and political influentials should also be included.

While the intent is to develop a general picture of the community healthcare system, this process represents an opportunity to identify the major issues from the perspective of those interviewed. The issues that are driving the planning process in particular should be identified, since these may provide focus for subsequent assessment activities. This process should also identify some key informants who might serve as useful resources later in the planning process.

The background research should also identify the decision-making process for the community's healthcare system, at least to the extent that it can be isolated. How are decisions made with regard to the expenditure of public healthcare funds? What healthcare organizations are politically influential? Who has the grassroots support of the community? What government agencies are involved in the coordination of health services?

Any potential barriers to the planning initiative should be identified as part of this process. Individuals or organizations that are clearly resistant to the planning process should be identified at this point. Immutable patterns of behavior that must be considered should also be identified. These understandings with regard to barriers become a part of the assumptions that drive the process.

ENVIRONMENTAL ASSESSMENT

Once a basic understanding of the community and its healthcare system has been established, a number of other data collection activities can be initiated. The first step in the formal data collection process involves an environmental assessment. "Environment" here is viewed in the broadest of terms, encompassing any aspect of society at any level that could be construed to have implications for community planning activities. The assessment should begin at the national level and be carried down to the level at which the planning is occurring. Thus, the analysis should include the national level, the regional level (if appropriate), the state level, and ultimately the level of the community under study.

Societal Trends

Broad societal trends should be analyzed and their implications for the local environment considered. These societal trends should include demographic trends, economic considerations, lifestyle trends, and even shifts in attitudes. Examples of pertinent trends abound. For example, the most significant demographic trend characterizing U.S. society at the beginning of the 21st century is the overall aging of the population, coupled with the movement of the large baby boom population into the middle-age range. This national trend has major implications for the delivery of care nationally, and there are few local communities that will not be affected by age-related demographic trends. Another example of a society-wide demographic trend with implications for healthcare is the growing racial and ethnic diversity characterizing U.S. society.

Broad economic trends are also a consideration, since one's economic circumstances influence both health status and health behavior. Periods of economic prosperity have different implications for healthcare than periods of recession or economic downturn. Similarly, a state of full employment affects healthcare differently from a situation of high unemployment. These economic conditions have implications for health status, health behavior, and the ability of the population to pay for healthcare.

Changing national lifestyles are another trend with implications for healthcare. A current example involves the health and fitness consciousness characterizing much of the American population. The fitness "craze" that began in the 1980s has created an unprecedented demand for health clubs, health food, athletic goods, and sports medicine. Following fast on its heels is the interest in alternative therapies, including an emphasis on herbal medicines.

Trends in consumer attitudes are another area of inquiry, and even changes in these attitudes at the national level may have implications for local communities. A case in point involves home healthcare. Until the 1980s the general public considered home care a less-than-desirable alternative to hospital care. However, over the past decade or so home care has come to be seen by many as the setting of choice wherever possible.

Health Industry Trends

Developments in the healthcare industry should be examined to identify any trends at the national or state levels that are likely to affect the local community. These could include trends in financial arrangements (discussed below), changing organizational structures within the delivery system, or the introduction of new treatment modalities. The trend away from inpatient care in favor of outpatient care continues to be a major factor in the healthcare arena. Recent examples of other industry trends include the rapid growth of cosmetic surgery and the current interest in rehabilitation.

Another recent industry trend with implications for the provision of healthcare is the emergence of large national for-profit chains that exert substantial influence on the healthcare system. Recent years have also seen the emergence of employers and employer coalitions as key players in the healthcare environment.

Regulatory, Political, and Legal Developments

To a great extent what happens inside the healthcare industry is influenced by developments outside of healthcare. At the federal and state levels, a number of regulatory functions exist and, with the stroke of a pen, the healthcare environment can be dramatically altered. Federal regulations governing the operation of the Medicare and Medicaid programs are an important case in point. On the other hand, states have primary responsibility for licensing health facilities and personnel. Almost over night, state agencies could enact provisions that dramatically alter the playing field. Examples abound in which a state agency has placed a moratorium on nursing home construction or home health licensures or an agency has determined that nurse practitioners should be allowed to write prescriptions. While these may involve narrow bureaucratic directives, such decisions can have a life-or-death effect on many healthcare organizations.

The political environment clearly has both direct and indirect implications for the operation of the healthcare system. Even though no legislation was enacted as a result of the Clinton administration health reform initiative in the early 1990s, the environment that was created as a result of the national debate encouraged many healthcare organizations to position themselves in anticipation of possible reform initiatives. The handling of the certificate-of-need process for a new health facility by a state agency—indeed, whether there is a C-O-N process at all—reflects the political environment of the state.

Legal activities at the national, state and local levels also have implications for the local healthcare system. There are numerous examples of recent legislation at the national level that have influenced physician referral patterns, the length of stay for women undergoing childbirth, and the ability of patients to sue health maintenance organizations. Even more legal issues are dealt with at the state level and these often have important implications for the local healthcare system.

Technology Developments

Developments in the area of technology can exert a major influence on the course of the healthcare system. The history of healthcare has, to a great extent, been a history of technological developments. While few major technological breakthroughs have occurred in recent years, a variety of refinements in available technology have influenced the course of the healthcare system. The introduction of new drugs has changed the manner in which behavioral health problems are addressed, refinements in biomedical equipment have made home care more feasible for a range of conditions, and microsurgical techniques have contributed to the shift of care from the inpatient to the outpatient setting.

The next major technological development is likely to be in the area of information management. Efforts on the part of communities to develop community health information management systems (CHIMS) for sharing patient data are indicative of the trend toward more sophisticated information management.

Reimbursement Trends

A strong argument could be made that the financing arrangements available for the provision of care are the major factor in determining the nature of a healthcare system. Most of the major watersheds in the history of U.S. healthcare can, in fact, be traced to financing-related events. Notable among these are the introduction of health insurance, the enactment of the Medicare and Medicaid programs, and the introduction of the prospective payment system by HCFA during the 1980s. In more recent years, the emergence of innovative financing arrangements involving health maintenance organizations, preferred provider organizations, and other entities has changed the healthcare landscape. Managed care is now driving the future direction of the healthcare system.

Financing issues may be impacted by all levels of government as well as by private sector third-party payors. Specific examples of the impact of changing regulations are found in the areas of ambulatory care and physician reimbursement. Changes in reimbursement that encouraged the use of outpatient services rather than inpatient services have had a tremendous effect on the operation of the healthcare system. Changes in the procedure through which Medicare reimburses primary care physicians relative to specialists have had a number of implications for medical practitioners.

Local financing issues may be as important as trends in national programs. The safety net that serves the medically indigent is likely to be locally funded. A reduction in funding for the public hospital or the community's charity clinics may have an immediate and disturbing effect on care for the medically indigent. Changes in a state's Medicaid program could have equally devastating effects on the availability of care for the affected populations.

BASELINE DATA COLLECTION

The environmental assessment establishes the backdrop against which further analysis takes place. The next step in the data collection process involves developing baseline data on the community. These baseline data provide the foundation for the planning process, the basis for any future comparisons, and the yardstick by which the success of the planning effort will be measured. This process identifies the who, what, when, where and how of the community and its healthcare system.

Profiling the Community

In most cases, the delineation of the "community" will be obvious, in that it is the geographic unit that comes under the jurisdiction of the government entity that is involved in planning. There may be situations, however, when the boundaries of the community are not clearly defined. For example, a regional planning authority may be established to address the needs of an area that cuts across state lines and involves a number of counties. The delineation of the boundaries of the "community" in this case requires a different approach. Techniques developed for determining the service area for a specific healthcare organization might be used in these cases. (These techniques are discussed in Chapter 7.)

As part of this community profiling process, the regional setting should be taken into consideration. Different regions of the country have their own cultural patterns, and these seem to have persisted despite the rapid "massification" of U.S. society. Different regions report varying levels of prevalence for certain health problems, and the variation in utilization of health services is now well documented (Center for Evaluative Clinical Sciences, 1999). At the very least, regional variations must be considered when health services demand is being estimated or projected for a particular community.

The *community type* should also be a consideration when collecting baseline data. Whether the dominant community type within the planning area is urban, suburban or rural will have important implications for both health status and health behavior. Not only will the circumstances surrounding the health of the population be different for different community types, but the challenge of planning for different community types exists.

The community assessment process should consider local *environmental factors* to the extent that they impact health status. There is growing evidence that aspects of our environment account for as much as 20 percent of the difference in health status. High levels of environmental pollutants, the presence of toxic waste dumps, and issues related to drinking water all have implications for the health status of the population under study.

In profiling the community, the temporal dimension is an important issue. Whether determining the needs of the population or the resources available to meet these needs, three time-horizons must be taken into consideration. The current inventory of needs and resources (the present) is a starting point. However, it is also important to develop a sense of the historical trends (the past) that are affecting the community. Is the population growing or declining? Are the characteristics of the population different today than they were five years ago? Is the trend toward closing of hospitals or adding more beds?

The most important timeframe, however, is the future, since planning by definition is futuristic. In fact, one of the factors contributing to the failure of past planning efforts has been the tendency to plan for today or, worse, for yesterday's issues. A plan should address tomorrow's issues and, to this end, the process should identify to the extent possible the future characteristics of the population, its future health service needs, and likely future developments with regard to resources.

Profiling the Population

The population of the community must be profiled along a number of dimensions. The common type of data utilized in the profiling process are described below.

Demographic Data

Demographic data serve as the foundation for most health planning activities. Not only are demographic data important for profiling the community, but they serve as the basis for the calculation of a number of statistics relevant to the planning analysis. While an understanding of the demographic composition of the target population is important in its own right, this information is also essential for identifying the prevalence of health conditions and determining utilization patterns within the community.

From a health planning perspective, it is useful to categorize demographic traits into *biosocial* variables and *sociocultural* variables. Biosocial characteristics are clearly distinguished as demographic variables by their link to biological traits. The demographic variables included in this category are: *age*, *sex* and *race*. (*Ethnicity* is sometimes included because of its close relationship to race.)

Age is probably the best single predictor of the utilization of health services. Age is related not only to levels of service utilization but to the type of services utilized and the circumstances under which they are received.

The *sex* of the consumer is another factor influencing utilization rates in U.S. society. Females are more active than males in terms of health behavior and are heavier users of the healthcare system. They tend to visit physicians more often, take more prescription drugs, and, in general, use other facilities and personnel more often.

The *population pyramid* is a useful way of simultaneously graphically depicting the age and sex structure of a population. A population pyramid involves a presentation of the age-sex distribution of a population by means of a bar graph where each bar represents one age-sex group. Female age cohorts comprise one side of each bar and males the other, and the ages are typically presented in five- or ten-year intervals. The "shape" of the pyramid discloses a great deal of information about the population in question, and this information can be converted into estimates of the demand for health services. (Figure 6-1 presents an example of a population pyramid.)

Racial and ethnic characteristics influence the demand for health services, and, as a result of recent trends, this aspect of population composition is becoming

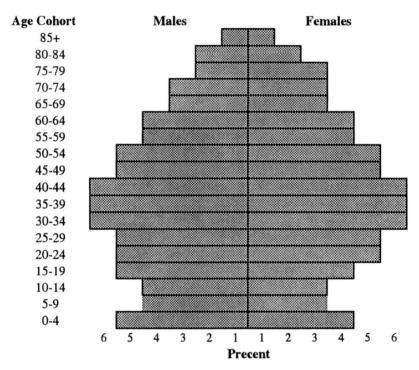

Figure 6-1. Population Pyramid.

increasingly important for health planners. Detailed information on the racial and ethnic characteristics of the population should be compiled, including qualitative data on attitudes and preferences. While differences in utilization may be traced to differences in the types of health problems experienced by these populations, many of the distinctions reflect variations in lifestyle patterns and cultural preferences. Because the public sector plays an important role in addressing the healthcare needs of minority populations, data on race and ethnicity are critical.

Sociocultural traits are important in profiling the population because of their correlation with health status and health behavior. The sociocultural variables discussed below include: marital status and related attributes, education, income, occupation/industry, and other sociocultural factors. Additional information on insurance coverage, psychographic categories, and community attitudes is included.

Marital status, household structure and, to a degree, *living arrangements* are all of interest to health planners. Marital status refers to one's current legal status with regard to marriage. Household structure refers to involvement in the physical household—i.e., where one actually lives. Living arrangements refer to the relationship between those sharing a household—i.e., roommates, married with children, unmarried relatives. For community health planners, marital status and household structure may have implications for the types of health problems that exist and the patterns of health services utilization.

Education is an important factor to consider during planning, since the educational level of the population is closely correlated with both health status and health behavior. This information is often important for the development of services that are compatible with the level of sophistication of the target audience. Certainly from a social marketing perspective, the level of education needs to be taken into consideration.

Income and related variables, such as poverty status, are obviously critical for any planning at the community level. Income, measured in terms of annual household income or per capita income, is an important predictor of both the level of morbidity within the community and likely patterns of health services utilization. The overall level of community affluence will influence both the healthcare "wants" of the population and the level of resources available.

Occupation and *industry* are important variables in profiling a community. Not only do individuals in different occupations and industries have differing consumer behavior habits, but the occupational or industrial mix of an area is an excellent indicator of the mix of healthcare services and products required by the target population. Distinctive patterns of healthy and unhealthy behavior have been correlated with different occupations and industries. Further, the occupational structure is likely to determine the extent to which employer-sponsored health insurance is available.

There are other sociocultural characteristics that might be important in different communities. *Religion* is a characteristic of the population that is difficult to quantify and has, in fact, played a limited role in community-wide planning. However, there are occasions when knowledge of a community's religious preferences may be appropriate for health services planning, especially if there are strong ties to church-affiliated health facilities in the community under study. The language spoken by the community population or sub-populations may also be a factor influencing healthcare communications and the efficient delivery of services.

The *insurance coverage* characterizing a community's population is an increasingly important topic for consideration by planners. While the community's "payor mix" may be more relevant to specific healthcare providers, the means of financing healthcare is not an unimportant issue for community health planners. It could be argued, in fact, that the utilization patterns within the community are to a great extent a reflection of the payor mix.

In analyzing the community's ability to pay for healthcare, the proportion of residents covered under various forms of insurance is an important consideration. Commercial (or private) insurance has typically included both group and individual coverage. This category has historically included the not-for-profit Blue Cross/Blue Shield plans and, increasingly today, managed care plans.

Other major payor categories include those covered under the federally-sponsored Medicare and Medicaid programs. Medicare coverage is primarily for the elderly, but it does include a growing proportion of disabled enrollees. Medicaid coverage reflects the participation of the medically indigent in the joint federal-state Medicaid program. In some communities, many Medicare enrollees may also be enrolled in Medicaid.

There are miscellaneous categories of government coverage that should be considered, although their size is usually negligible. These would include other federal programs for categorical conditions, state programs for specific diseases, and coverage under military-related programs such as the CHAMPUS program.

A residual category that remains after the other payor categories have been identified is generally referred to as the "self-pay" category. This involves a wide range of population segments that typically have little in common except for a lack of insurance coverage. This category includes uninsurable individuals who, due to past medical histories, can not obtain insurance. It includes the working poor who do not qualify for Medicaid yet do not have access to or cannot afford private insurance. This category also includes the homeless whose lifestyles mitigate against any type of permanent situation and the independently wealthy who prefer to pay out of pocket for healthcare should it be necessary.

The self-pay category is small in relative terms, but the growth in the number of uninsured individuals has served to swell its ranks. Recent estimates place the number of uninsured Americans over 40 million (or more than 15 percent of the population). This number appears to be growing as a result of cutbacks and/or cost increases in private insurance. The high unemployment rate among the U.S. workforce as we enter the 21st century has also had an impact on the availability of health insurance.

In community health planning, much of the emphasis is placed on the Medicaid and self-pay categories. These are populations that tend to be the most vulnerable in the face of health problems and are the most likely to place demands on the public health system. While the numbers of non-paying patients are small in the overall scheme of things, the burden of dealing with indigent patients can be considerable in communities where they constitute a significant portion of the population.

Psychographic Characteristics and Attitudes

It has become increasingly common to profile consumers in terms of their *psychographic characteristics* and assign them to lifestyle clusters. Psychographics refers to the values, attitudes and lifestyles that characterize a defined population segment. Lifestyle segmentation systems have been developed by a variety of vendors but they have only recently come into use in healthcare. The approach involves dividing the population up into a large number of segments (usually 50–60) that can then be profiled in terms of various characteristics including health status and health behavior. Psychographic factors are particularly important in examining attitudes towards one's health and the likelihood of involvement in healthy or unhealthy behaviors.

Psychographic analysis can help determine the likely health priorities and behavior of a population subgroup. This is important because groups that are similar demographically may be different in terms of their lifestyle-influenced health behavior. For example, one category of elderly healthcare consumers may prefer general practitioners for their primary care needs, while another category prefers physicians trained in internal medicine. While psychographic characteristics are considered more important for organization-level planning, knowledge of the psychographic clusters characterizing a community provides a useful perspective for community health planning.

The *attitudes* characterizing the population being planned for is another dimension that must be considered. "Attitudes" may encompass perceptions, preferences and expectations. The attitudes displayed by consumers in the community are likely to play a significant role in the direction the planning process takes, what is actually accomplished through the process, and, in fact, whether the process is carried out at all. In the community-wide context, planning initiatives are likely to rely heavily on health education programs and preventive actions that depend on appropriate consumer attitudes for their success.

The community's attitudes, for example, may reflect a pro-physician or pro-hospital stance. In other cases there may be strong positive or negative perceptions (whether based on fact or not) with regard to various institutions or providers. There may be preferences for certain types of practitioners or methods of treatment over others. Some communities may be very traditional in their attitudes toward healthcare, while others may be quick to embrace alternative treatment modalities.

Another important consideration is the *cultural preferences* of the target population. These cultural preferences (often reflected in lifestyles) may not be directly related to health behavior although many are. Social group preferences for marital status or family size may affect the health status of the population. More directly, dietary habits, exercise patterns, and patterns of unhealthy behavior (e.g., smoking and alcohol use) affect the health status of the population and ultimately the demand for health services. To the extent that healthy or unhealthy behavior is encouraged by the individual's cultural context, this is an important consideration for planners.

Noteworthy examples abound with states like Louisiana and Nevada cited for cultural preferences that could be detrimental to health status, while Utah is cited as a state whose cultural preferences promote good health and longer life. The fact that Wisconsin and Puerto Rico forfeited federal highway construction dollars in the past rather than raise the legal age for alcohol consumption reflects the prevailing cultural preferences in those locales.

Identifying Health Characteristics

A number of dimensions must be considered in examining the health characteristics of the population. This involves the collection of data on a variety of health indicators that can be used to determine the health status of the population and, in turn, the population's healthcare needs. This information should be supplemented with data on health behavior, including existing utilization patterns and informal health practices. Indicators of morbidity and mortality are of direct importance to health services planners. Indirect indicators such as fertility patterns also should be considered.

Fertility Characteristics

Fertility characteristics refer to the attributes and processes related to reproduction and childbirth. Fertility behavior should be considered by the planning analyst because of its effect on population size, growth, and composition. Fertility patterns exert a major influence on both current and future patterns of health services utilization. The most direct link involves the healthcare needs of mothers and children prior to, during, and after birth, with each phase involving unique service and facility needs. Other requirements emerge when the various stages of the reproductive process are considered. For example, healthcare providers and clinic facilities are major sources of contraception-related services. Disorders related to the male and female reproductive systems place additional demands on healthcare providers, and infertility treatment is a growing component of the healthcare system.

   In community-wide planning, many of the health-related issues can be linked to the level of "problem" pregnancies within the community's population. Trends in infant mortality, low-birthweight babies, births to adolescents, and births to unwed mothers all have implications for the healthcare needs of the community.

Morbidity Characteristics

Morbidity, or the level of sickness and disability within a population, is a major concern for health planners. Morbidity analysis involves identifying both the static and dynamic aspects of sickness, as well as how those patterns affect mortality. Several measures have been developed and adopted that are commonly used in morbidity analysis. Although little success has been made in establishing an overall measure of morbidity for individuals or populations, indicators for specific conditions are frequently used. These indicators include incidence statistics for specific conditions, symptom checklists, and various measures of disability. "Reportable" conditions are of particular interest to public health officials, since they relate to conditions that have the potential to spread to epidemic proportions.

   Some health conditions are monitored through reports from health facilities, sample surveys, and ongoing panel studies. Federal health agencies conduct periodic surveys of hospital inpatients and ambulatory patients in clinics and other outpatient settings. In addition, databases have been established for the systematic compilation of data on inpatient utilization and, to a lesser extent, outpatient utilization. These data collection efforts allow for the identification of cases for a wide variety of conditions and the monitoring of the level of these conditions over time. While this information is invaluable, coverage is far from complete at this point. Further, these compilations include only reported cases. If individuals afflicted by various disorders are not diagnosed and treated, they do not show up in these statistics.

Another approach to the development of morbidity indicators is the use of symptom checklists. A list of symptoms that has been statistically validated is utilized to collect data from a sample of the population in order to calculate a morbidity index. These system checklists are utilized to derive health status measures for both physical and mental illness. Individual scores may be summed to create a community-wide index. This can be very useful in comparing the health status of residents of various subareas of the community.

Another group of morbidity measures is referred to as disability measures. Like other aspects of morbidity, disability is difficult to measure within a population. While it would appear simple to enumerate the blind, deaf, crippled, or otherwise handicapped, the situation is actually quite complex. Many individuals who are legally or technically considered disabled may function normally, thereby blurring the lines between those who are disabled and those who are not.

Assuming that adequate data are available, various measures of morbidity can be calculated. Two of the most useful measures are incidence and prevalence rates. An incidence rate refers to the number of new cases of a disease or condition reported over a certain time period expressed as the number per 1,000, 10,000, or 100,000 people at risk. A prevalence rate refers to the total number of persons with the disease or condition in question at a specific point in time expressed as the number per 1,000, 10,000, or 100,000 people at risk.

The prevalence rate always exceeds the incidence rate, since the former is a component of the latter. The only time the two rates are comparable is when the condition under study is acute and of very short duration. For example, the incidence rate would almost equal the prevalence rate at the height of a 24-hour virus epidemic, since victims recover almost as quickly as they are affected.

Incidence and prevalence rates are both important for profiling the target population. If the analyst knows, for example, that the incidence rate for a certain medical condition is 17 per 1,000 population aged 65 years and over (and it is assumed that the incidence rate for that procedure will remain constant for the next five years), then the number of cases can be projected five years into the future if the size of the population of persons aged 65 and over for the service area in question is known. The incidence rate is simply multiplied by the projected population to determine the expected number of cases. The prevalence rate can be used in much the same way when the condition is a chronic one. This is precisely the way in which many hospitals and other healthcare providers forecast the demand for their services.

Mortality Characteristics

Mortality refers to the process of population attrition through death. Mortality analysis includes the study of those who die as well as the health conditions that contribute to their deaths. Mortality studies investigate the who, how, why, and when issues related to dying.

The most basic way to measure mortality is simply to count the number of deaths. Compiling death counts over a period of years has helped identify trends with regard to increases or decreases in mortality. Further, deaths can be cross-classified by the medical, social, and economic characteristics of the deceased. Two of the most useful of these characteristics to planners are the cause of death and the age at which death occurred.

The simplest measure used in mortality analysis is the crude mortality rate (CMR). This rate expresses as the number of deaths as a rate per 1,000 population. The fact that not all of the population is at the same risk of death, however, limits its usefulness. As a result, age-specific death rates (ASDRs) are often generated.

It may also be useful to decompose the CDR into cause-specific components and to calculate the percentage of total deaths attributable to each cause. These figures, which are derived by dividing the number of deaths from one cause by the total number of deaths, represent the proportion of population dying of a specific cause. A cause-specific mortality rate may provide some perspective on the morbidity characteristics of a population in the absence of more direct morbidity statistics.

Although mortality remains an important health status indicator for health planners, its usefulness is somewhat limited in contemporary society. Relatively few deaths occur each year and these tend to be clustered among the elderly who are dying from conditions associated with aging. Further, the chronic conditions that have become predominant in U.S. society are typically not directly associated with mortality. Individuals suffering from chronic conditions (e.g., hypertension) are likely to die from some other, more proximate cause (e.g., heart failure). Therefore, the designated cause of death may not be an accurate indicator of the health status of the deceased. For these reasons, mortality patterns are less useful for profiling the health status of the population than morbidity data.

Health Behavior

Health behavior can be defined as any action aimed at restoring, preserving, and/or enhancing health status. Both formal activities such as physician visits, hospital admissions, and prescription drug consumption and informal actions on the part of individuals such as diet, exercise, and risk-taking should be considered. A number of indicators are used to quantify health behavior and the most common ones are described below.

Hospital admissions is one of the most frequently used indicators of health behavior. The terms "admissions" and "discharges" are used to refer to episodes of inpatient hospital utilization. The hospital admission/discharge rate is generally stated in terms of the number of admissions or discharges per 1,000 population. For example, the hospital admission rate for the United States in 1995 of 120 admissions per 1,000 population might be expressed in terms of 12 out of every 100 residents (or 12%) being hospitalized during that year.

The hospital admission rate serves as a proxy for a variety of other indicators, since hospital admissions are correlated with tests conducted, surgeries performed, and related services and products. For more specificity, admission rates may be broken down by patient category. For example, hospital admissions rates by age group, place of residence, or diagnostic category might be calculated. In fact, the planner is more likely to be interested in diagnosis-specific rates than in overall rates.

Patient days refers to the number of hospital days generated by a particular population and are calculated in terms of the number of patient days generated per 1,000 residents. This indicator refines hospital admissions to reflect the utilization of resources, since measuring patient days serves to adjust for variations in length of stay. Changes in reimbursement procedures, in fact, have made the patient day more of a standard unit for measuring resource utilization than the admission episode. Two hospitals with comparable admissions levels may generate quite different numbers of patient days because of differences in their patient mix. Like admission rates, patient days may be calculated in terms of diagnosis, type of hospital, patient origin, and payor category.

Another indicator related to hospitalization is the *average length of stay* (ALOS). This is typically reported in terms of the average number of days that patients remain in the facility. For example, the average length of stay at a general hospital in the mid-1990s was around 5.5 days. On the other hand, the ALOS for a maternity hospital might be around two days and for a psychiatric facility around 45 days. This indicator provides a good measure of resource utilization. In fact, many healthcare plans reimburse hospitals on a per diem rate.

There are several other facility indicators that might also be mentioned. While none of these has the significance of hospital admissions, each is important in its own way. Utilization rates may be calculated for nursing homes, hospital emergency rooms, hospital outpatient departments, emergency departments, mental health centers, urgent care centers, freestanding surgery centers, and freestanding diagnostic centers.

Perhaps one of the most useful indicators of health services use is the level of physician utilization as measured by *physician office visits*. The physician is the "gatekeeper" for most other types of medical care, and physician use is a more direct measure of utilization levels than hospital admissions, since virtually everyone uses a physician's services at some time.

Analysts usually calculate physician utilization in terms of annual visits per 1,000 population. For example, a community of 30,000 might be expected to generate 120,000 physician visits per year, given the fact that residents average three physician office visits annually. Since physician utilization varies by specialty, rates for physician visits may be figured separately for the various specialties. Primary care physicians are likely to be generate more patient visits from a particular population than any particular specialty. In community-wide planning, access to physician services is almost always an issue, making quality data on physician supply and demand critical.

There are other types of personnel for whom utilization rates might be calculated. Most of these, like physicians and dentists, are independent practitioners who practice without the supervision of other medical personnel. Examples include optometrists, podiatrists, chiropractors, and increasingly nurse practitioners and physician's assistants, as well as various mental health counselors and therapists. Physical therapists, and speech therapists are other categories of healthcare personnel for whom utilization rates might be developed if, for example, the analyst were involved in planning for rehabilitation services. Utilization rates might be calculated in terms of visits per 1,000 population, the average number of visits per person annually, or the proportion of the population using the particular type of therapist.

As the importance of home healthcare are grown in recent years, the volume of *home health visits* has taken on more importance. Home care utilization is typically measured in terms of visits by various types of personnel. Thus, a population might be considered to have a certain number of home nurse visits or home physical therapist visits as indicators of utilization. Alternatively, the number of residents (i.e., the rate per 1,000) receiving home care might be calculated.

Community Resources Inventory

Once the healthcare needs and utilization patterns have been determined, the available community resources should be identified. "Resources" are viewed in the broadest sense here, ranging from facilities to personnel to sources of funding for health services. The focus here is on the resources involved in the direct provision of care. Although they may be important for some purposes, this discussion does not deal with "retail" establishments (e.g., pharmacies, opticians), rental services (e.g., durable medical equipment), or support services (e.g., laboratories, blood banks). The most important types of community resources are described below.

Facilities

A major component of resource identification involves an inventory of the facilities available for meeting the healthcare needs of the population. For community-wide planning, the broadest possible definition of "facility" is utilized. These include all types of facilities devoted to the treatment of physical or mental illnesses. The following are representative of the types of facilities that must be inventoried:

Hospitals

The central role of the hospital in the provision of care warrants a careful inventory of the area's inpatient facilities. This includes not only general hospitals but any specialty hospitals that might serve the population. Some categories of hospitals may ultimately be eliminated from the analysis (such as military hospitals or others that serve small, selected populations), but all should initially be included. The number of available hospital beds should be determined, with careful attention paid to operational versus licensed beds.

Area hospitals should be profiled in terms of admissions, occupancy rates, specialty areas and any other relevant characteristics. Market share should be calculated to the extent possible, trends in these indicators identified and, of course, the physical location of hospitals and other facilities with regard to population concentrations needs to be considered. Any identifiable trends in the characteristics of local health facilities should be noted.

Clinics

The number of clinics providing health services should be determined, particularly since this is the setting in which most clinical encounters occur. ("Clinic" here refers to any freestanding outpatient facility that dispenses medical care.) The key category, of course, is the physician-based clinic, and these clinics should be inventoried in terms of size, specialty, and any other relevant characteristics. Most of these will be private practices, but community-based clinics (such as federally qualified health centers) should be included as well and counted toward the overall resource base. Other types of clinics (non-physician) that should be considered include mental health centers and other behavioral health practices, dental clinics, eye care clinics, chiropractic clinics and podiatric clinics. Urgent care centers should be included as well.

Nursing Homes

The other major institutional facility besides hospitals is nursing homes, and nursing home access has become a growing issue as the number of elderly has increased. The number of nursing homes should be determined, along with the number of beds, occupancy rates, and the categories of clients served. The type of reimbursement accepted is also an important consideration with regard to nursing home access.

Residential Treatment Facilities

Another form of institutional care involves residential treatment centers. Typically reserved for behavioral health and substance abuse patients, residential treatment centers represent "inpatient" facilities in the sense that their clients remain overnight at the facility. They do not necessarily have the around-the-clock intensive clinical support that a hospital would provide. The types of clients that these facilities cater to is an important consideration in the inventory, as well as the type of reimbursement that is accepted.

Home Health Agencies/Hospices

Home health agencies have come to play a major role in the delivery of health services, particularly as the emphasis has shifted from inpatient care to outpatient care. These are technically not facilities in that they actually provide the care in the client's home. The range of services provided in a home setting has steadily grown and, in communities that suffer a shortage of physicians, home health agencies may represent an important source of care. The inventory should identify home health agencies in terms of the services they provide and the type of reimbursement they accept. They should also be identified in terms of organizational structure, such as freestanding/independent agency, affiliate of a national chain, hospital-based program, etc.

Hospices typically do not involve physical facilities but constitute a program of care that is implemented in the patient's home (although some hospice services may be provided in a hospital or some other setting). Although hospice services will not be a major factor in the overall operation of the delivery system, they are necessary to assure a comprehensive ranges of services.

Mental Health Centers

Mental health services (increasingly referred to as behavioral health services) have often been overlooked in inventories of healthcare facilities due to the bias toward physical medicine. However, a growing proportion of the U.S. population receives some type of mental health services, and the demand is expected to grow as lifestyle- and stress-related conditions proliferate. Mental health centers should be identified in terms of their volumes, the types of clients they serve, and their sources of reimbursement.

Diagnostic Centers

As a result of the effort to move care out of the inpatient setting, a number of freestanding facility types have emerged, including outpatient diagnostic centers. These may be multipurpose diagnostic centers or they may focus on a particular diagnostic category such as radiology. The number and types of freestanding diagnostic centers should be determined as well as their organizational affiliation.

Surgery Centers

Freestanding outpatient surgery centers have been another product of the shift from inpatient to outpatient care. As various specialties have shifted their surgical load form the inpatient setting to the outpatient setting, outpatient surgery centers have been the primary beneficiaries. As with other facilities, the type of patients, volume of services, reimbursement arrangements, and organizational affiliation should be determined as part of the inventory.

Urgent Care Centers

Urgent care centers (called by a variety of names) have become increasingly common sources of basic health services. Initially developed to as an alternative to emergency room care and as an option for off-hours care, urgent care centers have become a mainstay for segments of the population that do not have a regular source of care. They are, however, designed for one-time episodic care and technically do not serve as true primary care centers. The number of centers, their volumes, and their acceptable reimbursement should be determined, along with their organizational affiliation.

Programs and Services

A distinction is often made between "programs" and "services", with the former typically referring to a multipurpose operation that integrates a number of functions. The latter typically refers to a specific treatment modality that might be offered in a stand-alone fashion or as part of a program. Thus, an agency that provides personal assistants for the home might be considered to offer a service, while a home health agency that offers a full-range of nursing services, rehabilitation services, and home infusion, in addition to personal assistance aides, would be considered to have a program.

To a great extent, the services available parallel the facilities that are available. Similar institutions, however, may offer quite different services and these distinctions must be identified. Services are often divided into the categories of inpatient and outpatient (or ambulatory) services. Inpatient services are typically provided by hospitals, but nursing homes, residential treatment centers and some other institutional settings may be considered to provide inpatient services. Outpatient services (i.e., care not involving an overnight stay) may be provided by these same facilities, but are more likely to be offered by clinics, physician offices, and other freestanding facilities.

Other services that might be considered are emergency medical services, home health and hospice services, long-term care, and various community-based services. In addition, alternative therapy services should increasingly be considered as a category to be inventoried.

The identification of programs and services separate from health facilities and personnel is perhaps more important than it seems on the surface. This is primarily because services define the facility more than the facility defines the services in many cases. Further, healthcare consumers and referral agents are more likely to be seeking a particular service and may not care what type of facility provides it. For example, someone seeking treatment for an eating disorder will be searching for that type of service and it probably does not matter whether it is located at a hospital, a residential facility, or an outpatient facility. It would be rare for a consumer to select a hospital and *then* determine if it had the required service. (The exception would be cases where one's insurance restricted the use of facilities.)

Equipment

An inventory of the biomedical equipment available to the community should be included in the baseline data collection process. The availability (or lack thereof) of various types of equipment may become a major issue in the planning process. In fact, much of the planning effort should involve determining the appropriate complement of equipment to serve the population of the planning area. This inventory should take into consideration the type of equipment available, the level of utilization, the age and condition of the equipment, the ownership arrangements, and the types of reimbursement accepted.

In situations where critical equipment is lacking (e.g., a community without a magnetic resonance imaging machine), the unmet needs of the population in this regard must be considered. On the other hand, there are situations in which there is a surplus of certain types of equipment. This duplication of effort may result in unnecessary costs, underutilization of expensive equipment, and other situations detrimental to the system. The recent concern over possible bioterrorism activities has raised awareness concerning the need for specialized equipment for use in the event of a nuclear, chemical or biological attack.

Another important equipment category involves information technology. Any number of health initiatives at both the community and organization level have failed in recent years due to deficiencies in the information infrastructure. Healthcare continues to lag behind other industries in the adoption of contemporary information management technology, and many of the inefficiencies in the operation of the healthcare system can be attributed to this situation. An inventory and assessment of the information management technology available among the community's healthcare organizations is critical for effective community-wide planning. At the organization level, it is difficult to imagine the effective operation of any healthcare organization in the future, much less the initiation of planning initiatives, in the absence of an adequate information management infrastructure.

Personnel

It could be argued that the availability of clinical personnel within a community is the most important indicator of resource adequacy. The treatment capabilities available to the population are more a reflection of the personnel available than the facilities available. Personnel should be identified in terms of type, number, characteristics and distribution.

Physicians

The physician remains the pivotal player in the healthcare system, despite the shifts in control that have occurred in recent years. For this reason, as precise an inventory of physician resources as possible should be carried out. Physicians should be inventoried as a group and in terms of their distribution by specialty. To the extent possible, other characteristics should be identified as part of the profile. These include subspecialty areas, ages, type of practice (e.g., office-based, hospital), level of effort, hospital affiliation, and so forth. It is becoming increasingly important to determine the health plans with which a physician is affiliated (although that is probably more of an issue in private sector planning than for community-wide planning).

Developing an accurate inventory of the physician pool is one of the more challenging tasks in the community assessment process. There are no standard directories of physicians, and available sources such as the local medical society roster are typically far from complete and current. Recent trends involving frequent changes in group affiliation, the opening of secondary and tertiary offices, and increasing physician employment have made the determination of physician full-time equivalents even more challenging. If there is a medical school in the community, many physicians may be splitting their time between patient care, teaching and research. While medical residents at these institutions may represent a resource, it is difficult to know how to count them in terms of their effort.

A basic distinction that should be made in this inventory between primary care physicians and specialty physicians. In general, the two categories of physicians perform separate functions within the medical community. The primary care physician is responsible for basic services and, as such, family practitioners, obstetricians, pediatricians, and general internists are considered the first line of response for the healthcare system. Increasingly, they serve as the "gatekeepers" who channel patients into the system.

Community health planners are particularly interested in the adequacy of primary care services. An inherent component of any community health plan is the assurance that basic services are provided for. For this reason, community-wide plans always include standards for the level of primary care. The adequacy of the physician pool can be determined by applying such standards. The most common measure utilized is the physician-to-population ratio. For primary care, this approach has been formalized by the Health Resources and Services Administration

(HRSA) which publishes an annual report on areas that are underserved in terms of primary care.

Nursing Personnel

Nurses have historically served as the backbone of the healthcare delivery system, while constituting the largest category of health personnel. While the number of nurses practicing in a community may be more a function of demand than supply, the existing nurse staffing patterns provide an important perspective on the delivery system. Increasingly, nurse practitioners, nurse clinicians, and other highly trained nursing personnel are practicing independently. In fact, such personnel, usually practicing under a physician's supervision, may provide the bulk of the primary care in certain underserved areas.

As of this writing, the U.S. is in the midst of an unprecedented nurse shortage. The average age of active nurses is increasing rapidly, and replacements are not being trained at a fast enough rate to replace those that are leaving the field. In 2002 there were several hundred thousand nursing vacancies nationwide. While an inventory of nursing resources may not have been a priority for community-wide planners in the past, it is a major consideration in today's environment. Even among planners at the organization level, the availability of nurses within the community often becomes an issue.

Other Independent Practitioners

Several categories of independent practitioners should be inventoried as part of this process. These include dentists, pharmacists, optometrists, chiropractors, and podiatrists. These practitioners typically occupy specific niches within the delivery system, usually supplementing but sometimes competing with the services of physicians. In fact, in an era of managed care, it has become common to substitute "lower" level services from optometrists, chiropractors, and podiatrists for the more expensive physician services of ophthalmologists, neurosurgeons and orthopedic surgeons.

Mental Health Personnel

Mental health personnel are frequently overlooked when community assessments are conducted. Their position at the fringes of mainstream healthcare has historically prevented them from being effectively inventoried in such projects. The community assessment should identify and inventory the variety of practitioners that provide psychological, behavioral health, and psychiatric services to the community. These practitioners are likely to be especially important when the needs of the community's vulnerable populations are considered, and the increasing prevalence of behavioral health problems should draw them more into the mainstream of health services delivery.

Alternative Therapy Providers

A new category of practitioners that now requires inclusion is the variety of alternative therapy providers that practice in the community. Until recently, such practitioners where considered outside the mainstream of conventional medical care. Today, however, it is realized that consumers spend as much of their healthcare dollar on alternative therapies as they do on conventional medical care. Alternative therapists are used both as adjuncts to conventional care and as substitutes. Thus, the community's complement of acupuncturists, herbalists, homeopaths, nutritional therapists, and so on should be identified along with the more conventional practitioners. This is especially the case in communities with large ethnic populations that are likely to maintain certain forms of traditional medical practices.

Networks and Relationships

A thorough inventory of community health services should include a review of existing networks and relationships within the delivery system. This aspect of the research is particularly challenging, since no "directories" of relationships are likely to exist for the community. Some of these relationships may be formal and totally overt; others may take the form of "gentlemen's agreements" and be not widely appreciated by the general public. In an era of managed care and negotiated contracts for health services, the existence of networks and relationships has taken on added importance. The significance of such situations cannot be overestimated and it could be argued that the presence or absence of certain relationships has been the main barrier to effective health services planning in many communities.

The assessment of community facilities should consider the relationships that exist among various organizations. Health systems with multiple facilities in the community should be identified, as well as facilities that are affiliated with or owned by facilities or health systems outside the community. The extent to which hospitals have diversified into other areas such as home health and hospice, urgent care centers, or fitness centers, for example, needs to be determined.

A similar process should be utilized with personnel to determine the relationships that exist. In most communities provider networks have been established by hospitals, health plans or some other entity. By virtue of participating in certain networks, health personnel may be restricted in terms of the hospitals and other facilities that they can use or the health insurance plans they can accept.

In some communities, business coalitions have been established by major employers to negotiate directly with healthcare providers and/or insurance plans. These relationships may involve exclusive contracts between major purchasers of care and local health systems that must be taken into consideration during the planning process.

An important aspect of this analysis involves referral relationships. "Referral patterns" is used broadly here to include actions that channel consumers toward the use of a service or the purchase of a product. It is increasingly important, for example, for hospitals to know which physicians are admitting patients (and who is referring to their admitters), for specialists to know what primary care physicians are referring patients to them, and for urgent care centers to know how their patients found out about them.

Referral patterns in the community-wide planning context are probably most important in relation to public health services and community clinics. The planner needs to develop a clear understanding of the processes by which consumers come to access publicly-supported services and the extent to which the safety net protects the medically indigent.

Sources of Funding

An understanding of the manner in which health services are funded within the community represents an important aspect of the analysis. The payor mix discussed earlier is clearly a starting point for determining how the community pays for healthcare and, ultimately, the population's relative ability to pay for services. The extent to which health services reimbursement relies on government funding in the form of Medicare and Medicaid is important. The level of commitment of funds for public health and charity services is also an important consideration. Any unique sources of funding, such as state programs for categorical disease treatment, should be identified. The sources of funding for mental health services also should be determined, since these typically are reimbursed under a different system than physical health services.

The approach to planning is likely to be quite different for communities with a high proportion of commercial insurance, a large Medicare population, or considerable numbers of Medicaid and uninsured patients. Indeed, the payor mix of the population must of necessity be topmost in the minds of planners at the organization level.

ASSESSING HEALTH STATUS AND HEALTHCARE RESOURCES

Once the community's needs and resources have been identified and inventoried, they must be evaluated. A number of approaches can be utilized in this regard, although all ultimately involve some type of comparative analysis. The assessment of an indicator of health status, for example, could involve a comparison with that same indicator at some previous point in time, a comparison with the indicator for a comparable community or the national average, or a comparison with some standard that has been established. In fact, an indicator should probably be assessed from all of these perspectives. Thus, if the indicator in question is infant mortality, the current infant mortality rate would be compared with historical rates (and hopefully a trend established), with the rates reported for a comparable community or a meaningful average (e.g., that for the state or the nation), and with established standards (e.g., the target infant mortality rate specified in the Healthy People 2010 program).

The number of factors that can be used to assess the healthcare system is almost limitless and too numerous to be listed. They can reflect demographic characteristics (e.g., dependency ratio, sex ratio), socioeconomic characteristics (e.g., poverty level, employment status), health status (e.g., premature births, preventable deaths), health behavior patterns (e.g., immunization level, prenatal care participation), health services utilization (e.g., mammography rate, physician visit rate), ability to pay for health services (e.g., uninsured population, Medicaid enrollment), facilities and personnel supply (e.g., physician-to-patient ratio, bed-to-population ratio), and so forth. As noted below, many of these factors can be utilized to create a community-wide health status index.

Health Status Indices

The development of a health status index is often carried out in the course of a community assessment. The objective of the index is to provide a single number that can be viewed as an indicator of the health status of the community in question. This is done by combining data related to a number of relevant characteristics to create an index. The categories of data from which variables may be drawn include demographics, vital statistics, utilization measures, personnel levels, and various incidence and prevalence measures.

While this index by itself might not mean much, it can be used to compare sub-communities within the population to each other, to the community average, or to some other "standard". It can also be utilized to monitor changes in the community's health status over time or to compare the community to some national average or to an established standard of some type.

Various organizations have identified indicators that they think are important in the development of a health status index. Among these are the National Committee for Quality Assurance, the Institute of Medicine, and the Health Resources and Services Administration within the U.S. Department of Health and Human Services. (See Box 6-1 for a more detailed discussion of health status indices.)

SUMMARIZING THE COMMUNITY ASSESSMENT

A number of different techniques can be utilized to assess the system at this point. Some would apply to selected aspects of the analysis, such as demographic analysis. Others, such as a gap analysis, would allow for a more comprehensive assessment of the needs/resources situation. (Some of the most important techniques are discussed in Chapter 11.)

BOX 6-1
The Health Status Index

For health planners, an important but elusive measure has been an acceptable health status index. Beginning with the social indicators movement of the 1960s, periodic interest has been expressed in the development of an index that could be used to represent the health status of a population or a community in either absolute or relative terms. There is renewed interest in the concept today due to the revitalization of community-wide planning.

A health status index is a single figure that represents the health status of a population or a community. It involves an attempt to quantify health status in objective and measurable terms. A health status index is constructed by combining a number of individual health status indicators into a single index. This index can then be utilized to compare the level of need from community to community. It can be used as a basis for setting priorities and evaluating the worthiness of proposed programs. It can also serve as a basis for allocating resources and as a tool for evaluating the effectiveness of existing programs.

A number of conceptual problems surround the development of health status indices. These problems begin with the question of what indicators to include. To this are added the issues of quantification and measurement. Further, the question of how to weight the various component indicators is also raised. There are no simple means for resolving these issues. Every analysis must address them in the best manner possible and carefully document the process that is used in developing the index.

A variety of indicators can be utilized in the creation of a health status index. Many of the indicators that might be included—e.g., death rates—are fairly obvious. Others, such as certain demographic indicators, might not be. Nevertheless, it is common to use demographic traits such as the racial composition, the dependency ratio, and educational attainment as component indicators in a health status index. Some of these are referred to as "proxy" measures of health status, in that they are not direct indicators of health conditions but can be assumed to indirectly indicate the level of health status within a population.

The major categories of health status indicators commonly utilized include morbidity indicators, outcome indicators, utilization indicators, resource availability indicators, and functional status indicators. Morbidity measures are obvious indicators of health status, since they reflect the prevalence and/or incidence of various conditions, as well as the level of disability within a population. Thus, the extent to which a population is affected by various acute and chronic conditions constitutes an important component in any health status index. (Unfortunately, it is difficult to obtain actual data on morbidity and, although extremely important, this remains a problematic area in health status index construction.)

Outcome measures are so called because they ostensibly reflect the extent to which the healthcare system is effective. Outcome measures include such indicators as death rates, infant death rates, life expectancy, and potential years of life lost. Of these measures, the infant mortality rate is probably the most useful as a component of a health status index, since it represents far more than just the rate as which infant deaths occur; it speaks volumes about living conditions, nutritional levels, domestic violence and a number of other dimensions of socioeconomic and health status.

Utilization measures are also used as components of a health status index. This includes indicators such as the hospital admission rate, the rate of emergency room visits, the physician visit rate, and so forth. These measures tend to be among the more controversial, since it could be argued alternately that these are positive or negative indicators.

Resource availability entails another important set of indictors. These include the ratio of hospital beds to the population, the ratio of physicians to the population, and other measures of resources. The rationale for the use of such indicators is that the level of resource availability should be correlated with higher health status. Although this, too, is controversial, such indicators are frequently employed in index construction.

Measures of functional state constitute an additional category of health status indicators. These include a range of measures such as days of work lost, days of school lost, bed-restricted days, activity-restricted days, and so forth. The use of these measures reflects the notion that individuals who are limited in their functional abilities reflect poor health status (regardless of the source of the limitation).

Health status indices can be calculated for any level of geography for which data are available. However, the smaller the unit of geography the finer the distinction that can be made. Many health planning agencies conduct analyses down to the census tract level, while others utilize the zip code or county as the unit of analysis.

The following sample indicators might be considered in the construction of a health status index:

(continued)

Annual population change

Population under 15 years

Population over 65 years

Sex ratio

African-American population

Other racial/ethnic populations

Median household income

Households below poverty level

Female-headed households

Unemployment rate

Fertility rate

Death rate

Infant death rate

Premature births

Adolescent births

Out-of-wedlock births

AIDS cases

Physician-to-population ratio

Once the indicators have been chosen, values must be assigned to each indicator for each unit of geography being analyzed. A number of different methodologies can be utilized for this process, and the important factor is to come as close to both scientific rigor and face validity as possible. Assuming that all indicators are to be equally weighted, one approach might be to score each indicator on a scale of 1 to 5 for each geographic unit. Negative characteristics would be scored closer to 1 and positive characteristics closer to 5. The scores for each indicator could be summed and then divided by the number of indicators to provide an average score for each geographic unit somewhere between 1 and 5. It should be noted that the absolute number generated through the process means little; its value is derived from the ability to compare it with other figures. This index number could be used, for example, to compare one community to another or track the health status of a particular community over time.

The community assessment process should produce a document that summarizes the characteristics of the community and the issues relevant to health planning. The summary should describe the demographic and socioeconomic characteristics of the community and anticipated trends in these characteristics. It should summarize the community's health status and indicate any particular issues in this regard. The summary should describe the prevailing healthcare practices of the community including patterns of referral and utilization. It should also include an inventory of available health services and an assessment of their characteristics.

A critical determination in any planning process is the extent to which existing resources address the needs of the population. The findings in this regard will inform the remainder of the planning process. Identifying mismatches, maldistributions, and shortages or surpluses in healthcare resources provides the basis for much of the planning activity that follows. The ultimate objective is to identify unmet healthcare needs within the community and address them through the planning process.

The overall condition of the community should be described, with special attention to the gap between needs and services. These unmet health needs, along with other identified issues, provide the basis for the subsequent planning activities that take place. This "state of the community" document provides the starting point from which all future conditions are measured.

While those developing plans for organizations have historically not focused on the community assessment process, some consideration of the broader community is becoming increasingly common. Not only does the community assessment provide a context for any planning initiatives that the organization may undertake, but some level of community assessment is a prerequisite for implementing the population-based planning initiatives that an increasing number of healthcare organizations are pursuing.

References

Center for Evaluative Clinical Sciences (1999). *The Dartmouth Atlas of Healthcare.* Hanover, NH: Center for Evaluative Clinical Sciences.

Additional Resources

Dever, G.E.A. (1991). *Community Health Analysis.* Gaithersburg, MD: Aspen.

Mitchell, Arnold (1984). *The Nine American Lifestyles.* New York: Warner Books.

7

The Planning Audit

INTRODUCTION

When planning is carried out at the organization level, the data collection process is often referred to as a "planning audit". The planning audit can take a variety of forms and typically includes an internal audit and an external audit. The nature of the audit will depend on the type of planning that is being undertaken. The audit for a strategic planning project will be different from that for a marketing plan. On the other hand strategic planning and marketing planning emphasize the external audit over the internal audit, while financial planning, human resource planning and facilities planning may place more emphasis on the internal audit.

As with the community assessment, there is no one way to conduct a planning audit. Thus, this chapter does not attempt present a definitive model for conducting a planning audit but a generic version that can be applied to virtually all situations and modified for a particular setting as appropriate.

STATING ASSUMPTIONS

Here, as elsewhere, an important task involves the stating of assumptions. Assumptions should be stated at the outset of the project and may be modified or expanded as information is collected on the organization, the market, and the competitive situation. Assumptions can relate to many aspects of the process and several are likely to be formulated. In fact, assumptions might be stated about the process itself indicating, for example, which issues can and cannot be considered during the planning process.

As assumptions are being formulated, the mission of the organization should be reviewed. If no mission statement is currently in place, one should be developed, since the mission statement serves as the organizing principle for the planning process. Although the mission statement may ultimately be revised during the course of the process, it provides a starting point for planning.

PREPARING FOR THE PLANNING AUDIT

The planning audit will take place after the initial information gathering effort has been carried out. The analysts should have reviewed copies of any previously developed plans, research reports or consultant studies as a starting point for more formal data collection. Interviews with knowledgeable individuals within the organization may have already been conducted. In many cases, key informants outside the organization may have been interviewed as well.

These initial information gathering activities should have familiarized the planner with the key institutional players, major decision makers, and opinion leaders within the organization. This process should have also uncovered the major issues from the perspective of the respondents. While these issues are likely to be refined during the planning audit, they serve as "talking points" to get the process started.

As part of this process, any barriers that might impede the planning audit should have been identified. These barriers may include individuals who are likely to be resistant to the process, sensitive data that the analysts may not have access to, or deficiencies in information management systems that may present challenges for the audit. This information helps form the assumptions that will inform the planning audit.

As part of preparations for the planning audit, the planner should develop a project plan for this component of the planning research. This plan will specify the activities that will be carried out as part of the planning audit. It will identify individuals and departments within the organization (and, to a lesser extent, without) who must be involved in the audit. It will also specify the types of information that will be required for each activity and lay out the sequence of events that must be followed in order to complete the audit.

An important final step in the preparation process involves alerting those in the organization that a planning audit is going to be undertaken and disclosing what will be involved. While the audit involves a systematic and objective process of data collection and analysis, some within the organization might consider it a quest for their "dirty linen". For this reason, it is important that everyone involved is aware of the nature of the audit and that the threat represented by this process is minimized for the individuals within the organization.

PLANNING AUDIT DATA COLLECTION

The planning audit involves two major categories of data: internal data and external data. Knowledge of the internal characteristics of the organization is critical for the planning process, and a great deal of effort is likely to be exerted developing a detailed understanding of its internal operations. (This type of analysis is rare in community-wide planning, since multiple organizations are involved in that process.) Data on the external environment is equally critical for the planning process, particularly if strategic planning, marketing planning, or business planning is being undertaken. For more introspective planning exercises (e.g., financial planning, facilities planning), the external environment must still be taken into consideration.

This section describes some of the types of internal and external data that are important in the planning audit. Additional information is provided on the sources of such data in Chapter 12.

The Internal Audit

All healthcare organizations have immediate access to a "gold mine" of information–their own internal records. Healthcare organizations routinely generate a large amount of data as a by-product of their normal operations. The types of data that can typically be extracted from internal records include patient characteristics, utilization trends, and sources of revenue, among others.

These data may be acquired through the performance an *internal audit*. The internal audit can be broken down into a number of functional areas. An internal audit examines the organization's *structure*, its *processes*, its *customers*, and its *resources*. The structural analysis involves an examination of the "organization of the organization", identifying which personnel are responsible for which functions and, in the case of a hospital or physician group, profiling the medical staff or group partners.

This analysis of the organization's processes investigates the flow of customers through the system and the accompanying flow of paper. It identifies and evaluates the lines of communication, from the decision-making process at the top to the transfer of operational minutiae at the bottom of the organization. The process analysis also involves a review of financial trends, including the price setting process. The components included and the attention accorded different aspects of the operation will depend on the nature of the planning engagement.

The following categories of information are typically included in the internal audit.

Management Processes

The internal audit should examine the management processes that are in place, since these impact so many of the other dimensions of the organization. The audit should review the organizational structure, examine the policies and procedures that are in place, and assess to the extent possible the level of efficiency and productivity characterizing the organization. The decision-making process needs to be understood and the readiness of management to participate in the planning process determined. The buy-in of management is essential for a successful planning initiative.

Information Technology

Today, one of the first components of the internal operation that is likely to be considered is the organization's information technology. In the first place, the information management capabilities of the organization are going to influence the amount and quality of the data that can be generated for the planning analysis. More important, however, is the fact that information systems provide the foundation for performing most other functions within the organization. The efficient processing of customers, effective billing and collections, and the tracking of marketing activities are just some of the uses for information technology.

While many healthcare organizations in the past have gotten by without adequate information management capabilities, that will not be possible in the future. The demands for data are growing every day, and organizations that cannot respond will be at a competitive disadvantage. Detailed information must be available, for example, in order to negotiate managed care contracts. In fact, in the future managed care plans are not likely to contract with providers that do not have the level of information management that the managed care plan demands.

Recent information management developments in healthcare related to the Y2K issue and, now, to HIPAA regulations are bringing information management needs to the forefront. The growing interest in the paperless office and the need to efficiently manage patient data will keep the attention on information management issues for some time to come.

Services/Products

An early step in the internal analysis is typically the identification of the services and products offered by the organization. In some cases, the "product" may be obvious, in others it may not be. An organization offering a single service or product may be easily profiled, but this situation seldom exists in healthcare. Most healthcare organizations provide a range of services and/or products, but they are not likely to have thought of them in terms of specific products. This step typically requires more effort in healthcare than in other industries, since scant attention is likely to have been devoted to specifying the nature of the services and products offered by the organization. Each service and product should be profiled not only in terms of the defining characteristics of the service or product, but also in terms of packaging, presentation, and any other factor that might influence the ability to market it.

Customer Characteristics

The customer analysis should identify and profile *all* of the organization's customers. These may be very specific (as in the case of a medical supply company whose only customers are blood banks) or very diffuse (as in the case of a general hospital that has multiple customer groups). For healthcare providers, patients are typically the customer group that receives the most attention. A basic profile of existing patients includes demographic and socioeconomic characteristics, case mix (e.g., diagnosis, procedures), payor mix, and place of residence. With this information, one can evaluate the "quality" of the current patient population, determine which segments are more "desirable," and identify the categories of patients one would like to target.

Utilization Patterns

An analysis of the level of utilization of the organization's services and products is a critical component of the internal analysis. Current levels of utilization in terms of admissions, office visits, procedures performed, or products sold provide the starting point for understanding the operation of the organization. The utilization measures emphasized in the audit will depend on the nature of the organization and the type of planning process.

Planners may categorize utilization in terms of a number of dimensions including clinical category (e.g., cardiology, orthopedics), patient characteristics (e.g., age, sex), payor category (e.g., Medicare, private insurance), and the geographic origin of the patients in terms of their home ZIP code or county.

Utilization analyses not only provide a "snapshot" of the organization's current status, but are particularly important for tracking organizational performance. Thus, the analysis must examine past trends in utilization and include projections of future utilization patterns. Changes in utilization over time provide information on the changing status of the organization in relation to the market.

Financial Data

Data on the organization's financial status has become a critical component of the planning audit. Financial information has direct implications for product and service development, promotional activities, and competitive analyses. The relative financial performance of members of the medical staff may contribute directly to strategic marketing initiatives, and the mix of profitable and unprofitable services and products will affect the organization's bottom line. As managed care negotiations become a more common aspect of organizational life, financial information will become increasingly important.

The internal audit should consider sources of income and the manner in which income is expended, especially since the organization's likely future payor mix will be a major predictor of its profitability. Billing and collection processes should be reviewed and an understanding of compensation arrangements developed.

Staffing and Other Resources

Staffing data represent a valuable information resource for virtually every health-care organization. Personnel databases may provide information on the residential location of the organization's staff, the match between those treating patients and the patients' characteristics, the inventory of skills and experience available, and opportunities for the marketing of services to the organization's employees. For hospital planning, internal databases are likely to contain extensive information on the characteristics of the medical staff.

The planner requires this information to evaluate the strength of various specialty areas, identify gaps in the medical staff or other personnel, anticipate future specialty shortfalls (e.g., an aging staff), and develop marketing programs that focus on particular specialty areas. For physician groups, especially larger ones, internal information on physician characteristics, their activity patterns, and their productivity levels provides important knowledge for assessing the group's position within the current market and determining how well it is positioned for the future demands of the market.

Referral Patterns

In an era of increasing competition, the identification of the various sources of customers becomes critical. It is particularly important to identify referral sources and track their activity. Hospitals need to know which physicians are admitting patients (and who is referring to their admitters), specialists need to know what primary care physicians are sending them patients, and urgent care centers need to know how their patients found out about them.

The term "referral" is used broadly here to include any process that channels customers toward the use of a service or the purchase of a product. Healthcare organizations may collect information on referral at the time of patient intake, or this information may be a routine part of the paperwork for some organizations. Many organizations do not systematically collect this information and are forced to perform primary research to determine where their customers are coming from.

Indirect methods of determining referral sources may also be used, particularly patient origin studies. A specialty group with a multi-county service area may find, for example, that certain counties are underrepresented in terms of referred patients and others are overrepresented. This would suggest that referral relationships are weak in some areas and strong in others.

Pricing Structure

The pricing structure for a product or service has become increasingly important for planning purposes. Not only is price a basis for differentiation between providers but the pricing structure for a service may constitute a marketing device in its own right. The internal audit should determine how prices are determined and review the existing price structure in the context of industry averages.

For many healthcare organizations, the internal audit will include a fee structure analysis. This analysis reviews the charges being levied by the organization and identifies fees that are too high or too low based on some objective external standard.

Marketing Activities

All marketing activities that the organization has in progress should be identified. Although this may appear to be an external concern, the internal structure for promoting the organization's services and/or products is as important as external marketing efforts. In addition, the status of internal marketing should be reviewed. This involves the manner in which customers are processed, the way staff interacts with the customer, and internal procedures for tracking customer activity. All marketing resources currently deployed should be identified.

The External Audit

The external audit is comparable to the environmental assessment performed in community-wide planning. The external audit is particularly important in organization-level planning because of the emphasis placed on the characteristics of the market in many types of plans. The analysis should begin at the national level and be addressed at the regional level if appropriate. The assessment should clearly be extended to the state level and ultimately brought down to the level of the market area in which the organization operates.

Societal Trends

As was the case with the community assessment, broad societal trends should be analyzed and their implications for the local environment considered. These include trends in demographics, economic conditions, lifestyles and attitudes. The types of trends that are emphasized will depend on the nature of the organization and the type of planning that is to be conducted. Most analyses will include a review of broad demographic trends as a means of setting the context for planning.

Broad economic trends are also a consideration, even for an organization operating in a local market. The state of the economy has implications for the demand for health services and the ability of consumers to pay for care. A state of full employment involves different implications for healthcare than does a situation with high unemployment, particularly with regard to insurance coverage. National healthcare chains are particularly susceptible to shifts in the national economy.

Trends in lifestyles may be very pertinent for certain healthcare organizations. Developments like the emergence of the two-income household, the increase in childlessness, and the fitness movement may have implications for a wide variety of organizations. The growing interest in alternative therapies and other trends will continue to reshape healthcare going into the twenty-first century.

Changes in consumer attitudes at the national level may have implications for local market areas. The emergence of the baby boomers as a major force in society has been accompanied by a significant change in consumer attitudes. Baby boomers are clearly characterized by different outlooks from previous generations, and this "new consumer" is affecting all aspects of healthcare. These new attitudes have made possible the success of urgent care centers, freestanding diagnostic centers, health maintenance organizations and many other innovations in healthcare.

Health Industry Trends

Trends in the health industry itself should be analyzed to identify developments that are likely to affect the local market area. These could include trends in reimbursement, changing organizational structures within the delivery system, and the introduction of new treatment modalities. Current examples include the consolidation of firms in many sectors of the industry and the rise of alternative therapies. The emergence of new concepts such as post-acute care, assisted living facilities, and long-term acute care facilities may have an impact on organizations in the local market. Other industry trends include the continued influence of large national for-profit chains and the emergence of employers and employer coalitions as key players in the healthcare environment.

Regulatory, Political and Legal Developments

The regulatory environment exerts a significant influence over healthcare organizations. At every level of government, regulatory functions exist that have important implications for healthcare organizations. Federal regulations governing the operation of the Medicare and Medicaid programs are an important case in point. At the same time, states have primary responsibility for licensing health facilities and personnel. State agencies may directly or indirectly exert influence over the provision of care. A seemingly innocuous new government regulation could easily prove to be a boon or a bane for various healthcare organizations.

The political environment clearly has both direct and indirect implications for the operation of the health system. Presidential mandates or Congressional directives could have an impact that trickles down to the local market. At the state level, the certificate-of-need process may have a significant impact on the ability of healthcare organizations to expand their operations or add new facilities, equipment or services.

Legislative activities at the national, state and local levels also have implications for the local healthcare system. Examples abound of recent legislation at the national level that has influenced physician referral patterns, length of stay for women undergoing childbirth, and the ability of patients to sue health maintenance organizations. State legislative activities may have even more impact at the local market level. The actions of city and county governing bodies may have implications for local healthcare organizations, with those in the public sector most likely to be affected by these actions.

Technology Developments

Developments in the area of technology have major implications for health services providers and ultimately influence the demand for various health services. Advances in medical and surgical treatment modalities, pharmaceuticals, biomedical equipment, and information management all affect certain healthcare organizations. The introduction of new drugs has changed the manner in which behavioral health problems are addressed, refinements in biomedical equipment have made home care more feasible for a wide range of conditions, and microsurgical techniques have contributed to the shift of care from the inpatient to the outpatient setting. In the late 1990s, the introduction of a new drug for impotence, for example, became a major development within the healthcare system.

Reimbursement Trends

The type of reimbursement available for the provision of care has come to be a major consideration for healthcare organizations. The reimbursement picture is complicated by the variety of payors that potentially fund any healthcare provider. A provider's patient mix is likely to represent a variety of payors and many patients may have their care reimbursed by more than one payor. The emergence of managed care with its special reimbursement arrangements has further complicated the picture. For this reason, healthcare providers have had to increase their claims management capabilities.

Healthcare providers are faced with having to carefully control their solicitation of customers in order to avoid attracting non-paying customers and slow-pay or low-pay third-party payors. The reimbursement arrangements involved in managed care have become a major factor driving business decision making in healthcare.

Financing issues may be introduced by agencies at all levels of government, as well as by private sector third-party payors. Changes in reimbursement under federal insurance programs such as Medicare and Medicaid play an important role in altering practice patterns, and new "industries" have emerged in healthcare as a result of these changing reimbursement patterns. Similarly, the services that private insurers do or do not cover can have a major implications for healthcare organizations.

SPECIFYING THE MARKET AREA

An important step in planning at the organization level involves the identification and profiling of the market area. This is particularly the case when such activities as strategic planning, marketing planning, and business planning are involved. The more the process involves the external environment, the more important the market area analysis is.

The market area in the organization plan is comparable to the service area in the community-wide plan. A "market" can be defined in a variety of ways. The definition utilized depends on the purpose of the analysis, the product or service being considered, the competitive environment, and even the type of organization conducting the research. Five different ways of conceptualizing a market are discussed below.

Geographically based definitions of the market are probably the most commonly used approach to specifying markets on the part of health planners. Most planning research, in fact, focuses on a census tract, ZIP code, or county (or a group of any of these units) as the basis for analysis. The market area is typically delineated in terms of the boundaries of the geographical units chosen for analysis. (See Box 7-1 for a discussion of the geographic units utilized in market research).

In actuality, few markets (for healthcare or anything else) neatly follow political, statistical, or administrative boundaries. In fact, markets virtually always change faster than their formal boundaries, so there will invariably be some slippage between geographically-based market area boundaries and the actual market area. Nevertheless, market areas are often "gerrymandered" to conform to geographic boundaries that represent a reasonable approximation of the service area under study. The primary reason for this, of course, is the fact that the available data are usually organized on the basis of existing geographic units.

The market may be defined at any geographic level by a healthcare organization. While providers tend to serve local markets, the emergence of national healthcare chains has clearly affected this situation. Certainly, national pharmaceutical and medical supply companies serve national and even international markets. Many national organizations conduct their planning on a regional basis. Since health plans are regulated by the various states, they are likely to develop plans at the state level.

Second, a market may be defined in terms of a *population segment* or some other component of the population. Planners often define the "market for product x" in terms of demographics, psychographics or some other characteristic. Examples of markets defined in this manner are women of child-bearing age or a psychographically-defined segment such as "yuppies".

Markets conceptualized in terms of population segments can be exceedingly broad or quite narrow. If older Americans are considered the market, this obviously cuts a broad swath through the U.S. population. Thus, the market for an AARP-sponsored health plan is likely to be broad and diffuse. On the other hand, if the senior population that requires nursing home care is depicted as the market, this is obviously a much narrower segment of the population. Similarly, the study could involve the market for a broad range of services (e.g., comprehensive inpatient services) or for a narrowly defined individual service (e.g., outpatient eating disorder treatment).

Another type of market may be viewed from the perspective of the service itself—i.e., a market defined by *consumer demand*. For example, healthcare organizations may seek to identify geographic areas where there are large concentrations of potential patients for a particular service. In this instance, markets are defined in terms of their healthcare needs. Examples of markets defined in this manner are the population in need of geriatric services or the one in need of behavioral health services. A hospital may consider virtually the entire population within its defined service area as part of its "market", while a home health agency may envision a narrowly defined subsegment of the population as its potential market.

Fourth, markets may be defined in terms of the healthcare *opportunities* adjudged to exist in a given area. A given location could be viewed with interest because there is a shortage of providers or a lack of facilities. An area that is characterized by a lack of competition obviously offers an opportunity for some organization. In other cases, the numbers of providers may be adequate, but the fragmentation of providers may offer an opportunity for an organization that can appropriately "package" its services. This approach might be thought of in terms of addressing the *effective* market.

Additional opportunities may be offered by areas that are characterized by a high level of "unmet" healthcare needs. These would include areas (or populations) that appear to need a certain level or type of services but, for whatever reason, are not receiving them. For example, a given population, according to a demand model, should receive a certain number of mammograms per year based on its size and composition. If the number of mammograms being performed annually on this population is significantly lower, this may indicate an unmet need. (Note that many unmet needs exist in populations with limited resources; depending on the type of organization performing the research, these populations may or may not be appropriate candidates for targeting.)

Similarly, opportunities may exist in areas where a "gap analysis" indicates a shortfall in services or a mismatch between needs and services. The number of physicians or hospital beds that a given population is able to support can usually be determined utilizing various predictive models. If the number of physicians and/or hospital beds located in the area falls below the "expected" number, there may be opportunities in that market.

There is yet a fifth way to define a market, although in this case the term a "market without walls" might be appropriate. Increasingly, certain markets are no longer defined in terms of geographic units or population segments. For example, the markets for contact lenses, health food supplements, and certain home testing products have become less dependent on location, since they may be purchased by mail order or through television or Internet shopping services. In addition, the advent of telemedicine allows a specialist in one location to receive electronically-transmitted test results for a patient in a different location. The introduction of on-line pharmacies and even on-line physician diagnostic capabilities has contributed to a rethinking of what constitutes a market.

While markets are typically thought of in terms of the end-user, markets may also be framed in terms of health professionals of one type of another. Physicians as a group constitute a market for many products and services, and the marketing efforts of pharmaceutical companies with regard to physicians are legendary. Hospital chief information officers may constitute the market for information technology vendors, while physician practice managers may represent the market for many products and services.

One final basis for market delineation is in terms of disease characteristics. Many organizations are "categorical" in their approach in that they only serve certain clinically defined categories of patients. When organizations view a market area in this manner, the do not actually "see" the total population but focus on a particular segment. This segment may be characterized by those affected by arthritis or diabetes, those requiring psychotropic drugs, or those undergoing organ transplantation. The market may also cut across demographic, psychographic and payor groups. Thus, considerable planning research focuses on identifying the market in terms of disease categories.

Delineating Geographically Defined Market Areas

Effective planning requires an in-depth understanding of a healthcare organization's market area. The nature of the organization and the type of planning both contribute to a determination of the area to be targeted. Not surprisingly, the delineation of the current market area for the organization for which the planning is being performed is an early step in the planning process. The organization in question may be a hospital, a physician practice, or any other type of healthcare organization. There are a number of methods that can be used to specify the market area, and the method will vary with the type of service involved. For many organizations, it may be important to identify the primary, secondary and even tertiary market areas.

The planner must first decide on the unit of geography to be used for the analysis. The choice of geographic level depends on the amount of detail required and the type of market served. For a hospital or specialty group that serves multiple counties, the county is likely to be an appropriate unit for analysis. On the other hand, if the market is restricted to a particular county, it will probably be necessary to approach the analysis at the ZIP code or even the census tract level. Thus, the market area for a neighborhood clinic or for a solo family practitioner is likely to be less extensive than a county and should thus be defined in terms of a smaller unit of geography.

One method for delineating a market area involves determining the source of origin for the organization's patients. If appropriate, the residences of recent patients could be plotted on a map. The distribution of these patients should indicate the general market area for the organization, with the geographic area (e.g., ZIP code, county) from which 75 percent of admissions are drawn constituting the organization's primary market area.

A complex organization like a hospital may exhibit multiple market areas. The market area for general hospital services may be different, and much smaller, than that for more specialized offerings. Therefore, multiple market areas may exist for organizations that provide multiple services. The delineation of market areas should also account for patients who do not come from their residences, but from other facilities such as places of employment, nursing homes or industrial sites (Pol and Thomas, 2001).

Alternatively, market penetration rather than volume could be utilized to define the service area. It might be determined, for example, that the organization maintained high market penetration as measured by market share within selected ZIP codes. All ZIP codes in which the organization maintained a market share of 25 percent or more might be identified as the market area. It may turn out that these ZIP codes do not necessarily correspond with the ZIP codes identified in terms of patient volume. The planner must make a decision here as to which basis of market area delineation best suits the purposes of the project.

A third method for market area delineation involves establishing the maximum distance or driving time that consumers are willing to travel for a given health service. Computer software is available to perform this task, though in rapidly changing areas driving times can be significantly altered over a relatively short period of time. In general, this "drive time" method simply involves identifying the location of the service or facility and allowing the software to establish boundaries using the distance and travel time data specified. The represents a very pragmatic means of defining market area boundaries.

In some planning projects, the task may involve the delineation of a market area for a service or services not yet offered. Delineating these boundaries is much more difficult and usually requires multiple techniques. Initially, the residential distribution of patients using similar services should be plotted. If another organization is offering the same or similar services, then its market area boundaries should also be estimated. Distance/driving time data must be evaluated as well. However, a more subjective approach may be required because the service in question is new to the area. Data on the same service offered in a different market area may be available through professional networks. These data could help to establish time/distance parameters. Surveys of potential consumers of these services (e.g., physicians and patients) may also provide valuable information.

Once delineated, market area boundaries must be continuously monitored for change. Traffic patterns and driving times change, and market area boundaries may be significantly altered over a short period of time. Changes in tastes and preferences for services either on the part of physicians (e.g., increased interest in home infusion therapy) or patients (e.g., increased demand for outpatient services) must also be monitored to determine their affect on market area boundaries, as should the entrance or exit of competing organizations.

There may be situations, incidentally, in which the existing market area is not in keeping with the objectives of the organization. It may be that the composition of the identified market area is changing, as reflected in the characteristics of resident healthcare consumers. Or, the organization's clientele may have moved away from the facility, as in the case of an inner-city hospital whose patients have moved to the suburbs but continue to patronize the facility. The question to ask becomes: Is this the appropriate market area to use as a framework for planning?

In establishing "target" market areas for specific goods and services, there are certain established rules that should be applied. Targeted markets must be amenable to being ranked, they must be realistic in size, the targeted customers must be reachable, and the targeted customers must have some minimum level of response potential. Assuming that the market is of adequate size, another consideration becomes the potential number of cases is the actual geographic distribution of prospective customers within the service area. The importance of customer distribution varies with the type of service and the characteristics of the population. Some services are supported by a local population and others by a more far flung population. On the other hand, some populations are much more mobile than others or are otherwise more or less sensitive to travel times and/or distances.

BOX 7-1
Units of Geography for Health Services Planning

Virtually all health planning activities are linked to a particular geographic area. Planning agencies typically have a specific geographic area over which they have authority. Private sector healthcare organizations typically plan for "markets" that are delineated based on geography. Even when the target audience is a population segment rather than a geographic unit, this audience will ultimately be linked in one way or another to geography.

For our purposes, the geographic units used in health services planning can be divided into three major categories: political/administrative units, statistical units, and functional units. Each category is described below.

POLITICAL/ADMINISTRATIVE UNITS

Political or administrative divisions are the most commonly used geographic units for planning purposes. This is partly due to the fact that many organizations involved in community planning have jurisdictions that coincide with political boundaries such as cities, counties, or states. Further, it is convenient for private sector organizations to use standard political or administrative units to establish their boundaries. Political units also are useful in spatial analysis, since many statistics are compiled for political units. The following political and/or administrative units are frequently used by planners.

Nation

The nation (in this case, the United States) is defined by national boundaries. Although a few national chains may be interested in data at the national level, most healthcare organizations focus on lower levels of geography. However, national averages (e.g., mortality rates) are often important as a "standard" to which other levels of geography might be compared.

State

The major subnational political unit is the state, with data collected for 50 states, the District of Columbia, and several U.S. territories. Because the individual states have responsibility for a broad range of administrative functions, many useful types of data are compiled at the state level. In fact,

(continued)

state agencies are a major source of health-related data. However, each state complies data independently of other jurisdictions, resulting in uneven data reporting from state to state.

Counties

The county (or, in some areas, townships or parishes) represents the primary unit of local government. The nation is divided into over 3,100 county units (including some cities that are politically designated as counties). The county is a critical unit for health services planning, since many healthcare organizations view their home county as their primary service area. Further, states typically report most of their statistics at the county level, and the county health department is likely to be a major source of planning data. Even healthcare organizations with regional markets are likely to consider the county as the building block for data collection.

Cities

Cities are officially incorporated urban areas delineated by boundaries that may or may not coincide with other political boundaries. Although cities typically are contained within a particular county, many city boundaries extend across county lines. Because cities are incorporated in keeping with the laws of the particular state, there is little standardization with regard to boundary delineation. For this reason, cities do not make very useful units for planning analyses. In many cases, however, city governments are involved in data collection activities that may be useful to health services planners.

Congressional Districts

Congressional districts are established locally and approved by the federal government. These districts are typically delineated by means of political compromise and may not correspond with any other geographic boundaries. Limited amounts of data are collected at the congressional district level, and the boundaries tend to change over time, making these units not particularly suited for use in health services planning.

State Legislative Districts

State legislative districts have similar characteristics to congressional districts. They are drawn up by the states based primarily on political compromise. Very little data are collected for these political units and their boundaries are subject to frequent change. For these reasons, they are not very useful as units for health services planning.

School Districts

School districts are established for the administration of the local educational system. Although theoretically reflecting the distribution of school-aged children within the population, other factors may play a role in determining the configuration of school districts within a community. While school districts may be sources of data useful in developing population projections, few health-related statistics are generated for this unit of geography.

Statistical Units

Statistical boundaries are established for a variety of purposes, but they are primarily created to allow various agencies of government to aggregate data in a useful and consistent manner. The guidelines for establishing most statistical units are promulgated by the federal government. The most important statistical units for planning purposes are discussed below.

Regions

Regions are established for statistical purposes by the federal government by combining states into logical groupings. Four regions have been established by grouping states based on geographic proximity and economic and social homogeneity. Health statistics are sometimes reported at the regional level by federal health agencies. (The term "region" is also used informally to refer to a group of counties or states delineated for some other purpose than data compilation.)

Divisions

For statistical purposes, the federal government divides the nation's four regions into nine divisions. Each division includes several states, providing a finer breakdown of the nation's geography. Divisions are seldom used as a basis for health services planning.

Metropolitan Statistical Areas

Metropolitan statistical areas (MSAs) are delineated by the federal government as a means of standardizing the boundaries of cities and urban areas.

Since each state has different criteria for the incorporation of cities, the MSA concept provides a mechanism for creating comparable statistical areas. An MSA includes a central city, a central county, and any contiguous counties that could logically be included within the urbanized area. A significant amount of data is available on MSAs, and this unit is often used to designate a healthcare service area.

Urbanized Areas

An urbanized area as defined by the Census Bureau includes the entire densely settled area in and around each large city, regardless of whether or not the area is within the corporate limits. Although limited amounts of data are available for urbanized areas, knowledge about urbanized areas is important in developing a full understanding of the population distribution within a metropolitan area.

Census Tracts

Census tracts are small statistical subdivisions of a county established by the Census Bureau for data collection purposes. In theory, census tracts contain relatively homogeneous populations ranging in size from 1,500 to 8,000. For many purposes, the census tract is the ideal unit for health services planning. It is large enough to be a meaningful geographic unit and small enough to contribute to a fine-grained view of larger areas. The Census Bureau collects extensive data at the census tract level, although this information is only available every ten years from the decennial census. Much of the emphasis in community-wide planning is on the census tract level of geography.

Census Block Groups

Census tracts are subdivided into census block groups that include approximately 1,000 residents. A tract is composed of a number of block groups, each containing several blocks. This provides an even finer picture of a community at the tract level, although fewer data elements are likely to be compiled at the block group level.

Census Blocks

Census block groups are subdivided into census blocks, the smallest unit of census geography. The term "block" comes from the fact that the typical block is bounded on four sides by streets, although some other visible feature (e.g., railroad track, stream) or nonvisible feature (e.g., city limits) may serve as a boundary. Census blocks tend to be the most homogeneous of any unit of census geography, with the average block housing approximately 30 persons. Only a limited amount of data is available for census blocks.

Block Numbering Areas

In areas that were not divided into census tracts, the Census Bureau historically divided territory into block numbering areas (BNAs). These tended to be rural areas in which BNAs served the same purpose as census tracts. However, with the 2000 census, the two systems were combined and block numbering groups were phased out. BNAs remain useful when retrospective data collection is necessary.

ZIP Code Tabulation Areas

ZIP Code Tabulation Areas (ZCTAs) are a new statistical entity developed by the U.S. Census Bureau for tabulating summary statistics from the 2000 census. This new entity was developed to overcome the difficulties in precisely defining the land area covered by each ZIP Code used by the U.S. Postal Service (see below). Defining the extent of an area is necessary in order to accurately tabulate census data for that area. ZCTAs are generalized area representations of U.S. Postal Service ZIP Code service areas. ZCTAs are built by aggregating the Census 2000 blocks, whose addresses use a given ZIP Code, into a ZCTA which gets that ZIP Code assigned as its ZCTA code. They represent the majority USPS five-digit ZIP Codes found in a given area. For those areas where it is difficult to determine the prevailing five-digit ZIP Code, the higher-level three-digit ZIP Code is used for the ZCTA code. The Bureau's intent was to create ZIP code-like areas that would maintain more stability from census to census.

FUNCTIONAL UNITS

A number of other geographic units are used in health services planning, particularly by private sector healthcare organizations. These units are often more suited to business development activities than are political or statistical units. However, the "custom" geographies that are delineated for planning purposes may take these units into consideration.

(continued)

ZIP Code

Unlike the geographic units previously discussed, ZIP codes do not constitute formal government entities. ZIP codes tend to be much larger than census tracts, sometimes including tens of thousands residents. Their boundaries are set by the U.S. Postal Service and are subject to change as population shifts occur and/or the needs of the postal service dictate. This lack of stability often means that ZIP codes have limited value for historical analyses or for tracking phenomena over a long period of time. Further, ZIP codes seldom coincide with census tracts or other political or statistical boundaries, making the synthesis of data for various geographies extremely difficult.

Nevertheless, the ZIP code is a useful unit for defining the market areas of smaller physician practices, smaller hospitals, and even specialty niches for larger health systems. Commercial vendors compile a great deal of information at the ZIP code level. Perhaps more important, healthcare organizations typically maintain ZIP codes for virtually every consumer they come in contact with, making this an accessible geographic identifier linked to every customer record.

Markets

"Market" is a generic term for the target area or population identified by a healthcare organization. From a geographic perspective, it refers to the area that is included within the sphere of influence (however measured) of the healthcare organization. Frequently, the market area is constituted from individual ZIP codes or counties, thereby creating a custom geographic unit. In other cases, the market may conveniently coincide with an existing political boundary (e.g., a county).

Areas of Dominant Influence

Taken from media advertising, the area of dominant influence (ADI) refers to that geographic territory (typically a group of counties) over which a form of media (e.g., television, newspaper) maintains predominance. This concept has been adapted for healthcare and could be thought of as the "effective" market for a particular healthcare organization.

Since the level of need within the target population may not correspond with the level of interest, it is important to determine the extent to which the population really *wants* the service. This is a point in the process where primary research may be required. Although it may be possible to conduct a psychographic analysis of the market area and, from that, develop an idea of the level of interest in a particular service, many situations will demand a survey of some type. Ideally, no new program or service should be introduced without a consumer survey and the newer the service or the more unfamiliar the market being entered, the greater the need. Many new programs have failed because the actual level of interest of the target population was much less in reality than it was on paper.

The delineation of a market area often requires the calculation of an organization's overall market share or its share based on specific services or products. This could involve a hospital's share of the total area admissions, an orthopedic surgeon's share of all hip replacements, or a health plan's share of total health plan enrollment. Market shares can be calculated by dividing the organization's number of cases (e.g., admissions, office visits, procedures performed) by the total number of cases for the identified market area.

The organization's internal records of procedures, discharges, or diagnoses, for example, can serve as the numerators for market share calculations. Denominators are derived in one of two ways. First, in some markets, the denominator data are available as the result of publicly sponsored record collection activities. For example, hospital discharge data are often collected by state health departments and aggregated at geographic levels such as the county. A simple calculation divides the number of discharges from Hospital x in County y by the total number of discharges in County y.

The second way to gather data for rate denominators is to estimate the number of procedures and discharges using population and incidence information. The number of diabetes cases in Market Area z can be estimated by multiplying national or regional incidence rates by population data specific to age or other enumerated factors known to differentiate the probability of being diagnosed with diabetes. The reason for estimating the incidence is that in many instances there is no market-specific count of procedures, discharges or diagnoses that can serve as the market share denominator.

It is not unusual to divide the market area into a primary market area, a secondary market area and, often, even a tertiary market area. The techniques utilized above to specify the market area can be refined to create these sub-markets. For example, it might be determined that the geographic area from which the "closest" 50 percent of patients originate will be considered the primary market area and the area from which the next 25 percent of patients originate will be the secondary market area. All other locations that contribute patients are considered part of the tertiary market area. Varying planning or marketing approaches might be developed for the respective sub-markets.

PROFILING THE TARGET MARKET

Once the market area has been demarcated, the population of the identified area must be profiled. This process follows much the same steps as that for the community assessment. However, the factors taken into consideration in profiling the population for organization-level planning are likely to be much more focused than for community-wide planning.

In profiling the community, the temporal dimension is very important. Whether determining the needs of the target market or identifying competing services, three time horizons must be taken into consideration. Obviously, the current inventory of needs and resources is a starting point. However, it is also important to develop a sense of the historical trends that are affecting the community. Is the population growing or declining? Are the characteristics of the population different today than they were five years ago? Are the numbers of competitors increasing?

The most important timeframe, of course, is the future, whether this means two, five or ten years. A plan should identify the future characteristics of the population, the future health service needs of that population, and likely future developments with regard to competitive forces.

As with the community assessment process, the regional setting should be taken into consideration. Different regions of the country have their own cultural patterns, and these seem to have persisted despite the rapid change that has swept U.S. society. Different regions report varying levels of prevalence for various health problems, and the variation in utilization of health services is now well documented (Center for Evaluative Clinical Sciences, 1999). Thus, regional variations should be considered when health services demand is being estimated or projected for a particular market area. National healthcare organizations in particular must take regional variations in practice patterns into consideration in their planning activities.

The type of community is also a consideration when collecting baseline data on the market. Whether the dominant community type within the market area is urban, suburban or rural will have important implications for both health status and health behavior. Consumer attitudes are also likely to be different for the various community types, and the existence of sub-markets within the market area may be a complicating factor in the planning process.

As with the community assessment, the first type of data typically compiled is demographic data, including biosocial and sociocultural traits. At a minimum, the analyst would examine the population in terms of age, sex, race/ethnicity, marital status/family structure, income and education.

The situation of the target market with regard to insurance coverage is an important consideration in the external audit. The emphasis on insurance coverage will vary depending on the nature of the organization. The "payor mix" of a market area (and for the organization being planned for) is perhaps more directly significant to specific healthcare providers whose financial viability is a function of their payor mix. While many providers attempt to limit the number of self-pay patients they serve, there is a multi-billion dollar market for elective services that are not typically covered by insurance plans.

The entire vanity market involving facelifts, tummy tucks and other cosmetic procedures is strictly driven by "uninsured" patients. Another example is the alternative therapy "industry" that has emerged to challenge mainstream medicine, built almost entirely on out-of-pocket payments.

The demographic analysis is often accompanied by an assessment of the psychographic characteristics of the market area population. Information on the lifestyle categories of the target audience can be used to determine the likely health priorities and behavior of a population subgroup. *Consumer attitudes* is another dimension of the population that is typically considered at this point. The attitudes displayed by consumers in a market area are likely to have considerable influence on the demand for almost all types of health services. At the organization level, the attitudes of a wide variety of constituents besides direct consumers must be taken into consideration.

Identifying Health Characteristics

The health status of the market area population can be examined along a number of dimensions. Indicators of morbidity and mortality are of direct importance to health services planners, and indirect indicators such as fertility patterns also should be considered. These were discussed in some detail in the previous chapter, so they will only be summarized here.

Fertility characteristics refer to the attributes and processes related to reproduction and childbirth, and the importance of these characteristics varies depending on the type of organization and the type of plan. The number of births as well as the characteristics of those births, along with the attributes of the mothers and fathers of the children, form the basis for fertility analysis.

Historical patterns of fertility exert a major influence on current patterns of health services demand. A wide range of service and product needs revolve around childbearing. Childbearing also triggers the need for such down-the-road services as pediatrics and contraception-related services. The demand for treatment of the male and female reproductive systems and the heightened interest in infertility treatment are by-products of the reproductive process.

The level of *morbidity* within a population is a major concern for health services planners. Incidence and prevalence rates can both serve a useful planning purpose, and both may be employed as part of a planning analysis, depending on the nature of the project. This category includes disability indicators along with measures of morbidity in terms of the level of sickness. To the extent possible, planners need to project rates of incidence and prevalence into the future in order to plan for coming developments.

The study of *mortality* examines the relationship between death and the size, composition, and distribution of the population of the market area. Organization-level planners typically have less interest in mortality analysis than those involved in community-wide planning, since the latter are more concerned with the overall health status of the community. Nevertheless, mortality data is always examined to determine what it can tell us about the health status of the community.

Specifying Health Behavior

Health behavior, as noted earlier, involves any action aimed at restoring, preserving, and/or enhancing health status. This includes both the formal utilization of health services and informal actions on the part of individuals that are designed to prevent health problems and maintain, enhance or promote health. Organization-level planners are likely to have a much more focused interest in health behavior than do community health planners. As at the community level, the analyst will examine health behavior in terms of both formal and informal actions, focusing on those indicators most relevant to the organization in question.

In terms of formal activities, the potential indicators include hospital admissions, patient days, average length of stay, utilization of other facilities besides hospitals, physician office visits, visits to non-physician practitioners, and drug utilization. Among the indicators that have become important more recently are the utilization of freestanding medical facilities and various types of alternative therapies.

THE COMPETITIVE ANALYSIS

Most external audits involve some type of competitive analysis. The planning research should not only determine the position of the organization within the market but also its position relative to its competitors. In the absence of competitive data it is difficult to gauge one's status in the market and even more difficult to measure change over time. In addition, many types of planning depend on the competitive analysis to establish the framework for developing strategies.

An important first step is a determination of the nature of the competition. Certainly the competitive environment in healthcare has become cloudier as a variety of new forms of healthcare organizations have emerged. In simpler times, hospitals knew that other hospitals were their competition, cardiologists knew that other cardiologists were their competition, and so forth. Today, the environment has changed and competition can take a number of forms. In the case of hospitals, many types of organizations besides hospitals have begun competing with their services. These are not always "outside" interests, in fact, since their own medical staffs may set up competing operations. The boundaries of specialty practice have become blurred as aggressive specialists seek to expand their range of services. The purveyors of alternative therapies have emerged to challenge mainstream physicians on many fronts.

The degree of detail involved in the competitive analysis depends on the nature of the organization and the type of planning that is being initiated. Ideally, the research process should develop the same body of knowledge on competitors as on the organization itself. Admittedly, complete access to internal records of competitors is not likely to be available, but much information will be a matter of public record and, therefore, accessible. Depending on the nature of the competitor, information will be needed on services and products, pricing, volume or utilization, and staffing. In the case of hospitals a medical staff profile should be developed as well). It will also be important to identify the locations of competitors' facilities.

Much of this information may be available from public sources, but it depends on the type of organization as well as reporting requirements in the state where it operates. Many healthcare organizations are required to file reports with the state on their operations. They may also be required to submit applications for various licenses or certificates. Certificate-of-need applications may be required for healthcare organizations adding facilities or services. Publicly-held corporations must file a variety of reports that can be accessed, and many privately-held healthcare organizations publish annual reports. Recipients of Medicare reimbursement must file costs reports with the Center for Medicare and Medicaid Services. These types of reports are generally accessible to the public.

Certain information will inevitably be difficult to obtain. It would be helpful, for example, to know something about the financial status of competitors, their business plans, the contracts they have obtained or the relationships they are developing within the community. Information of this type is not as readily available, but may be gleaned from interviews with key informants in the community.

In addition to this quantitative data, there is a qualitative aspect that should not be ignored. It might be important, for example, to determine the status of competing physicians with regard to their practices. While on the surface it might appear that there is a significant number of competing general surgeons in the community, closer inspection may indicate that one is practicing part-time due to some impairment, another is reducing his patient load as he transitions into retirement, and another is dissatisfied with his group affiliation and is considering moving out of town to practice. This type of qualitative information may require unorthodox research techniques but it can usually be obtained.

Patients and former employees of competitors can be useful sources of market intelligence. Patients of competitors may be found among the organization's current customers or they may be uncovered through a random survey of the community. More aggressive analysts might even attempt "exit interviews" with patients leaving the competitor's facility. Competitors' patients may be a useful source of information on referral patterns, community perceptions and preferences, and customer satisfaction levels. Heightened concerns over the confidentiality of patient records demands the careful handling of any data of this type.

Former employees of competitors provide a perspective of a different type. They have been inside the organization and will be familiar with its internal operation. They may be able to provide that qualitative dimension that offers insights into the strengths and weaknesses of a competitor. While it would be inappropriate to violate any confidentiality agreements, former employees typically freely offer valuable information if given the opportunity.

Finally, other practitioners, especially those involved in some type of referral relationship are likely to be useful sources of information. Physician practices might start with their referring physicians as a source of information. From them it may be possible to determine their referral patterns and the reasons for choosing the specialists for referral that they use. It may also be possible to obtain a comparative perspective from these informants. Perhaps even more important is the information that can be obtained from those with whom there is no referral relationship. The reasons for existing referral patterns and any perceived deficiencies attributed to the organization may be identified from these sources.

MARKET AREA PERCEPTIONS AND ATTITUDES

Another dimension that is particularly important in organizational planning is the perceptions and attitudes of the population of the market area. The population here is defined in the broadest sense to include any group whose opinion of the organization may have an impact on its success. The most important of these groups is the organization's customers. While this constituent group is easily recognized in most industries, the nature of the customer is complicated in healthcare. The patients of a specialty physician practice, for example, may be considered its customers at the same time that practice is entirely dependent on referrals from other physicians, thereby placing referring physicians in a customer category.

In addition to the organization's customers, the groups from which it might worthwhile to obtain information during the planning process could include the general public, the medical community, competitors, referral agents, local employers and business coalitions, health plan representatives, legislators and other policy setters, and the organization's own employees. Depending on the nature of the organization and the type of planning initiative, the perspectives of some or all of these groups could be critical.

SUMMARIZING THE PLANNING AUDIT

The planning audit should produce a document that summarizes the internal characteristics of the organization and its position within its market area. The summary should describe the demographic and sociocultural characteristics of the market and report anticipated trends in these characteristics. It should describe trends in demand for the organization's services and review the competitive situation. The perceptions of various groups should be described and the organization's strengths and weaknesses outlined.

The summary should describe the opportunities that exist in the market and the steps necessary to take advantage of them. These opportunities should be tempered by the threats to the organization that exist in the environment. This "state of the organization" document provides the starting point from which all future planning will ensue. (Chapter 11 presents techniques for conducting research on the market area.)

References

Center for Evaluative Clinical Sciences (1999). *The Dartmouth Health Care Atlas*. Hanover, NH: Center for Evaluative Clinical Sciences.

Pol, Louis G., and Richard K. Thomas (2001). *The Demography of Health and Healthcare*. Burr Ridge, IL: Irwin Professional Publishing.

Additional Resources

U.S. Census Bureau. URL address: www.census.gov.

8

Strategic Planning

INTRODUCTION

Strategic planning is a well-established activity in most industries and, to many, it has become synonymous with corporate planning. Strategic planning has come to be seen as a prerequisite for any business activity, and in many ways it represents the epitome of contemporary business planning. Strategic planning is *a formal, on-going process for developing goals and implementing actions for positioning the organization in the market while matching available resources with market opportunities.*

This definition implies that planning is a "process" that involves both the development and the implementation of a systematic plan. This process focuses on "positioning", indicating the important relationship between the organization and its environment. It also recognizes the importance of matching available resources to opportunities, as this is the ultimate goal of any planning exercise.

THE FUNCTIONS OF STRATEGIC PLANNING

In today's healthcare environment the importance of strategic planning cannot be overemphasized. The notion of planning as a framework for decision making applies to strategic planning more so than to any other type of planning. Rational choices in healthcare require a context that sets out objectives to be met, as well as agreed-upon criteria for decision making.

The strategic plan serves as a mechanism for adapting to an ever-changing environment. The emphasis that it places on "positioning" vis-à-vis the market sets it apart from most other types of planning. Indeed, the nature of strategic planning equips it for adapting to the moving target that the healthcare arena has become. Ultimately, a strategically oriented organization is one whose actions are aligned with the realities of the environment.

The strategic plan should provide an edge for the organization, making it better informed and better organized than its competitors. If the challenge is to "get there first" in healthcare today, the strategic plan should provide an advantage in this regard. If one cannot be first for some reason, the objective should be to be the best. This objective, too, is supported by the strategic plan.

The strategic plan should be the basis for resource allocation, particularly when scarce resources are being dispensed. Inherent in the definition is the matching of internal resources with opportunities within the market. If outside capital is required, few sources of capital will make major commitments in the absence of a strategic plan. Any joint venture partners or strategic development partners are going to inquire about "the plan" early in the discussions.

The strategic plan should also provide the basis for relationship development in an environment that is increasing being driven by networks of providers, integrated delivery systems, and referral relationships. The plan should address the appropriateness of existing linkages and identify potential additional relationships.

Most importantly, the strategic plan should be a call to action. Indeed, many healthcare organizations have spun their wheels for years waiting for a clear direction to present itself. The strategic plan should, as the name implies, embody the organization's strategy. More than that, it should convey the vision of the organization and lay out the scenario for what it should be when it reaches "maturity".

THE NATURE OF STRATEGIC PLANNING

Strategic planning has a number of attributes that set it apart from other types of planning and illustrate its unique characteristics. Strategic planning is *lateral* in that it cuts across the various divisions of an organization. As such it requires coordination across organizational lines and demands more open cooperation across structure and function than other types of planning. Coordination is critical for both the development and implementation of the plan.

Strategic planning is *relative* in its orientation. Conceptually, strategic planning only exists as it relates to the external environment and other players in that environment. In a traditionally product-oriented industry, the relationship with the external environment is limited. In a service-oriented industry, like healthcare has become, the external environment is the *raison d'être* for strategic planning.

Thus, the internal focus characteristic of traditional types of planning is deemphasized. After all, the real issues are "out there" in the environment.

Strategic planning is *long-term* in its orientation (or at least longer term than traditional forms of planning). Theoretically, strategic planning should include long-term goals, intermediate term strategies, and short-term tactics. Five- or ten-year time horizons should typically be observed.

Strategic planning should be *creative* in its orientation. This represents a major distinction between strategic planning and most other types of planning. Creativity in budget planning or facilities planning may not be seen as a virtue. With strategic planning, however, creativity is *de rigueur* if the plan is to address the issues posed by the environment. The strategic planning orientation demands that conventional wisdom be left at the door of the conference room. This means no more "business as usual" and no more introspection. Strategic planning demands "thinking outside the box".

The strategic mindset also discourages a tactical focus. This short-term approach to planning is not appropriate in a context where longer-range strategies are demanded. Tactics are more often than not reactive. The question should *not* be: "How do we counter a move by one of our competitors?" Strategic planning should be proactive in its approach. It should not be distracted by current circumstances but should focus on likely developments within the environment five years or more down the road.

Since strategic planning is about *positioning*, the vision of the strategic plan should reflect how the organization sees itself positioned within the environment five or ten years into the future. This is the scenario from which the intermediate steps should be derived.

Strategic planning deals with the *business side* of the organization. The only other type of plan that is more focused on the business aspects is the business plan itself, and this should be a subcomponent or spin-off from the strategic plan. The objectives that are specified in the strategic plan are likely to be business objectives.

Strategic planning is typically not a component of community-wide planning, although it would be inappropriate to contend that it should be totally excluded from planning at the community level. In fact, there is growing conviction that the goals of public sector organizations operating within the context of the community-wide plan cannot be reached without following strategic planning principles. This realization has prompted an unprecedented interest in strategic management among public sector healthcare entities.

THE STRATEGIC PLANNING PROCESS

Planning for Planning

The first step in the strategic planning process involves planning for planning. This often starts with the question: Why are we doing planning? It should be realized that strategic planning is virtually never done because it is the right thing to do. It is almost always prompted by a problem or perceived problem related to the organization. Further, the perceived problem is often not the real issue but, upon investigation, is found to be symptomatic of other issues. For that reason, the approach that is followed is more often a function of the desires and interests of those initiating the plan.

Much of the early activity in the strategic planning process is organizational in nature. It involves identifying the key stakeholders, decision makers, and resource persons that must be taken into consideration in the process. This is the first step in developing an understanding of the organization and serves to generate the list of key informants to be utilized later in the data collection process.

This phase also involves establishing a planning team that will guide the process. The nature of this team will vary from situation to situation, but its establishment is clearly a prerequisite for moving forward. Much of planning for planning involves determining who is to be involved in the process and, more important, who is to lead it. While there is no foolproof combination of team members that assures success, certain categories of participants must be involved. These include representatives of the various stakeholders, key decision makers, opinion leaders, and representatives of all constituent groups. The team should also include those representing various substantive areas within the organization. While it is not unusual to employ an outside consultant to assist in the development of the plan, the plan must ultimately be a product of the organization's staff. Therefore, it is imperative that the right personnel be engaged at the initiation of the project.

It is clearly important to develop planning competence within the organization as well. This is an important first step is the development of a strategic mindset and, in most organizations, this represents a significant challenge. Inculcating a strategic mindset does not happen overnight, and it takes education and reeducation before it becomes established. For this reason, outside resources may be relied upon heavily during the organization's initial efforts at strategic planning.

The question often arises at this point as to who should do the planning. If this question is directed toward internal resources, the choice must be made by the organization. If the question refers to internal staff versus outside experts it is a different matter. There are options with regard to the internal versus external resource debate. (See Box 8-1 for a discussion of internal versus external resources for planning.)

Stating Assumptions

One of the critical steps at the outset (and actually at any juncture in the planning process) is the stating of assumptions. Assumptions might be made considering the players involved in the local healthcare arena or about certain health care "facts of life". Assumptions also should be stated with regard to the nature of the market

BOX 8-1
Choosing Between Internal and External Resources

Few healthcare organizations have the internal resources readily available to develop a strategic plan. Even those organizations that are fortunate enough to have an established planning or research department are likely to have to marshal additional resources for the major undertaking of formulating a comprehensive strategic plan. When this issue comes up, a question is typically raised with regard to the use of internal versus external resources. That is, should the process rely primarily on staff and resources that exist within the organization or should much or most of the planning activities be outsourced to a consultant?

There are clearly advantages and disadvantages to each of these approaches. There is a natural tendency on the part of administrators to prefer to use existing resources to the extent possible, although this preference may not be shared by the staff that are already stretched thin by other responsibilities. Several arguments could be made for the use of internal resources. Obviously, staff is already in place and they are familiar with the territory. Existing personnel are aware of the history of the organization and know how it operates. They are aware of existing personnel and other resources and in a position to access and/or mobilize them. Given the desire to keep information on the organization "close to the vest" (and current concerns over confidentiality of clinical data), an argument could be made for keeping the data "in the family" lest it fall into the wrong hands. The argument is further made that the cost of the planning can be minimized by using people who are already on the payroll, an issue that will be revisited below.

One argument that is not always made but should be for the use of internal resources relates to the transition from planning to implementation. Developing a strategic plan is one thing; implementing it is another. When it comes time to transition from planning to implementation, the process often breaks down. Emphasizing internal staff in plan development allows for a smoother transition toward operationalization of the plan. Even if different departments pick up the implementation process, they will be interfaced in one way or another with those involved in planning, allowing for a reasonable degree of continuity. This is not likely to be the case with an outside consultant who coordinates the planning process but may be long gone when the time for implementation arrives.

(continued)

Many of the arguments for the use of internal resources for the planning process can also be viewed as disadvantages. In the typical setting, all personnel (including dedicated planning staff) will already have a full plate of responsibilities to which all of their time is committed. Carving out additional time for a major planning initiative is a logistical challenge and likely to be accompanied by a considerable amount of negativity on the part of the staff.

The fact that existing staff already know a lot about the organization and its operation can be viewed as a drawback to the planning process. Being "too close to the problem" has its dangers, and existing staff are likely to have biases concerning certain departments and activities as well as preconceived notions about the direction the organization should take. Strategic planning calls for thinking "outside the box" and invariably results in a restructuring of the organization's operations and staffing. Individuals who serve to gain or lose from these developments may not be the best ones to be determining the course of the organization. The need for complete objectivity can also make the use of internal resources problematic. Indeed, concerns of staff over the outcome of planning or the disclosure of certain information may make cooperation from various parties within the organization difficult to achieve.

The use of external resources also has several advantages. Outside consultants are likely to display a level of expertise not available within the organization. Even organizations with existing planning departments are not likely to have the capabilities of a consultant that specializes in plan development. The outside consultant is likely to have national experience and thus a perspective that internal staff are not likely to have. He will have been exposed to any number of strategic planning initiatives and have a broad understanding of both process and strategy. The consultant may have access to data sources, analytical techniques and other resources that may not be available to internal staff.

The outside consultant can be expected to offer a degree of objectivity that may not be possible with internal resources. He is likely to come into the situation without any preconceived notions and be open to options that would never occur to internal staff or, if they did, be rejected out of hand. The outside consultant has no vested interest in the outcome of the plan and does not have to worry about pleasing a boss or "stepping on toes". Analyses can be carried out and decisions made without fear of future negative consequences for the consultant.

The ability of outside consultants to obtain complete and accurate information from the organization's staff is often debated. On the one hand, there may be suspicion on the part of staff with regard to the planning process and the intentions of the consultant. There may be fears that the information provided will be used to the detriment of the one providing it at some point. There may also be a concern over the provision of sensitive information (including clinical data) to an outsider who may, in fact, work for a competitor at some point in the future. Many employees are skeptical about the motives of the consultants and may, sometimes based on past experience, consider the process a waste of their time.

On the other hand, outsiders can typically elicit information from staff that they would never disclose to their supervisors or coworkers. Their experience with other, similar situations may allow them to ask the right questions and more insightfully analyze the responses. Further, employees may welcome the opportunity to voice their complaints or put forth suggestions for which no previous opportunity for expression existed.

An outside consultant cannot be expected to be as familiar with the healthcare environment in which the organization operates as its staff are likely to be. In healthcare, there are often deep-seated relationships and patterns of interaction in the community that may not be obvious. There are also aspects of the community that cannot be understood in the short time period during which the consultant is on the job. Factors that may be obvious to local health professionals may be totally missed by an outside consultant facing a daunting amount of information for analysis.

The fact that the outside consultant is not likely to be around once the plan is completed is an issue for concern. Given that the process often breaks down at the point that the process passes from planning staff to management, the consultant's absence as implementation commences can be a serious drawback. A few consultants advertise their willingness to assist with the implementation process but, in the typical case, the consultant has moved on to another planning engagement when implementation begins.

The issue of cost is often a pivotal factor in the decision to use internal versus external resources. There is a belief that the use of existing staff is likely to be more cost-effective than an outside consultant since they are already on the payroll. Indeed, they are being paid a lot less per hour than an outside consultant would charge. Further, it may be felt that adequate data are available from internal resources that don't have to be purchased to support the planning process.

This perspective represents an unrealistic view of the situation for most organizations. In healthcare in particular, managers don't only manage but are also involved in "line" activities. Diverting their time and attention from

(continued)

clinical, technical or administrative duties means that those responsibilities are not fulfilled or, more likely, they will be carried out by less capable parties or by "agency" staff that carry a significant cost premium. Further, the cost and effort involved in mobilizing the necessary staff is likely to be significant. The need to initiate data collection activities incurs additional costs; starting from scratch to perform primary research, for example, is much more expensive than utilizing the existing processes of an outside consultant. Ultimately, reliance on internal resources is a very expensive proposition when direct and indirect costs are considered, and there is the possibility that this approach will not even yield the desired results.

Outside consultants are not inexpensive, and there is a tendency to evaluate their cost in relation to staff salaries. However, the consultant's hourly fee does not just cover an hour's labor, but it also pays for the expertise that the consultant brings to the project. It is difficult to place a price on insights that may never have surfaced without the input of the consultant. Given the significance of the strategic plan for the organization, it is hard to justify shutting off potentially critical options in order to save a few dollars. In the case of the consultant, they will not be fully compensated until they deliver the product; internal resources continue to be paid whether they produce a plan or not.

Ultimately, the choice between internal and external resources should not be an either/or decision. Indeed, the strategic direction must emanate from the organization's staff regardless of the level of outside involvement. For this reason as well as others, both internal and external resources are utilized in appropriate proportion in successful planning projects. Existing staff have a lot to contribute, and data resources are likely to be available within the organization. On the other hand, outside consultants have the perspective and the technical skills to build on the knowledge of existing staff and the available internal resources. This approach capitalizes on the advantages offered by internal staff and external resources.

(and its population), the political climate, the position of other providers, and any other factors that might affect the planning process.

Some assumptions can–and should–be stated at the outset of the planning process. Others will be developed as information is collected and more indepth knowledge is gained concerning the market, its health care needs, and available services. Although assumptions will undoubtedly be refined as the planning process continues, it is important to begin with general assumptions. For example, "Managed care will continue to exert a major influence on the local market" or "We're number four in market share and there is no way we will ever be number one."

Initial Information Gathering

The data collection process for the strategic plan begins with the gathering of general background information on the organization. This includes a review of any available organizational materials, such as publications produced by the organization (including annual reports), press releases, and marketing materials. It may even be appropriate to review the "vitas" of management and key clinical and technical personnel. Other potential sources of information include reports filed with regulatory agencies, business plans that have been presented to funding sources, grant proposals, and certificate-of-need applications. Certain internal documents, such as executive committee minutes, planning retreat summaries, and evaluation studies may also be useful.

It is important to review any previous planning studies or consultant reports that have been developed for the organization. These documents may provide valuable background information on the organization, supply baseline data that can be used for comparison purposes, and provide an analytical framework that can be readily updated. These documents provide the basis, along with other information compiled, for organizing the more formal aspects of the analysis.

Initial information gathering should include interviews with knowledgeable individuals within the organization. These should include a reasonable sampling of individuals within the organization who represent different functional areas, vested interests, and perspectives. For large organizations, these initial interviews may be restricted to key administrators and medical staff and perhaps one or more individuals with a handle on institutional history. Within a smaller organization such as a physician's practice, it will be possible to conduct initial interviews with medical staff, administrative staff, and perhaps other key individuals during initial information gathering.

What should the planner expect to learn from a review of these materials and the initial interviews? The *major issues* should be identified, remembering that these may not be the same issues that prompted the planning initiative. The list of issues at this point may be relatively long and unrefined. Narrowing down the list to the most relevant issues will be part of the planning process.

The *organizational structure* should be identified. This means not only the stated structure but the actual structure in terms of the manner in which the organization functions. This involves a review of the division of labor, the chain of command, and the internal communications channels.

The *key players* in the organization should be identified through this process and, when appropriate, any influentials external to the organization as well. The number of key players will vary depending on the size and complexity of the organization. Some key players are obvious, such as those in formal positions of authority. Division or department heads are also likely to be identified as key informants. Other critical participants may be those who are positioned to have access to critical information. These might include planning or marketing professionals, information technology professionals, the director of the medical records department, and the managed care liaison, for example.

Another category of key informant to consider would include those knowledgeable by virtue of their unique experience within the organization. These might include a long-term personnel director or individuals who have worked at various levels and/or for different departments within the organization. Others may be important due to their role (often unrecognized formally) as opinion leaders. Some employees may, by virtue of contacts, personality, knowledge, or other traits be considered "influentials." In some hospitals, for example, the union representative may have an influence far beyond his or her formal title within the organization.

This stage of the process should also identify the *key constituents* of the organization. Who, in effect, must the organization report to? If it is a tightly held private organization, there may be few outside the organization that matter. On the other hand, if it is a private, not-for-profit entity, there are likely to be board members, regulators and others to which the organization must be accountable. If it is a publicly-held company, the board of directors and its shareholders represent constituents of some importance as well. Other constituents to consider include patient groups, referring physicians, employee benefits managers, insurance plan representatives, and politicians. These must be identified during the initial stages of the analysis so this information can inform subsequent research.

Much of what is gleaned during initial information gathering could be considered to reflect the "corporate culture" of the organization. This term refers to the character of the organization's internal environment. There is now ample documentation of the manner in which the corporate culture affects the operation of the organization and determines the extent to which the environment is amenable to the planning process. The culture of the organization will influence both the planning process and the implementation of the plan.

This initial information gathering should also identify any potential barriers to planning. What are the organizational considerations that may impede planning? Will communication issues prevent cooperation? What individuals or positions are likely to be resistant to the planning process? The planner is not likely to have the complete answers to these questions at this point, but an appreciation of potential roadblocks should emerge as background information accumulates.

The planner should now be in a position to begin to think in terms of the assumptions that will drive the planning process. It is possible at this point to make assumptions concerning the support of various parties, the organization's structure, the corporate culture, the quality of communication, the decision-making process, and so on. These assumptions help set the parameters for the planning process.

Profiling the Organization

This initial information gathering should lead to a sense of "what" the organization is and which business it is in. This will involve examining the existing mission statement and goals of the organization. If these are not stated, the assumed mission and goals should be identified. One of the real turning points for any healthcare organization involves coming to grips with what business it is in. Hospitals who continued to think they were in the hospital business rather than the healthcare business found themselves at a competitive disadvantage with hospitals that realized they had a broader mission.

To this end, a couple of important questions must be addressed during the early stages of research. The first of these is: What is our product or products? This appears to be an easy question, but one few healthcare organizations can readily answer. This is partly because they have never thought in those terms, but also because there is usually no simple answer. Unless the organization's sole business is selling a healthcare "widget", the products and services offered are likely to be complex and not easily classified. What product does the specialty practice provide, for example? Health? Disease elimination? Prolonged life? Improved quality of life? Or looked at differently, is the product the individual procedure or diagnostic technique that is performed, or is it the holistic program of health care being offered? Regardless of the complexity involved, specifying the organization's products and services is an important step in developing a strategic mindset.

The second question is: Who are our customers? This issue is no less complex unless, again, the organization provides a very specific product to a very specific customer. The more multipurpose an organization, the broader the range of customers it will have. For a hospital, it could be argued that the list of customers includes: patients who receive services; family members and other decision makers who influence patient behavior; staff physicians; referring physicians; major employers and business coalitions; and insurance companies and managed care plans. In many cases, other providers of care may be customers; this is especially true with the emergence of networks of providers and integrated delivery systems. The list does not stop here, particularly if the hospital is tax exempt as a result of its not-for-profit status. In this case, other "customers" could include consumer advocacy groups, policy makers, legislators, regulators and the press. As with the product issue, the question of customers is complex. Clarification of the nature of one's customers is an important precursor to the development of a strategic mindset.

Prior to moving forward with additional research, it is usually worthwhile to present the planner's initial impressions to key decision makers. This provides an opportunity for all parties to get "on the same page" and to clear up any serious differences of perspective that may have developed. There are cases in which the findings from this initial stage of information gathering have resulted in a decision to not follow through with the planning process. There has also been the occasional courageous consultant who has pointed out that, unless certain changes were effected in the behavior or perceptions of top management, it would be futile to continue with plan development.

Every planning initiative, of course, requires the development of a project plan to guide the process. This is particularly important with strategic planning due to the frequent need to cross departmental lines and coordinate the activities of units that may not be used to working together. (Project planning is discussed in Chapter 5.)

BASELINE DATA COLLECTION

Assuming that there is consensus on moving forward with the planning process, data collection can now begin in earnest. Although the primary focus of strategic planning is the external environment, the process begins with a thorough self analysis.

The Internal Audit

The "internal audit" as described in Chapter 7 has perhaps its most thorough application within the context of strategic planning. The intent of the internal audit is to determine who does what within the organization, when and where they do it, how they do it, and even why and how well they do it. It is amazing how many times it is discovered that the reason for an activity is never questioned until an outside consultant points out the activity and staff members ask each other: "Why do we do that?"

The internal audit will involve additional interviews focused on specific aspects of the organization and its operation. It may require that questionnaires be administered to all or many of the staff. It will require access to a wide range of internal data describing operations, policies and procedures, staffing, finances, physical plant, information systems, and any other relevant aspect of the organization and its operation. The internal audit may even require the use of primary research methods to obtain certain information.

The planner quickly learns that there are at least four views of just about every aspect of the organization's activities. The first involves the written policies and procedures governing the process under study. The second involves the manager's version of what transpires. The third involves the employees' description of what happens. The fourth and final version reflects what actually does happen based on an objective assessment of the situation. While it is important that the actual process be identified, the other three versions are no less important to the planning process. Policies and procedures, as well as the perceptions of both management and staff, have implications for the direction the planning initiative takes.

The internal audit covers a wide variety of organizational features and can be incredibly detailed and thorough. The following list illustrates the aspects of the organization that might be addressed by means of an internal audit:

✓ Existing services and products
✓ Nature, number and characteristics of customers
✓ Utilization patterns for services
✓ Sales volumes for products
✓ Staffing levels and personnel characteristics

✓ Internal management processes
✓ Financial status
✓ Fee/pricing structure
✓ Billing and collections practices
✓ Marketing arrangements
✓ Locations of service outlets
✓ Referral relationships

The internal audit for a strategic plan will typically involve some type of operational analysis. This is likely to include at a minimum, analyses of patient flow, paper flow, and information flow. The operational analysis may also examine staffing patterns, physical space considerations, and productivity. This type of analysis can be highly technical and may require the use of outside resources.

The External Audit

The external audit in the strategic planning process begins with the same steps described in earlier chapters for assessing the organization's environment. The process starts with an analysis of the macro-environment and progresses through the various levels down to the micro-environment. Broad social trends are reviewed and developments within the economy are analyzed for their implications for healthcare. Health industry trends are reviewed, with attention paid to developments in the regulatory and reimbursement arenas.

The scope of the external audit will be determined by the nature of the organization and the issues being considered. For a major hospital or a health system many aspects of the healthcare environment will be important. For more specialized organizations, it may be possible to focus on those aspects of the external environment that have implications for that particular segment of the industry.

For most healthcare organizations, the analysis is carried down to the local market level. However, if the organization carrying out the planning is national is scope, the level of analysis may be different. Even so, most healthcare providers operate in a local environment. The "climate" of the community related to the range of issues addressed in the environmental assessment must be considered.

Defining the Market

The "market" for the organization can be defined in a number of different ways. The definition utilized depends on the purpose of the analysis, the product or service being considered, the competitive environment, and even the type of organization conducting the planning. Markets may be defined based on geography, demographics, consumer demand, disease prevalence, and so forth. The various bases for defining the market are discussed in detail in Chapter 5.

Profiling the Market Area Population

In the typical strategic planning initiative, a profile of the market area population is the first task. The type of information required on the market area population varies with the nature of the project. The first type of data typically compiled is demographic data, including biosocial and sociocultural traits. At a minimum, the analyst would examine the population in terms of age, sex, race/ethnicity, marital status/family structure, income and education. In the process, the situation with regard to insurance coverage is typically assessed.

The demographic analysis is often accompanied by an assessment of the psychographic characteristics of the market area population. Information on the lifestyle categories of the target audience can be used to determine the likely health priorities and behavior of a population subgroup. Consumer attitudes is another dimension of the population that is typically considered at this point. The attitudes displayed by consumers in a market area are likely to have considerable influence on the demand for almost all types of health services. At the organization level, the attitudes of a wide variety of constituents besides direct consumers must be taken into consideration.

Identifying Health Characteristics

The health characteristics of the population should be identified following the steps outlined in Chapters 6 and 7. The emphasis, of course, will be on those dimensions that are relevant to the needs of the organization.

The fertility characteristics of the population should be determined to the extent they are relevant. The number of births as well as the characteristics of those births, along with the attributes of the mothers and fathers of the children, form the basis for fertility analysis.

Historical patterns of fertility are a major influence on current patterns of health services demand. A wide range of service and product needs revolve around childbearing. Childbearing also triggers the need for such down-the-road services as pediatrics and contraception-related services. The demand for treatment of the male and female reproductive systems and the heightened interest in infertility treatment are by-products of the reproductive process.

The level of morbidity within a population is a major concern for health services planners. Incidence and prevalence rates can both serve a useful planning purpose and both may be employed as part of a planning analysis, depending on the nature of the project. This category includes disability indicators along with measures of morbidity in terms of disease incidence and prevalence. To the extent possible, planners need to project rates of incidence and prevalence into the future in order to predict healthcare needs.

The study of mortality examines the relationship between death and the size, composition, and distribution of the population of the market area. Organization-level planners typically have less interest in mortality analysis than those involved in community-wide planning, since the latter are more concerned with the overall health status of the community. Nevertheless, mortality data are usually examined to determine what they can tell us about the health status of the community.

The emphasis in most strategic planning initiatives will be on the morbidity profile of the population. The incidence and prevalence of various health conditions will drive much of the planning activity. For most organizations, the demand for health services derived from this level of need is what determines the market. Planners are likely to be interested in both the level of morbidity and the utilization patterns that it produces. As in other planning contexts, it is important to develop projections for these indicators of health status to assure that the plan is addressing future considerations rather than current ones.

Health Behavior

Health behavior involves such formal activities as physician visits, hospital admissions, and drug prescriptions, as well as informal actions on the part of individuals that are designed to prevent health problems and maintain, enhance or promote health. An understanding of the population's health behavior should supplement the information previously developed on the market area's need for health services and, in some cases, utilization data represent the best source of this knowledge.

Obviously, healthcare organizations will focus on those indicators of health behavior that are most relevant for their operations. Hospitals are likely to require information on almost all of the indicators described throughout this book. Other organizations of more limited scope are likely to focus on specific indicators of utilization in their analyses.

The strategic plan is likely to require more detail on health behavior than other types of planning. The following types of health behavior may be considered, depending on the type of planning being carried out:

✓ *Inpatient Admissions*
  Hospital admissions
  Nursing home admissions
  Residential treatment center admissions
  Mental health facility admissions
✓ *Outpatient Visits*
  Hospital outpatient visits

Hospital emergency room visits
Physician office visits
Other clinician office visits
Urgent care visits
Diagnostic center visits
Surgicenter visits
Mental health center visits
✓ *Other Service Utilization*
Home health visits
Physical therapy treatments
Alternative therapy treatments
✓ *Procedures Performed*
Diagnostic
Therapeutic
✓ *Prescriptions Written*

Many strategic planning initiatives require information on the informal aspects of health behavior as well. It may be important to determine the extent to which the market area population practices self-care, is involved in healthy lifestyles, or emphasizes prevention.

Competitive Analysis

The resource identification process characteristic of other types of planning takes the form of a competitive analysis in the strategic planning process. While there may be some reasons for identifying the full range of available health services within the market area, the focus will typically be on the organizations and/or services that are likely to be in competition with the entity doing the planning.

Options to consider for the competitive analysis are presented below, remembering that only selected ones may be relevant in a particular situation.

✓ *Healthcare Facilities*
Hospitals
Nursing homes
Physician offices
Community clinics
Non-physician clinical offices
Residential treatment centers
Assisted living facilities (and other seniors residential units)
Mental health facilities
Home health agencies/hospices

Urgent care centers
Freestanding diagnostic centers
Freestanding surgery centers
Specialty treatment centers (e.g., pain management)
✓ *Healthcare Equipment*
Biomedical equipment
Durable medical equipment
Information technology
Emergency services equipment
✓ *Health Personnel*
Physicians
Nurses
Nurse clinicians, physician assistants and other physician extenders
Dentists
Optometrists
Podiatrists
Chiropractors
Mental health professionals
Rehabilitation therapists (e.g., physical therapists, speech therapists)
Clinical support personnel (e.g., radiology technologists)
Administrative support personnel (e.g., medical records technicians)
Alternative therapists
✓ *Programs and Services*
Inpatient programs/services
Hospital outpatient programs/services
Emergency services
Ambulatory care programs/services
Long term care services
Community-based services
Home health services
✓ *Funding Sources*
Commercial insurance (including managed care)
Medicare (including Medicare HMOs)
Medicaid
Other federally-funded programs (e.g., Veterans Administration)
State funding sources (e.g., mental health services)
Local funding sources (e.g., public hospital subsidy)
✓ *Networks and Relationships*
Formal hospital alliances
Integrated delivery systems
Provider networks
Chain-operated facilities (e.g., hospitals, nursing homes)

Contractual relationships
Business coalitions for health

The final category, networks and relationships, has become increasingly important in the contemporary healthcare environment. A thorough inventory of health services should include a review of existing networks and relationships whether or not the organization is involved. In an era of managed care and negotiated contracts for health services, the existence of networks and relationships has taken on added importance. The significance of such situations cannot be overestimated and organizations must take the influence of these arrangements into consideration in their planning efforts.

An important aspect of this analysis involves referral relationships. As relationships have become more important, they are being increasingly emphasized in the strategic planning process. In fact, it can be argued that patients will utilize a provider in the future because of existing relationships, rather than the traditional approach of relationship development *following* utilization. The existence of networks, integrated delivery systems, and other relationships within the community should be fully addressed during the strategic planning process.

State-of-the-Organization Report

At this stage of the planning process, it is usually worthwhile to present a state-of-the-organization report. The nature of the report will reflect the various issues raised earlier, focusing on those of most relevance to the organization.

The state-of-the-organization report should include the following sections summarizing data collection up to this point:

✓ Overall societal/healthcare/service trends
✓ Market area delineation
✓ Market area population profile
✓ Market area population health characteristics
✓ Current position of the organization/product
✓ Customer profile
✓ Competitive situation
✓ Other likely future developments affecting the organization

This status report should include the strengths, weaknesses, opportunities and threats identified during the analysis. It should include an "issues statement" based on the results of the analysis to this point. The mission statement and the original assumptions should also be revisited at this juncture.

The state-of-the-organization report represents an opportunity to frankly describe the state of the organization. This allows all parties to "get on the same page" and to develop consensus with regard to the assumptions. This is the launching point for subsequent plan development.

Developing Strategies

This is an excellent point in the process to consider strategies. A strategy involves a generalized approach to be taken to the challenges of the market. At the organization level, the choice of strategy is critical. The strategy establishes the tone for subsequent planning activities and, in effect, sets the parameters within which the planners must operate. Examples of strategies that might be adopted by organizational planners included:

- ✓ *Dominance strategy* whereby the number one player in the market opts to focus on maintaining this position
- ✓ *Second fiddle strategy* in which the "runner up" in the market concedes this second fiddle status and plans accordingly
- ✓ *Frontal attack strategy* in which the organization decides to take on the market leader or major competitors head on
- ✓ *Niche strategy* in which the organization concedes it cannot be involved in the competition for the mainstream market, but instead concentrates on niche markets based on geography, population groups, or selected services.
- ✓ *Flanking strategy* in which the organization "outflanks" the competition by entering new markets, cultivating new populations, or offering fringe products

These are only some examples of the types of strategies that might be adopted, and the options are essentially unlimited. A complex plan may involve more than one strategy, in fact. For example, a hospital may concede a second-tier position as a general hospital, while actively striving to control major niches within the market.

DEVELOPING THE STRATEGIC PLAN

The effort expended up to this point provides the foundation for the actual development of the plan. If the initial work is properly carried out, the planning process should flow smoothly, at least from a technical perspective.

Setting the Goal(s)

The goal or goals that are established should reflect the information that was provided in the state-of-the-organization report and should be in keeping with the organization's mission statement. Goals tend to be relatively general in nature and lack the specificity of objectives and other components of the plan. They identify an ideal state that will serve as the target for future development. For a national medical products company, the goal may be to establish the firm as the low-cost provider of a certain product. For a local health services provider, the goal may involve positioning the organization as a niche player to take advantage of certain market opportunities. For the purveyor of a specific service, the goal may be to become recognized as the provider of choice for a certain segment of the market.

The number of goals to be established depends on the complexity and size of the organization and the nature of the issues at hand. If the focus is narrow, a single goal may be appropriate. On the other hand, the complexity of many healthcare organizations mandates the establishment of multiple goals. Goals may be established, for example, specific to particular service lines or units within the organization.

Setting Objectives

The objectives for a strategic plan are stated in such terms as: The hospital's orthopedic practice will recruit a sports medicine specialist within the next twelve months (in support of the stated goal of expanding the organization's orthopedic service lines). For every goal a number of objectives are likely be specified, with four or five objectives not being unusual. Multiple objectives are common since it is likely that action will be required on a number of different fronts in order to attain a specified goal.

As the planning team establishes objectives, any barriers to accomplishing the stated objectives of the organization should be considered, and these must be identified and assessed. The extent to which these barriers can be overcome must be determined. In the case of insurmountable barriers, an objective may have to be eliminated. It may be found, for example, that a lack of physical therapy personnel represents a potential barrier to expanding the organization's outpatient rehabilitation program. If it can be determined that there is, in fact, an untapped source of physical therapy staff, this may be diminished as a barrier. In another case, it may be found that the objective of expanding medical staff privileges at the other hospital in town is being thwarted by a competing practice that is well established at that hospital. This may turn out to be an insurmountable barrier.

Prioritizing Objectives

The prioritization of objectives becomes an important step in the process. There is no one procedure for prioritizing objectives, and the approach is likely to vary with the situation. However, some level of consensus must be developed beforehand on the process in order to systematically consider priorities. There are a number of questions that might be asked in this regard and these are spelled out in Chapter 6.

The challenge is to identify on the front end the criteria that are the most important for prioritization purposes. It may even be necessary to utilize different sets of criteria within one planning initiative due to the nature of the project. The process is also likely to result in the elimination of some objectives that are deemed less important once the criteria are applied.

The possibility of unanticipated consequences arising from the meeting of any of the objectives should also be considered. For each objective it is important to specify the likely consequences of carrying it out. This should involve both the intended consequences and potential unintended consequences. Virtually every action taken is going to result in negative consequences. While these cannot be eliminated, conceding their existence is the first step toward minimizing their impact.

For example, if the stated objective is to open an outpatient surgery center in the shadow of a competing hospital (in support of the goal of expanding surgical market share), both the intended and unintended consequences of meeting this objective should be considered. The intended consequences would include: increasing outpatient surgical volume (thereby improving market share), increasing surgical revenue, capturing some of the competitor's patients, providing an additional site for staff physicians to operate, and establishing a presence in "enemy" territory.

On the other hand, the potential unintended consequences might include: transforming a passive competitor into an active one, offending members of the competing hospital's medical staff, drawing patients away from existing surgical facilities while not attracting new patients, and so forth. Too often the positive aspects of the situation are examined in isolation from the negative consequences that could result from the actions.

Specifying Actions

The specification of the actions to be carried out is a critical step in the process. Having determined what should be done, it is necessary to indicate how it will be done. For each of the objectives that have been identified, a set of actions must be specified. In virtually every case, numerous actions must be performed to achieve an objective. These actions take a wide range of forms, from assuring that postage is available to support a direct mail initiative to developing a strategic partnership as a means of reaching an objective.

If the objective of a specialty practice is to recruit and deploy a new sports medicine physician in a satellite office within twelve months, a number of actions must be carried out. These include: identifying a recruiting firm, allocating funds for recruitment costs, setting up an internal screening committee; determining compensation terms, identifying a site for the new office, furnishing the new office, and so forth. Many of these actions imply a certain sequence and this is a point at which the original project plan might be further refined to specify the sequencing of the action steps.

IMPLEMENTING THE PLAN

An implementation plan is required to transform recommendations into actions. The planning process creates a road map, and now the organization has to use it to get where it wants to go. It is at the implementation stage that the process often breaks down. The fact that "the last plan is still sitting on the shelf" generally reflects a failure of implementation rather than any flaw in the plan itself. The transition from planning to implementation involves a hand-off from the planning team to the management team. It also requires implementation at several different levels and by different divisions within the organization. The implementation plan is likely to require significant change in many aspects of the organization, including management processes, information systems, and the corporate culture.

Steps in Implementation

In order to approach plan implementation systematically, both a detailed project plan and an implementation matrix should be developed. The implementation plan as initially described in Chapter 5 depicts the logical process that must be followed in order to carry out the objectives of the strategic plan. The fact that the process now shifts from the planning team to the organization's managers makes a well thought out implementation plan imperative. And, again, the need to coordinate various units within the organization further mandates a detailed approach to implementation.

The implementation matrix should specify who is to do what and when they are to do it. The matrix should list every action called for by the plan, breaking each action down into tasks, if appropriate. For each action or task the responsible party should be identified, along with any secondary parties that should be involved in this activity. The matrix should indicate resource requirements (in terms of staff time, money and other requirements). The start and end dates for each activity should be identified. Any prerequisites for accomplishing this task should be identified at the outset (and factored into the project plan). Finally, some milestones should be identified that allow the planning team to determine when the activity has been completed. (See Chapter 6 for an example of an implementation matrix.)

Requirements for Implementation

The resource requirements from the implementation matrix should be combined to determine total project resource requirements. For most strategic plans there will be a number of factors to consider. The amount of *capital investment* necessary to support implementation must be determined. Similarly, during startup and subsequent periods of operation the amount of *operating funds* that will be required must be determined. The implementation plan should indicate any *facilities* that will be required along with any and *equipment* needs. In addition, the *human resource* requirements for the initiative should be determined. This should include both commitment of existing internal personnel and additional human resource requirements. *Information system* requirements must be specified and their development coordinated with other information management initiatives. Any changes in *governance or management* will need to be specified, along with anticipated *marketing* needs.

When this process has been completed, the total resource requirements of the project will have been identified. It is not until this point that the burden that must be born by the various units of the organizations becomes clear. The extent of the requirements may have to be addressed in relation to available funds and any other fiscal constraints.

Means of Implementation

The means used to implement the plan will invariably involve various departments and units, and the impact of the project on them should be considered at this point. Processes that transcend departmental boundaries are likely to be controversial and, as with many types of change, resistance is likely to be exhibited.

Both direct and indirect means of implementation can be utilized. The direct means of implementation have been addressed to a certain extent through the development of the implementation matrix and the identification of resource requirements. Indirect means might include changes in *physical facilities*, modifications in *communications* within the organization, or *symbolic actions* that provide psychological support for the operationalization of the plan.

In many cases, the corporate culture will have to be modified in order for successful plan implementation. If a planning mindset does not already exist within the organization, this will have to be incorporated into the culture. If the culture emphasizes strict organizational divisions, a new way of thinking may have to be introduced in order to implement the strategic plan across divisional lines. Ongoing efforts toward inculcating a strategic orientation among organization staff should be instituted.

EVALUATING THE EFFECTIVENESS OF THE PLAN

The means for evaluating the success of the strategic planning initiative should be built into the planning process. This is important to those involved in the process, as well as to any parties that may be assessing the value of the planning initiative. For example, grantmakers and funders will usually want to know how many people were reached and served by the initiative, as well as whether the initiative had the community-level impact it intended to have. The organization's decision makers need to determine the effectiveness of the efforts in order to make mid-course adjustments. Individuals throughout the organization deserve to know how effective the planning initiative was in order to determine if their efforts in support of it were justified.

Evaluation should involve on-going monitoring of the strategic planning process, including benchmarks and/or milestones for assessment along the way. This will require the clarification of the objectives and goals of your initiative. As noted in Chapter 5, the evaluation process should address planning and implementation issues, the extent to which objectives were achieved, the impact of the process on participants, and the impact on the organization's constituents.

Process evaluation should assess the efficiency of the planning process, including the appropriateness of the structure, the frequency and adequacy of communication, and the extent to which the "ground rules" were followed. Outcome evaluation should assess the results of the planning exercise of concrete deliverables and more subjectively perceived outcomes.

Data collection and benchmarking are extremely important for measuring progress and quantifying benefits accruing to the community or to the organization. Documenting the process of community or organizational change is an ongoing task that should occur on a regular basis. (See Box 8-2 for a discussion of plan evaluation in the physician practice setting.)

THE STRATEGIC PLAN: A MOVING TARGET

While it may be convenient to conceptualize the strategic planning process as a discrete activity with a beginning and an end, this is often not realistic in today's healthcare environment. Planning should not be considered as a discrete activity, but should be merged with the other functions of the organization. Strategic planning in particular, with its emphasis on the external environment, should involve a process that is tied in with the operation of the healthcare organization. Rather than being an end in its own right, any plan should serve as a launch point for subsequent planning activity.

The strategic plan also represents a moving target due to the volatility of the healthcare environment. There was a time when healthcare organizations could expect a little breathing room between one major development in the healthcare arena and the next. For example, Medicare might have made a significant

BOX 8-2
Evaluating the Effectiveness of Strategic Planning:
The Medical Group Model

The challenges facing a physician practice have never been greater than they are today. Practice management has become increasingly complex and now calls for a range of skills beyond those usually available to any one person. Apart from the stresses of day-to-day operations, physician-managers and administrators are increasingly being confronted with questions like: Where will the practice be tomorrow, next month, or at the end of the year? What must the practice do to adapt to changing reimbursement patterns? What are the implications of changing demographics within the market area?

Given these types of question, there is pressure, on the one hand, to forge a long-term plan for the practice; on the other, there is concern with the immediate future. These are not unrelated issues, however, in that the immediate future impacts the five-year plan. Because the planning process helps the group identify itself, it forces the members within the group to "buy into" the plan, and, most important, it allows the group to focus on the process for allocation of its scare resources.

Before a practice can develop a plan it must understand the internal and external issues facing the group. For example, how does the world perceive the group? What are the practice's strengths, weaknesses, opportunities and threats? Planning should give the practice the ability to circumvent obstacles while maintaining forward momentum toward a recognized goal.

Some of the short-term issues that face medical practice physicians and administrators today include:

✓ The operational effectiveness and efficiency of their practice
✓ Satisfaction levels of patients and referring physicians
✓ Organizational responsiveness to patients
✓ Effective billing and accounts receivable processes
✓ Clinical outcomes monitoring
✓ Compliance and accounting audits
✓ Marketing management

The challenge for today's physician-manager is to address these disparate issues through a coherent plan that works for the group, its patients, its employees, and the countless other entities that interact daily with the

(continued)

group. This involves coordinating internal processes (like patient flow) with external processes (like marketing initiatives).

A strategic plan developed by a physician practice must be focused on meeting the needs of its customers, even more so than many other healthcare organizations. There are certain critical indicators of success that are shared by the better performing medical groups. In these medical groups, the patient flow process was analyzed from the time the patient made the initial phone call for the appointment until the last piece of paper was filed in the medical record of the patient's chart. A critical element in the success model derived from this analysis was the satisfaction of the patient with the flow.

The typical medical group thinks in terms of designing systems that streamline internal processes. This "internal" flow issue is related to "external" expectations on the part of the patient. In the better performing practices, the level of patient satisfaction is given equal weight with financial success. In addition to streamlined patient management processes, other factors identified as critical for superior patient satisfaction include: hours of operation, scope of services provided by the group, quality of care provided by the physician and the staff; the quality of communication between the physician/staff and the patient; the quality of communication between the physician back to the referral source and to the insurance company; and the quality of patient education offered by the group.

The lesson to be learned from these "best practices" is that, for practices to survive and thrive in the future, they must structure the practice to meet or exceed the needs of patients. The strategic plan determines the "interventions" required to create a system that meets the needs of the practice's customers. Once these interventions are in place, it is critical that the tools for evaluating their effectiveness be available.

The practice's performance review must measure the effectiveness of communication between the patient and the physician and the support staff, evaluating whether the quality of care provided by the physician and staff met the needs of the patient, and evaluating the level of responsiveness of the group overall to the needs of the patient. The most direct way to evaluate the effectiveness of the practice's strategic plan is through a benchmarking system. This involves evaluating practice performance on a monthly, quarterly, or semi-annual basis and subsequently developing action plans to improve performance. All medical groups are in a constant state of dynamic motion, and the practice should evaluate its situation and modify its processes to be more responsive to its internal and external environments on an almost daily basis.

Simply defined, a benchmark is an operating performance standard. It is an indicator of the relative strength or weakness of an organization at a departmental or cost accounting level. Typical benchmarks include such items as: number of days in accounts receivable, net fee-for-service collection percentage, new patient referrals, overhead percentage, and the ratio of full-time non-physician employees to full-time physicians. The only way to evaluate how well the practice is doing is through a comparison with some standard or benchmark.

Although it may be interesting to compare experiences with those of Dr. Smith in a different medical specialty with a different number of physicians operating in his facility, such comparisons are of limited value. A practice must compare its operations to physician groups in the same medical specialty and of comparable size. Then and only them can we meaningfully specify performance at the 25th, 50th, 75th or 90th percentile. Once that comparison is made, it is possible to state quantitatively that the practice is at a given point on the continuum and ranks in the specified percentile in terms of overall performance. This can be thought of as a monthly "report card."

Benchmarks should only be considered a guide; the actual benchmarks used in a practice must be developed based on the size of the practice, practice location, and specialty. Any benchmark used to measure the effectiveness of your practice must:

✓ Be clearly understood by the staff and the physicians in the practice
✓ Be agreed to by the group, the physicians and the employees
✓ Be trackable with data generated by the practice's systems

change in its reimbursement practices and little more would happen in this regard for a couple of years. Today, dramatic change comes fast and furious. For this reason, it is likely that the strategic plan will be modified before it is even completed. Developments related to reimbursement, technology, provider relationships, and managed care can occur almost over night. The planning process must be flexible enough to take into account fast-breaking developments in the environment.

A final factor to consider is the dynamics of the planning process itself. As the planning team carries out its activities, it will be in constant contact with various components of the organization. This interaction will involve the exchange of information, the solicitation of ideas, and the posing of potential strategies. Remembering that the value is in the planning and not in the plan, it is not uncommon for many of the plan's ultimate recommendations to be implemented before the

✓ Provide results that can be communicated to the participants
✓ Be a cause of celebration and rewards when targets are met

The benchmark system will generate baseline data that can be presented to the group to assist in its overall planning efforts. There can be no question about the effectiveness of the interventions called for in the strategic plan, if there are clear benchmarks against which they can be compared.

Needless to say, all of the activities described above require access to the necessary data, and another characteristic of the best medical groups is that they have adequate information processes in place. Quality data equates to better decisions.

Internal productivity reports and external benchmark survey data can also be used to provide meaningful feedback to physicians concerning their own level of productivity. Physicians can be paired with an "administrative partner", a nurse team leader or department manager, to review monthly reports. As a result, practicing physicians can remain well informed about their performance and the impact it has on the department, particular clinic site, or the group as a whole.

Ultimately, productivity will hinge on the ability of the practice to coordinate the range of internal processes with external considerations. Practices that fail to interface these "two sides of the coin" will be at a disadvantage in a competitive healthcare environment. Having a well thought out plan in place—and the ability to evaluate its effectiveness—is critical for the continued viability of any medical group.

Source: David K. Rea, M.P.A., F.A.C.M.P.E., Rea & Associates, Memphis, Tennessee.

plan is finalized. The ideas and proposals that are developed, as well as suggested changes in operational aspects, may be adopted by various parties within the organization at a faster pace than others. In fact, there are likely to be few original ideas developed during the strategic planning process; most of them have already been thought of by the organization's staff. The plan, however, provides the impetus for acting on some of these ideas, as well as validation of their worthiness and permission to move forward.

The plan may be modified many times before it is finalized. In fact, it may be best if it is never finalized. If it is properly constituted, the process and the plan both should be able to adapt to the changes that occur during the planning process. In this sense, the plan teaches the organization to swim rather than simply throwing it a life preserver.

Additional Resources

Bryson, John M. (1995). *Creating and Implementing Your Strategic Plan: A Workbook for Public and Nonprofit Organizations.* San Francisco: Jossey-Bass.

Cunningham, T. (1998). "Healthcare Strategic Planning: Approaches for the 21stCentury," *Journal of Healthcare Management*, 43(4): 378ff.

Goodstein, L. D., Nolan, T. M., and J. W. Pfeiffer (1992). *Applied Strategic Planning: A Comprehensive Guide.* San Diego: Pfieffer and Company.

Henley, R. (1999). "Plan for Lasting Success," *Healthcare Financial Management*, 53(10): 14ff.

Mintzberg, Henry (1994). *The Rise and Fall of Strategic Planning.* New York: The Free Press.

Rovinsky, M. (2002). "Physician Input: A Critical Strategic-Planning Tool," *Healthcare Financial Management*, 56(1): 36–38.

Sheldon, Alan, and Susan Windham (2002). *Competitive Strategy for Health Care Organizations.* Frederick, MD: The Beard Group.

Zuckerman, Alan (1998). *Healthcare Strategic Planning.* Chicago: Health Administration Press.

9

Marketing Planning

INTRODUCTION

While marketing planning is well established in other industries, it is a relatively new function in health care. Until the 1980s, healthcare providers typically did not engage in formal marketing activities, thereby obviating the need for marketing plans. While some sectors of the industry such as insurance, pharmaceuticals, and medical supplies have a long history of marketing planning, organizations involved in patient care have only recently become involved in marketing activities. The introduction of competition in the 1980s, probably more than any other factor, has driven the need to systematically approach the market for health services. Now, the contemporary healthcare environment demands that virtually all health care organizations have a marketing plan.

Marketing planning may be defined simply as *the development of a systematic process for promoting an organization, a service or a product.* This straightforward definition masks the wide variety of forms and the potential complexity that characterize marketing planning. Marketing planning may be limited to a short-term promotional project or comprise a component of a long-term strategic plan. It can focus alternatively on a product, service, program, or organization.

The Nature of Marketing Planning

While marketing plans share many of the characteristics of other types of plans discussed in this book, marketing planning is distinguishable from other types of planning along a number of dimensions. Of all of the types of planning discussed, marketing planning most directly relates to the customer. While other types of plans may reference "patients", "clients", or "consumers", marketing plans are single-minded in their focus on the customer. The emphasis on "promoting" in the definition above assumes that the organization or service is being promoted to someone. Whether the customer is the patient, the referring physician, the employer, the health plan, or any number of other possibilities, the marketing plan is developed in response to someone's needs.

Because of its emphasis on the customer, the marketing plan is probably the most externally oriented of any of the plans discussed. Although a concern for internal factors does exist (and "internal marketing" may be a component of many marketing plans), the marketing plan focuses on the characteristics of the external market with the objective of influencing change in one or more of these characteristics.

The marketing planner initially obtains much of the same information on the internal characteristics of the organization that would be done, say, for strategic planning. At the same time, the marketing planner has information needs above and beyond those required in other planning scenarios. A more indepth understanding of the organization's products and services and the manner in which customers are processed is required. Detailed information on existing marketing activities will be needed. The same type of information will typically be required on competitors in the market area.

Marketing planning is often, although not always, shorter in scope than other types of planning. In many cases, the desired outcomes in marketing planning are more immediate. Few strategic plans are expected to reach their goals in a matter of months, but a focused marketing plan may include the expectation that objectives (e.g., awareness of a new service) be met within six months or less.

The shorter timeframe reflects the fact that marketing planning is typically more narrow in its focus than other types of planning. In fact, the marketing plan is often a subcomponent of the strategic plan or the business plan. Although marketing plans geared toward changing the image of an organization are understandably broad, many marketing initiatives involve a particular product or service. As such, they are very focused and relatively narrow in scope.

One final, and important, difference relates to the manner in which outcomes are evaluated. While strategic plans are evaluated on the success of the plan in positioning the organization vis-a-vis its environment, the intent of most marketing plans is to affect change in consumer knowledge and/or behavior. Thus, the evaluation process is likely to measure changes in consumer awareness and attitudes or, even more concretely, through the monitoring of changes in patient volume, sales, revenues or market share.

Although marketing planning is often seen as a stand-alone activity, it should reside within the context of the organization's overall strategic initiatives. Thus, the objectives of the marketing plan should correspond with those outlined in the strategic plan. A marketing plan should be an inherent component of any formal business plan as well. Even if established relationships exist with customers for an existing product, a marketing plan is required; a plan is even more important if new customers are being sought or new services being introduced. In fact, potential investors reviewing a business plan are not likely to give much credence to the business proposition in the absence of a marketing plan.

Marketing planning is typically not a component of community-wide planning, although it would be inappropriate to contend that it be totally excluded from planning at the community level. In fact, there has been growing conviction that many of the goals of public sector organizations operating within the community cannot be met without the benefit of a well-crafted marketing plan, and the notion of "social marketing" is becoming increasingly accepted by not-for-profit healthcare organizations. The fact that *everyone* needs to market has been evidenced by the emergence of numerous "how to" marketing books published for not-for-profit organizations. (See Box 9-1 for a discussion of social marketing.)

Marketing planning is one of the few planning activities that may actually have a departmental "home" within the organization. Many large healthcare organizations have formal marketing departments, and this unit provides a base for the development of marketing plans. Strategic planning, on the other hand, tends to be more organization-wide and typically does not have a departmental base. Business planning activities tend to occur throughout the organization and not be restricted to any department. Thus, it is not unusual for a large health care organization to have more in-house expertise related to marketing planning than it does for other types of planning.

Organization versus Service Marketing

Marketing planning typically focuses on either the organization or a product or service offered by the organization. With organization-focused marketing, the intent is typically to promote the overall image of the organization. This may involve increasing awareness, creating a more positive image, clearing up misperceptions, or generally promoting the organization within the community. As such, this type of marketing is more general in its approach than marketing that focuses on a specific product or service.

The goals and objectives in marketing the organization will be relatively broad, as will the target audience. The intent is to convince essentially everyone that this is the best hospital, cardiology practice, or health plan. Thus, the approach used is likely to resemble traditional mass marketing more than the target marketing that has become common in recent years. The timeframe involved in marketing planning for the total organization is likely to be fairly lengthy relative to

---

BOX 9-1
Marketing Planning for Social Marketing

"Social marketing" is a form of marketing that is performed frequently within the healthcare field. While a variety of different definitions might be applied to social marketing, it typically refers to marketing by a not-for-profit organization—quite often a government agency—with the intention of promoting a program designed to bring about some type of social change. It is more likely to promote a cause than a particular service or product. It attempts to bring about social change through influencing the behavior of groups of individuals. At the same time, it is more targeted to the community than it is to the individual. In this regard, it attempts to influence public opinion in order to bring about some benefit to the general population.

Not surprisingly, the healthcare organizations involved in social marketing are those that are mandated to improve health conditions through programs geared toward society as a whole. These include public health departments (e.g., promoting prenatal care), government agencies (e.g., promoting seat belt use), and voluntary associations (e.g., anti-smoking campaigns). These programs utilize the mass media to promote their respective causes.

The development of a social marketing program involves the same marketing planning process that would accompany the marketing of a product or service. The marketing planner would examine the societal trends that are contributing to the issue being addressed and determine what factors play a role in the development and spread of the condition. This research approach was applied in the campaign to combat AIDS, for example, by identifying the distribution of HIV and AIDS within the population, determining its cause, identifying the affected populations, and determining the means of transmission. This information provided the foundation for the development of a social marketing program as one means of addressing the AIDS epidemic.

As with any planning process, a goal was formulated—in this case, reducing the spread of HIV. The objectives that were identified in support of this goal included: reducing the number of new cases during a specified time period; increasing awareness of the dangers of AIDS among at risk

---

service marketing, as changes in attitudes and perceptions cannot be effected overnight.

Finally, outcomes are evaluated much differently for organization-wide marketing than for the marketing of a specific service or product. Even though sales

populations, providing information and referral resources for the affected and at-risk populations; and encouraging behavior change among high-risk populations. The marketing planning process also involved identifying the barriers to the achievement of these objectives. These included such factors as ignorance as to the nature of the disease and its spread, fear on the part of those who might be affected, and the stigma associated with the disease.

The social marketing plan utilized the information to develop marketing initiatives aimed at the achievement of these objectives. A particular message was formulated and certain media were selected for the delivery of the message. The campaign involved the use of public service announcements on billboards, in print media (e.g., newspapers, magazines), and in electronic media (e.g., radio, television). It also involved community outreach programs in areas where high-risk populations were likely to be concentrated. These programs provided information for those at risk and encouraged the behavior changed necessary to combat the epidemic.

The social marketing initiative also involved a component geared to the general public. This component publicized the risk factors associated with the spread of HIV but, at the same time, attempted to demythologize AIDS and reduce misconceptions the general public held about the condition. Part of this campaign was intended to reduce the stigma associated with HIV and AIDS, thereby encouraging at-risk and affected populations to more readily present themselves for testing and treatment.

While social marketing was not the only approach used to combat HIV and AIDS, the efforts of various agencies contributed to reduction of infection within the target population. Social marketing contributed to the successful management of HIV within the initial target population, a population that was receptive to these types of marketing initiatives.

By the beginning of the 21st century, however, HIV had spread to new populations in the United States. No longer concentrated among white gay males, it began to spread rapidly among African-American and Hispanic populations and among heterosexual populations. These new populations may not be as receptive as the original affected population to social marketing. At the very least, a different message and different media are likely to be required to address the AIDS epidemic among these hard-to-reach populations.

volume, revenues, profits and other objective indicators may be considered as outcome measures, the real test is the extent to which the marketing initiative has resulted in increased name recognition, greater consumer awareness of its programs, higher ratings relative to its competitors, and/or more frequent selection by consumers as the provider of choice.

The process of marketing a product or service has essentially the opposite characteristics. The image of the organization is a secondary issue, since the objective is to make the public aware of a specific product or service. Or, in the case of an existing service, the intent will be to distinguish it from that of competitors and make it appear more desirable to consumers. The goals and objectives are, thus, much narrower and much more concrete. The target audience is also much narrower. Promotions geared for the general public would be a waste of resources and are not likely to achieve the desired effect. Not everyone is a candidate for the birthing center, even though obstetrical care is a fairly widespread need. The more specialized a service is, the more targeted the marketing must be.

While all planning activities should be time delimited, marketing plans are often obsessive in this regard. Clear-cut target dates are virtually always included, since the content of marketing campaigns is often time sensitive. There may be some slack in a strategic plan's time line for an objective related to increasing market share, but a marketing plan that calls for the establishment of consumer awareness prior to the opening of a new clinic does not allow much margin for error.

The outcomes in marketing a service will typically be measured in terms of sales, revenues, and profits. This is not to say that enhanced awareness, increased consumer preference, and other more subjective measures are not important. Ultimately, however, a marketing plan designed for a product or service is going to be measured in terms of concrete results.

Obviously, the approach to marketing planning is going to vary depending on the focus of the project. A lot depends on whether the plan is generated for a new organization or service or for an existing one. In the former case, the intent of the marketing plan is to create awareness, generate initial business, and establish a customer base. Thus, approaches to acquiring customers will be different from those used at a later stage to retain them. Since little may be known about the actual characteristics of prospective customers, general promotional principles are utilized.

For an existing organization or service the intent may be to enhance or improve the organization's image. On a more concrete level, the objectives may include changing existing customer behavior, such as convincing customers to switch to the organization or service from a competitor or encouraging the customer to consume more services. Since information on existing customers is available, the approach here focuses on capitalizing on this knowledge to derive as much business as possible from existing clients. This knowledge can also be used to expand the customer base to new clients.

When hospitals and other health care organizations first began formal marketing in the 1980s, much of the effort went into image advertising for promoting the overall advantages of the organization. These image campaigns were very expensive and generally did not accomplish their objectives. It was not unusual—and still isn't—for a hospital to be top of mind with the public and be rated as best on all important dimensions, but still not be the facility of choice with the general public. This is because many other factors than those addressed in a marketing campaign are likely to influence the individual's choice of hospital (even if they have a choice at all).

These initial attempts at marketing the organization fell well below expectations. Not only did an improved image (if that, in fact, did occur) not necessarily translate into increased business, but the hospitals that were most conspicuously involved in this type of advertising often generated considerable negative backlash due to their apparent extravagance.

Today, most advertising by health services organizations focuses on products or services. This is in keeping with the national trend in other industries to back away from an all-things-to-all-people approach and focus on specific products and specific target audiences. Thus, instead of General Hospital touting its virtues, you might find highly targeted campaigns promoting its outpatient surgery program, its home health agency, or its newly acquired lithotripter.

Who Needs Marketing Planning?

There are few organizations in healthcare today that cannot benefit from marketing planning. Most, in fact, are finding it a prerequisite for survival in an increasingly competitive environment. Although hospitals, physician groups, and other organizations involved in direct patient care have only been involved in marketing since the 1980s, growing numbers are now trying to develop marketing expertise.

The slowness of many health care providers to adopt modern marketing techniques can be attributed to the historical lack of need for marketing on the part of providers. Indeed, there has been a great deal of resistance to the notion of marketing on the part of many not-for-profit organizations. Physicians and some other providers were often prohibited ethically or legally from advertising and this was thought to limit all types of marketing.

Some private sector for-profit and not-for-profit organizations, however, have a long history of marketing and, hence, marketing planning. Perhaps the nation's pharmaceutical companies stand out in this regard, especially since the pharmaceutical industry is reputed to spend a greater proportion of its budget on marketing than any other industry. Other components of the industry that have a longer history in marketing and promotions include insurance companies and distributors of medical supplies and equipment. In fact, marketing on the part of insurance plans took on a new dimension when national managed care organizations became part of the picture.

Part of the residual resistance to this endeavor is a function of misperceptions as to what constitutes "marketing". Even today, many health professionals think strictly of advertising when the issue of marketing is raised. Most of them do not realize that they have been involved in marketing for most of their careers; they just didn't recognize it as such. Physicians who frequent clubs where other physicians are members or send a followup note to a fellow physician after a referral or agree to serve as the team physician for the high school football team are all involved in marketing activities. The challenge for marketers has been to demonstrate the scope of marketing and to fit existing activities within that framework.

THE MARKETING PLANNING PROCESS

Planning for Planning

The same notion of planning for planning applies here as it does with any other type of planning. Before the actual planning can commence, the spade work must be done with regard to the marketing framework (e.g., the relationship to the strategic plan), the identification of key players, the establishment of a marketing mindset, and so forth. These activities will vary depending on whether marketing planning is envisioned at the organization level or on behalf of a specific product or service.

The situation for marketing planning is somewhat different from that for most other types of planning. A planning structure is often already in place in the form of marketing staff and a procedure for developing marketing initiatives. Unlike strategic planning, for example, the lead planner is not going to have to recruit key members of the planning team *de novo* in order to start the planning process. It may be that additional resource persons are brought into the mix to develop the marketing plan for a new service line, for example. But this involves adding to the existing planning structure rather than starting from scratch.

Stating Assumptions

The stating of assumptions at the outset and throughout the planning process is important in marketing planning. For example, a major assumption in marketing planning may relate to the type of image that the organization wants to convey. There is a big difference between presenting the image of an aggressive, profit-seeking enterprise driven by hard-bitten business principles as opposed to an image of a humble community-based organization intent on serving the needs of the population. Other assumptions might relate to the type of approach or appeal that is to be considered.

Assumptions should be stated with regard to the potential consequences of the marketing initiative, and this is a situation in which marketing planning is unique. In today's reimbursement environment, for example, a health care provider does not want to attract all potential consumers for a product or service. The organization wants to attract those who can be reasonably expected to pay. At the same time, it should not appear that the provider is deliberately excluding certain classes of patients. This delicate balance plays a role in the development of assumptions.

The nature of the assumptions made at the outset reflects the extent to which a product or service is already in the market and has some level of awareness and utilization. In addition, the extent to which marketing activities are already underway will affect the assumptions that are made.

Initial Information Gathering

To the extent that a healthcare organization already has a marketing function in place, it may be unnecessary to perform many of the tasks associated with initial information gathering. The marketing staff will typically have already examined most aspects of the environment as part of their on-going market research activities and, at most, some updating of information on certain aspects of the environment will be necessary. In the case of a newly formed marketing department or the introduction of outside marketing resources, it may be necessary to carry out the type of comprehensive gathering of background information described in previous chapters.

The data collection process begins by gathering general background information on the organization through a review of any materials that have been prepared on the organization and on the particular product or service. Simply determining the attributes of the organization and/or its services may not be adequate for marketing planning, however. The planner really needs to know the extent to which the organization or service is different and the extent of these differences.

In a large organization such as a hospital, the marketing staff is not likely to be familiar with all services, especially if they had not been heavily marketed in the past. New services are frequently added by a hospital and some existing services may be marketed for the first time. These situations are likely to call for additional background information gathering.

This review of materials should be accompanied by interviews with knowledgeable individuals within the community, both inside and out of the medical establishment. A general understanding of the external market should be developed during this phase of information gathering as well.

Not surprisingly, much more emphasis is placed on identifying and assessing existing marketing activities in the marketing planning process than in other types of planning. An early step typically involves inventorying marketing resources and determining the extent to which current marketing activities relate to the proposed project. It is easy to overlook on-going marketing activities (especially if they are not labeled as such), but duplication of effort should be minimized. At the same time, the possibility of marketing activities operating at cross purposes with each other needs to be avoided. (A classic example would be the hospital that was promoting its emergency room as the place for *all* unscheduled health problems, while marketing its urgent care network as an alternative to emergency room care.)

As part of this process, potential barriers to the planning initiative should be identified. Individuals or organizations that are clearly resistant to any planning process will surface, although the development of a marketing plan may not be nearly as "intrusive" as that for a strategic plan. Immutable patterns of behavior should be identified, particularly if internal marketing is to be involved. Supporters of services within the organization that may considered in competition could become an issue, for example. The director of the emergency department may not react favorably to a marketing campaign meant to direct patients away from the ER to urgent care centers affiliated with the hospital. While some barriers can be surmounted, others might not be. These understandings become a part of the assumptions that drive the process.

BASELINE DATA COLLECTION

Marketing planners place considerable emphasis on the characteristics of the organization. The planner must understand the nature of the organization and develop a feel for its "character." This is particularly true if an image campaign is envisioned for the total organization. But it is also true if a specific product is being marketed. For example, a relatively unknown service might be differentiated from that offered by competitors by pointing out the support available from an organization that already has a positive image in the community. This "halo effect" may be used to advantage if this in fact is the situation. Thus, a new progressive birthing center could be promoted partly on the basis of the clinical backup available from the large staff of specialists in the med/surg units and the fact that extensive neonatal intensive care services are available as needed.

The first step in the formal data collection process here as elsewhere involves an environmental assessment. If the marketing planning focuses on the organization, the environmental assessment is likely to be broader than if it focuses on a specific product. Although marketing planning should involve an evaluation of the environment at all levels as would be done for other types of plans, the effort expended may not be as great due to the narrower focus of many marketing initiatives.

Obviously, a lot depends on the nature of the organization that is involved in marketing planning. A national organization that seeks a truly national market—e.g., a pharmaceutical company developing a direct-to-consumer marketing initiative—will probably perform an analysis involving substantial detail at the national level. On the other hand, a home health agency that is licensed to practice in a single county is not likely to need much detail with regard to national trends in order to develop a marketing plan. Regardless of the type of organization, the question should be: What external constraints are likely to affect this organization and what can be found out about them?

An added dimension related to marketing planning involves the collection of data on similar initiatives in other markets. The planner should be able to incorporate information about marketing approaches that have and have not worked when similar organizations or services were being marketing in other contexts.

The Internal Audit

In performing the internal audit for a marketing plan a number of different aspects of the organization should be examined. Among the components that are particularly relevant for marketing planning are the following:

Services/Products. What are the services that are provided and/or the products that are offered? What are the characteristics of these services and products?

Customer Characteristics. How many customers does the organization have and what are their charactersitics? Where do patients reside and what is the "reach" of the organization? What is the case mix of current customers? What are the financial categories of the patient base?

Utilization Patterns. What is the volume of services and products consumed by the organization's customers? How does this volume breakdown by service line or procedure?

Pricing Structure. How is pricing determined for the organization's services and products? How does this price structure compare with that of competitors, the industry average? How price sensitive are the goods and services offered?

Marketing Arrangements. What marketing programs are currently in place and how is marketing structured? What type and level of resources are available for marketing? Are there processes in place for internal marketing?

Locations. To what extent are operations centralized or decentralized? How many satellite locations are in operation and how were their locations chosen? Are there markets that are not being served by existing outlets?

Referral Relationships. How are customers referred to the organization? To what extent are there formal referral relationships?

THE EXTERNAL AUDIT

The external audit in the marketing planning process involves the same steps described in earlier chapters for assessing the organization's environment. The process starts with an analysis of the macro-environment and progresses through the various levels down to the micro-environment. Broad social trends are reviewed and developments within the economy are analyzed for their implications for healthcare. Health industry trends are reviewed, with attention paid to developments in the regulatory and reimbursement arenas.

The scope of the environmental analysis will be determined by the nature of the organization and the issues being considered. As noted below, the external audit for marketing planning addresses some additional dimensions.

As part of the environmental assessment, broad *social trends* should be analyzed and their implications for the market area considered. These societal trends should include demographic trends, economic considerations, lifestyle trends, and particularly shifts in attitudes. Many trends discussed elsewhere have implications for marketing planning, and, in many ways, marketing planning is more sensitive to changing societal patterns than are certain other types of planning.

Lifestyle trends are likely to be more important when it comes to marketing planning than for other types of planning. An example of changing lifestyles involves the health and fitness consciousness that characterizes many segments of the American population. The fitness movement that began in the 1980s has created an unprecedented demand for health clubs, health food, athletic goods, and sports medicine. It has not been uncommon, in fact, for a marketing plan to focus on the fitness-related attributes of a product or service that was never intended as a fitness aid.

Even changes in *consumer attitudes* at the national level may have implications for local communities. Until recently, for example, few healthcare organizations would openly market impotence treatment. Now, with more liberal attitudes in evidence, clever advertisements attract attention to these organizations and their services, and the marketing of an impotence medication took on a high profile in the late 1990s.

The same type of analysis should be applied to *health industry trends* to determine what developments are likely to affect the local community. The emergence of healthcare service lines in the 1980s, for example, influenced the marketing agenda. Further, a major marketing effort has been introduced by health maintenance organizations seeking to capture the indemnity insurance market. Trends like these two have profound implications for those involved marketing planning.

Of particular importance in marketing planning is the *industry or product life cycle*. A new product that is being introduced will be approached differently from an existing product that is struggling to differentiate itself. Both will be approached differently from an established product that is nearly at the end of its life cycle. (This important issue is discussed further in Chapter 10.)

Regulatory, political and legal developments should all be considered. Regulations enacted by a variety of governmental and non-governmental agencies set constraints on marketing activity. The political environment also has both direct and indirect implications for marketing planning. There is no doubt that the marketing plan for Columbia/HCA took a different turn in the mid-1990s after its activities came under federal investigation. Legal activities at the national, state and local levels also have implications for the local healthcare system. For example, marketing activities that could be thought to illegally encourage referrals or other questionable activities would be factors to consider here.

Developments in the area of *technology* can exert a major influence on the nature of the health caresystem. Not only should the marketing planning team be familiar with the technology surrounding a given service or product, but it must be familiar with other technology in the field. Promoting an organization's new procedure as cutting edge may be inappropriate if hundreds of other hospitals are already performing this procedure. It is also important to be aware of any technological developments on the horizon that may affect the positioning or perception of the product being marketed.

Reimbursement patterns may be influenced by all levels of government as well as by private sector third-party payors. Anticipated developments in reimbursement must be taken into consideration in marketing planning. To the extent that consumers with the ability to pay for the service are important, the reimbursement situation within the market must be considered. The marketing initiative, in fact, is likely to be tailored to appeal to a particular payor category. If price is an issue, information on the availability of insurance benefits is important.

Profiling the Market Area and Its Population

A logical first step in the marketing planning process is the identification and profiling of the market area to be considered. The market area could range from a very small geographic area served by a pharmacy, for example, to a national or even international market served by a pharmaceutical company. The "market" that is profiled should be in keeping with the scope of the organization being planned for.

There may be situations when the market area is not clear cut, and a certain amount of research may be required to identify the market that is to be cultivated. (See Chapter 8 for a discussion of the delineation of market areas.) In most cases, the market will be delineated by geography. Certainly local health care providers will be restricted to a relatively circumscribed geographic area. On the other hand, the market may actually involve broad population segments and, except for national boundaries, may not be related to geography at all. Thus, a retail pharmacy mail order business may have a national market defined in terms of population characteristics that exist independent of geography.

The type of information required on the market varies with the nature of the project. The first type of data typically compiled is demographic data, including biosocial and sociocultural traits. At a minimum, the analyst would examine the population in terms of age, sex, race/ethnicity, marital status/family structure, income and education. In the process, the situation with regard to insurance coverage is typically assessed.

The demographic analysis is often accompanied by an assessment of the psychographic characteristics of the market area population. Information on the lifestyle categories of the target audience can be used to determine the likely health priorities and behavior of a population subgroup. The attitudes displayed by consumers in a market area are likely to have considerable influence on the demand for almost all types of health services. At the organization level, the attitudes of a wide variety of constituents besides direct consumers must be taken into consideration.

Of these various characteristics of the market area population, attitudes probably receive more attention from marketing planners than from other types of planners. While there may be interest in the demographic or psychographic characteristics of the population, marketing planners often view these primarily as clues to the attitudes of the population. Since the thrust of many marketing plans involves changing attitudes, this category of information is critical and often requires primary research.

In situations in which the market is not closely linked to geography, data collection for the market profile will be addressed differently. For example, the market may be constituted of active, younger seniors or of women of child-bearing age. In either case, the characteristics of the market will be determined initially independent of geography (except for the limitation of national boundaries). Thus, the characteristics of younger seniors or women of child-bearing age will be identified in terms of the above dimensions and *then* linked to geography for the spatial dimension. Geographic areas with concentrations of young seniors or areas with concentrations of child-bearing age women would subsequently be identified.

Market Segmentation

Of particular importance in marketing planning is the market segmentation process. Most marketing initiatives are going to involve target marketing in which subsegments of the population are singled out for cultivation. Market segmentation can take the following forms:

Demographic Segmentation. Market segmentation on the basis of demographics is the best known of the approaches to identifying target markets. The links between demographic characteristics and health status, health-related attitudes, and health behavior have been well established. For this reason, demographic segmentation is always an early task in any marketing planning process. Demographically distinct subgroups are typically defined relative to various services and products.

Geographic Segmentation. An understanding of the spatial distribution of the target market has become increasingly important as healthcare has become more consumer driven. One of the implications of this trend has been the increased emphasis on the appropriate location of health facilities. The market-driven approach to health services has demanded that healthcare organizations take their services to the population, and the major purchasers of health services are insisting on convenient locations for their enrollees. Knowledge of the manner in which the population is distributed within the service area and the linkage between geographic segmentation and other forms of segmentation is critical for the development of a marketing plan.

Psychographic Segmentation. For many types of products and services an understanding of the psychographic characteristics of the target population is essential. The lifestyle clusters that can be identified for a population often transcend (or at least complement) its demographic characteristics. Most importantly, psychographic traits can be linked to the propensity to purchase various services and products, as well as to the attitudes, perceptions and expectations of the target population. (See Box 9-2 for a discussion of lifestyles and the use of health services.)

Usage Segmentation. A common form of segmentation long used by marketers is now being applied to healthcare. The market area population can be divided into categories based on the extent of use of a particular service. In the case of urgent care center usage, for example, the population can be divided into heavy users, moderate users, occasional users and non-users. This information provides a basis for subsequent marketing planning that can be tailored differently, for example, for existing loyal customers and non-customers.

Payor Segmentation. A form of market segmentation unique to healthcare involves targeting population groups on the basis of their payor categories. The existence of insurance coverage and the type of coverage is a major consideration in the marketing of most health services. Health plans cover some services and not others, and this becomes an important consideration in marketing. For elective services that are paid for out of pocket, a highly targeted marketing approach is required. The payor mix of the market area population has now come to be one of the first considerations for many marketing planning activities.

Identifying Health Characteristics

The health characteristics of the population will be identified following the steps outlined in Chapters 6 and 7. The emphasis, of course, will be on those dimensions that are relevant to the needs of the organization.

The *fertility* characteristics of the population need to be considered, and the importance of these characteristics will depend on the type of organization. The number of births as well as the characteristics of those births, along with the attributes of the mothers and fathers of the children, form the basis for fertility analysis. For marketers, the characteristics of those involved in child-bearing is important.

BOX 9-2
Lifestyle Analysis for Marketing Planning

Lifestyle segmentation systems have been used for decades in other industries but have never received wide acceptance in healthcare. Historically, healthcare provider organizations have depended on physicians or health plans to channels patients to them. They, in fact, had little interest in the characteristics of their patients. In the new health care environment, however, there is growing interest in customer segmentation. The market has become much more consumer driven, and individuals are taking a much more active role in healthcare decision making. Today, growing numbers of health plans, health services providers, and other organizations are expressing an interest in customer segmentation and target marketing.

Lifestyle segmentation is also of interest to health planners and others who are concerned about the distribution of healthcare phenomena within a population. Although variations in demographic and sociocultural characteristics serve to explain a lot of the differences found in health status and health behavior among various groups, there is growing evidence that lifestyle characteristics may actually transcend these standard dimensions for segmentation. Among the elderly, for example, it was customary to classify those over 65 into one monolithic category or at best three categories based on age breaks (e.g., 65–74, 75–84, and 85 and over). Lifestyle analysis indicates, however, that the 65–74 age cohort actually contains two or more lifestyle clusters that may have similar demographic traits but be different in terms of the lifestyles. For this reason, planners must consider the lifestyle clusters that characterize the population under study.

The first lifestyle segmentation systems—also referred to as psychographic segmentation systems—were developed in the 1970s. This new approach to segmenting the population was developed in response to some of the perceived deficiencies in demographic profiling. Marketers had come to realize that people in the same demographic category may fall into different groupings based on lifestyle despite being very similar on paper. Lifestyle research discovered that within this demographic category there were various lifestyle categories that had a greater impact on consumer behavior than age did.

The best-known early lifestyle segmentation system was developed by Stanford Research International (SRI) in the 1970s. It was called VALS for "values and lifestyle system" and inspired a variety of subsequent lifestyle segmentation systems. The VALS system was eventually overshadowed by more consumer-oriented approaches, and three later systems are widely used today. These are lifestyle segmentation systems developed by Claritas (PRIZM), Experian (MOSAIC), and CACI Marketing Systems (ACORN). While the various systems are built using similar methodologies, they differ in terms of the specific procedures utilized to create the categories.

The concept behind all segmentation systems is the use of geodemographic data in conjunction with data on consumer behavior, attitudes and preferences to establish distinct lifestyle clusters that cover the entire population. This allows researchers to classify healthcare consumers into distinct categories, each with its peculiar characteristics. Once the lifestyle segments have been identified for a population, it is possible to attach a broad range of characteristics to the respective categories.

The PRIZM developed by Claritas may be the best-known system, primarily due to the clever names it has given its lifestyle categories. Individuals may be classified as, for example, "Patios and Pools", "Shotguns and Pickups", or "Executive Suites" among the 62 PRIZM clusters. The PRIZM system is the only one that has been used extensively to date to link health characteristics to the lifestyle clusters. (This information, however, is proprietary and can only be obtained by becoming a client of Inforum, the data vendor that developed the health care links to the various clusters.)

U.S. MOSAIC is the latest version of the Experian lifestyle classification system. This system also includes 62 lifestyle clusters grouped into 12 major categories. The naming scheme is somewhat more straightforward than for the PRIZM system, with the "Upscale Singles Category" including such clusters as "High-income urban singles in apartments" and "Urban, upper-mid-income seniors in apartments".

CACI's ACORN is an acronym for "A Classification of Residential Neighborhoods". A number of multivariate statistical methods were applied to create this system. CACI analyzed and sorted the country's 226,000 neighborhoods by 61 unique lifestyle characteristics, such as income, age, household type, home value, occupation, education, and other key determinants of consumer behavior. Next, market segments were created by a combination of cluster analytic techniques. The techniques were selected to produce statistically reliable solutions and to handle an immense amount

(continued)

of information. This process resulted in the assignment of over 220,000 neighborhoods to 43 lifestyle segments.

Health planners involved with the development of marketing plans are increasingly emphasizing the importance of lifestyles for both health status and health behavior. It is a logical step to link various health characteristics to the respective lifestyle clusters. As the value of lifestyle segmentation becomes more obvious to health professionals, the range of health-related characteristics that are likely to be associated with the various lifestyle segments can be expected to grow.

A wide range of service and product needs revolves around childbearing, and childbearing also triggers the need for such down-the-road services as pediatrics and contraception-related services. The demand for treatment of the male and female reproductive systems and the heightened interest in infertility treatment are by-products are considerations.

The level of *morbidity* within the population can be determined from incidence and prevalence rates. Disability indicators should be considered along with measures of morbidity in terms of disease prevalence. To the extent possible, planners need to project rates of incidence and prevalence into the future in order to plan for coming developments.

Organization-level planners typically have less interest in mortality analysis than those involved in community-wide planning, since the latter are more concerned with the overall health status of the community. Nevertheless, mortality data is usually examined to determine what it can tell us about the health status of the community. Indeed, differences in hospital mortality rates are sometimes used as a basis for marketing campaigns.

The emphasis in most marketing planning initiatives will be on the morbidity profile of the population. The incidence and prevalence of various health conditions will drive much of the planning activity. For most organizations, the demand for health services derived from this level of need is what drives the market. Planners are likely to be interested in both the level of morbidity and the utilization patterns that it generates.

Identifying Market Needs

Marketing planning differs from other types of planning in the sense that the research component of the planning process may exert an inordinate influence on the focus of the plan. In strategic planning, in contrast, the process is informed by the research findings, but it is not likely that the strategic direction of the organization is going to be radically modified as a result of the research. With market research, on the other hand, the intent may be to determine what the needs and desires of the market are quite independent of the services that the organization is already providing. It is not inconceivable that the marketing research could result in a decision to develop a new service or a new business line that had not been considered before. This is the hallmark of a market-driven industry; the organization does not simply sell what it has to offer, but it goes to the market to determine what the opportunities are.

Identifying Consumer Behavior

Health behavior is likely to be conceptualized by the marketing planner in terms of consumer behavior and/or decision making. Consumer participate in such formal activities as physician visits, hospital admissions, and drug prescriptions, as well as informal actions that are designed to prevent health problems and maintain, enhance or promote health.

An appreciation of the nature of consumer behavior is much more important for marketing planning than for other types of planning. Since marketing is driven by consumer needs, an appreciation of the behavioral dimension of any target population is essential. It is ultimately this behavior that the marketing plan seeks to influence.

A basic understanding of the process that consumers go through in the purchase decision-making process is important for marketing planning purposes. The following steps in the consumer purchase model should be taken into consideration in the development of a marketing plan (Hillestad and Berkowitz, 1991). The point at which the target market is located in the consumer behavior progression will determine the focus of the plan.

Awareness. Awareness refers to the initial exposure of the target population to the product or service being marketed.

Knowledge. Knowledge refers to the point at which the potential consumer understands the nature of the product or service.

Perception. Perception develops at the point at which the consumer develops an opinion of the product or service.

Contract access. Contract access is a step unique to health care, in that many services or products will not be considered for purchase if the provisions of the consumer's insurance plan do not cover them.

Location. The geographic availability of a service may become a factor once a consumer expresses interest in the product or service.

Preference. Preferences develop at the point that the consumer expresses a tendency for one type of product or service (e.g., a podiatrist rather than an orthopedic surgeon) and/or decides between different providers of the same service (e.g., Podiatrist A rather than Podiatrist B.)

Choice. This is the decision point at which the consumer eliminates other options and decides to buy a particular product or utilize a particular service.

Usage. This is the point at which the consumer actually buys the product in question or utilizes the service.

Satisfaction. The consumer subsequently displays some level of satisfaction with the product or service and this influences future utilization.

Advocacy. The successful marketing initiative will ultimately create an advocate for the product or service, thereby extending the impact to the initiative.

One other consumer dimension of importance to the marketing plan involves the bases on which consumers differentiate various services and products in the market. This might be thought of as the "hot buttons" characterizing the target market. It is important to determine if the target population is most interested in, for example, *quality* or *value* in a service. Or, is it the case that, for a particular service, *location* or *convenience* is the most important consideration. In other cases, *price* may be a determining factor in consumer behavior.

The bases for differentiation may not be obvious from baseline data collection, and this is an area in which primary research may be required. Regardless of the effort required, this is critical information. This knowledge will not only shape the marketing strategy, but it has implications product/service design, packaging, distribution, and pricing.

One other unique characteristic of healthcare that has implications for the marketing plan is the fact that the end-user of a service may not be the ultimate target of a marketing initiative. In fact, healthcare marketers have identified a number of other categories of target audiences that may be more important than the end user. For example, various categories of *influencers* have been identified. These could be family members, counselors, or other health professionals that encourage consumers to use a particular product or service. The role of various *gatekeepers* might also be considered. These could include primary care physicians, insurance plan personnel, discharge planners, and others who have responsibility for channeling consumers into certain services.

Another category involves the *decision makers* who make choices for the consumer. These could be family members, primary care physicians, or caregivers who act on behalf of consumers for various reasons. Finally, there is a category of *buyers* of healthcare services that includes employers, business coalitions, and other groups that might indirectly control the behavior of consumers by determining which services they can and cannot utilize.

Competitive Analysis

The resource identification process takes the form of a competitive analysis in the marketing planning process. The focus will typically be on the organizations and the services that are likely to be in competition with the entity involved in marketing planning.

In actuality, competition takes place at two levels in the healthcare market. At the level of service provision, the content of the services provides a basis for competition. At the marketing level, however, the *perceptions* that exist within the target audience constitute another battleground for competition. In many ways, the battle for the "hearts and minds" of the customer is waged independently of the competitive activities based on actual product attributes.

The review of *facilities* in marketing planning will typically be restricted to those facilities that are directly applicable to the project. A facility competing in terms of a narrowly defined service may be interested only in those facilities that offer that service. Marketing planning for a full-service hospital, on the other hand, will require a very broad review of facilities. This would include not only the hospitals that compete with the facility, but also the variety of non-hospital organizations that compete in a particular market area with the hospital.

The same approach would be followed with regard to *products and services.* The programs and services to be analyzed will typically be those of immediate concern to the organization. The more complex the organization and the more comprehensive its services, the wider the net that will be cast in terms of competing programs and services.

Although a competitive advantage in terms of *equipment* is typically not thought of as a marketing angle, there are numerous examples in healthcare in which hospitals or other facilities compete directly on the basis of the technology they have to offer. If the technologies are comparable, the marketing challenge is to somehow differentiate, for example, one hospital's imaging capabilities from another's. In some cases, the technology may be truly unique (as with the first organization to acquire the latest laser technology for eye surgery). The marketing approach will be different in this case than it would if everyone's technology was comparable.

In many ways, healthcare organizations, particularly those involved in direct patient care, succeed or fail based on the characteristics of their *personnel.* Certainly in developing an image campaign, the qualities of the organization's personnel will be displayed. Even for a particular program or service, the presence of a "name" physician or access to the only retina surgeon in the market constitutes a basis for differentiation. The planner will want to determine the number, type and characteristics of the personnel within the organization for these purposes.

The inventory of market area services should include a review of existing *networks and relationships* within the delivery system. This aspect of the research is particularly challenging, since no directories of "relationships" are likely to exist for the community. In an era of managed care and negotiated contracts for health services, the existence of networks and relationships has taken on added importance.

An important aspect of this analysis involves referral relationships, since much of the marketing plan research will focus on identifying sources of customers. The research should identify both existing referrers and non-referrers to the program. It should also identify potential referral source types that are not already being tapped. Ultimately, a consideration of referral relationships is critical for most marketing plans.

Inventory of Marketing Resources

Data collection for marketing planning includes a component related to the organization's existing marketing resources. This information indicates the resource base on which the marketing planner can build. This inventory includes information on the role of the marketing department within the organization and, more specifically, its role with regard to the service or product in question. The analysis should also determine the level of marketing expertise that currently exists within the organization. It is important to determine the extent to which marketing is built into the operation of the organization, with this information helping to determine the extent to which a marketing "mindset" exists.

Obviously, the planner needs to determine if there is an existing marketing plan and, if so, what its characteristics are. At the same time, any on-going marketing evaluation activities should be identified. The nature and location of any marketing activities need to be determined. Marketing planners are likely to be more concerned about internat marketing issues than most other types of planners.

Consumer Awareness

Of particular importance in the marketing planning process is the degree of consumer awareness that exists with regard to the organization and/or product under consideration. Information on awareness of and perceptions concerning competing organizations and their services and products is important as well.

This is an area where there is likely to be little existing information, unless a substantial market research process is in place. In the typical case, primary research will be required to determine the extent to which consumers are familiar with the organization or its products, the image held by consumers, this level of knowledge, and this propensity to utilize various services. Similar data should be collected on consumer perceptions of competitors and their services.

It may be necessary to develop an understanding of the degree of awareness characterizing different segments of the market. A high level of awareness may exist among segments of the market area population that are not likely to be heavy users, while the segments with the greatest customer potential may exhibit a low level of awareness.

Market Share Analysis

The market share for the organization or the specific product or service is an important consideration in the marketing planning process. This information not only provides an indicator of the current position of the organization or service in the market, but serves as an important basis for evaluating the success of a marketing initiative.

If the organization is the focus of the marketing initiative, the market share the organization holds within the market area should be determined (e.g., the hospital's share of total hospital admissions). Overall market share may not be as important, however, as market share for the various service lines or specialty areas. Certainly the planner will want to know how the overall market share is split among the various programs. It may be less important to know that the hospital holds a 25 percent market share of admissions within the market area than it is to know that the share for obstetrics is 35 percent and for cardiology is 15 percent. Realistically, it is difficult to change overall market shares for hospitals in established medical markets. It makes more sense, then, to think in terms of the market shares characterizing component programs.

If a specific product or service is the focus, obviously the planner will want to determine the market share held by that product or service. If the service line is outpatient surgery, for example, a first step is to determine the extent to which the surgery center controls the market. Again, it will probably be worthwhile to break this down into component procedures, since the overall outpatient surgery figure may not be very meaningful.

When dealing with national corporations, it is likely that the market shares they hold can be easily determined. Sales volumes for pharmaceuticals, medical supplies, and equipment are closely tracked, and market share data are likely to be readily available. However, determining the share held by a product or service at the local level may be more of a challenge.

Despite the challenge, market share must be determined to the extent possible. This may require some primary research or, at the very least, some creativity in "massaging" available data in order to obtain the necessary information. The fact that market share is likely to be a critical benchmark for determining the effectiveness of a marketing plan mandates that every effort be made to establish the baseline market share and track it during the course of the marketing campaign.

The market share analysis is comparable to the gap analysis performed in community-wide planning and strategic planning. The "gap" is in effect the difference between the market share held by the organization or product and the overall market or volume for that product. Thus, a 25 percent market share indicates that the organization is failing to capture 75 percent of the potential business. It becomes important to analyze this 75 percent to determine how the rest of the market is divided up. If the other 75 percent is controlled by a single competitior, the marketing approach will be a lot different than if the remainder is divided among a dozen small players. Other considerations might include whether the competitors are small local players or large national concerns. Further, are we considering well established organizations or are a lot of new players entering the market?

STATE-OF-THE-MARKET REPORT

At this stage of the process, it is usually worthwhile to present a state-of-the-market report. The nature of the report will depend on such issues as whether an organization or a product is being marketed, whether it is a new product being introduced or an old one that is being revived, and whether the target is existing customers or new ones.

The state-of-the-market report should include the following sections summarizing the data collection up to this point:

- ✓ Overall industry/product trends
- ✓ Market area delineation
- ✓ Market area population profile
- ✓ Market area population health characteristics
- ✓ Current position of the organization/product
- ✓ Competitive situation and market share
- ✓ Likely future developments

This status report should include the strengths, weaknesses, opportunities and threats identified during the analysis. It should also include an "issues statement" based on the results of the analysis to this point. This is also a point at which the mission statement and the original assumptions should be revisited to verify that the marketing direction is in keeping with the intent of the organization.

This is an opportunity to frankly describe the state of the market and the organization's position in it. This provides a means for getting all parties on the same page and confirming assumptions. This should be the launching point for subsequent plan development.

DEVELOPING STRATEGIES

Marketing strategies set the tone for subsequent planning activities and in effect set the parameters within which the planner must operate. The strategy that is chosen will influence the nature of the plan that is ultimately developed.

The development of strategies for a marketing plan is often different from that for other types of plans in that the focus may be narrower, say, than for a strategic plan. Indeed, the marketing strategy should ideally be derived from the organization's overall strategy. The strategy options are almost unlimited and could include an educational initiative, a public relations rather than an advertising approach, a soft-sell versus a hard-sell approach, and so forth. Ideally, the strategy employed for a marketing initiative will support the organization's mission statement and reflect the strategies embodied in the organization's strategic plan. Thus, if the organization's strategy involves positioning itself as the "caring" organization, marketing initiatives should support this approach. Of course, there are occasions in which a particular marketing situation may call for a departure from the established approach. For example, a hospital that has been content to live in the shadow of a more powerful competitor and pursued a "we're Number Two" approach may develop a world class program in a particular area and decide to take a much more aggressive approach in the marketing of this service than for the organization in general.

DEVELOPING THE MARKETING PLAN

The effort up to this point provides the foundation for the actual development of the plan. If the initial work is properly carried out, the planning process should flow smoothly, at least from a technical perspective.

Setting Goals

The goal or goals that are established for the marketing plan should reflect the information that was provided in the state-of-the-market report. As in other planning activities, the goal should be in keeping with the organization's missions statement.

The number of goals to be established depends on the complexity and size of the organization, the nature of the issues at hand, and the type of planning being undertaken. If the marketing focus is narrow, a single goal may be appropriate. On the other hand, the complexity of many healthcare organizations mandates the establishment of multiple goals related to various components of the organization.

The goal of the marketing plan would be stated in a form such as this: To establish Hospital X as the top-of-mind facility in the market area. Or, for a service oriented initiative, it might read: To capture the market niche for occupational medicine.

Setting Objectives

For every marketing goal a number of objectives may be specified, since it is likely that initiatives will be required on a number of different fronts in order to reach the specified goal. Marketing objectives are stated in such terms as: The proportion of the general population for whom Hospital X is top of mind will be increased from 10 percent to 25 percent within six months (in support of the stated goal of making Hospital X top of mind in the community.) Or, for service marketing: The occupational medicine program will capture 25 percent of the industrial market within six months.

Barriers to marketing objectives could arise for a variety of reasons. There are some types of barriers that are more or less unique to marketing planning.

For example, there may be ethical or legal considerations associated with some types of marketing, including situations in which advertising may be prohibited for certain health professionals. There are also issues of appropriateness and taste that may be a consideration. It may be found that the educational level of the target audience is a barrier to introducing a new high-tech procedure or that a new procedure is considered "experimental" by the public, thereby making potential patients apprehensive.

Prioritizing Objectives

The prioritization of objectives may not be as important an issue in marketing planning as it is for some other types of planning. However, there needs to be some consensus developed beforehand on the process in order to systematically consider priorities if that becomes necessary. The challenge is to identify on the front end the criteria that are the most important.

One approach that might be used for prioritizing the objectives of a marketing plan involves the traditional "four p's" of marketing: product, price, place and promotion. The decision could be made, for example, to focus on the product in the marketing initiative, at the expense of the price, place and promotion. Thus, objectives that are most directly related to promoting the characteristics of the product would be emphasized. Or, it might be appropriate to capitalize on the price advantage of the product, thereby encouraging an emphasis on objectives that focused on the pricing dimension.

Specifying Actions

The next step in the marketing planning process is the specification of the actions to be carried out. It is one thing to indicate what should be done, it is another to specify how it should be operationalized. For each of the objectives that have been identified a set of actions must be specified. These actions take a wide range of forms, from assuring that postage is available to support a direct mail initiative to enlisting a celebrity spokesperson as a means of reaching an objective.

If the objective of a specialty practice is to raise the awareness of its new sports medicine program, for example, a number of actions must be carried out. These may include: selecting an advertising agency, allocating funds for marketing, "packaging" the program, calling on potential referrers, and so forth. Many of these actions imply a certain sequence, and this is a point at which the original project plan might be further refined to specify the sequencing of the action steps.

The action steps developed for a marketing plan may be more standardized than those for other types of plans. It is likely that marketing initiatives are already underway (unlike a strategic plan that is being developed for the first time), and this type of activity may be frequently carried out by the organization. A reasonable understanding of the resource requirements is likely to have been previously established, and there may be resources available that could be redirected toward the planning initiative.

IMPLEMENTING THE MARKETING PLAN

Planning is ultimately only an exercise, albeit a meaningful one. The payoff comes in the implementation of the plan. The planning process creates a road map that the organization must use it to get to where it wants to go. To a certain extent, planning is talk, but implementation is action.

Marketing planners typically have the advantage that the hand-off from planning to implementation is likely to be smoother than it is for other types of planning. Indeed, the same parties are likely to be involved in both activities. This is in contrast to strategic planning, for example, in which the planning team transfers responsibility to management once the plan has been developed.

Steps in Implementation

In order to approach plan implementation systematically, it is important to develop both a detailed project plan and an implementation matrix. The project plan has been discussed elsewhere, and standardized approaches are likely to be in place for the implementation of a marketing plan.

The implementation matrix should list every action called for by the plan, breaking each action down into tasks, if appropriate. For each action or task the responsible party should be identified, along with any secondary parties that should be involved in this activity. The matrix should indicate resource requirements (in terms of staff time, money and other requirements). The start and end dates for this activity should be identified. Any prerequisites for accomplishing this task should be identified at the outset (and factored into the project plan). Finally, some benchmark should probably be established that allows the planning team to determine when the activity has been completed.

The resource requirements from the implementation matrix should be combined to determine total project resource requirements. When this process has been completed, the total resource requirements of the project will be identified for the first time. The extent of the requirements may have to be addressed in relation to available funds and any other fiscal constraints.

In marketing, there are well established techniques for implementing a marketing plan. The different approaches that might be utilized include advertising, public relations activities, and community outreach efforts, among others. The implementation plan may focus on a traditional media campaign with heavy advertising or it might emphasize direct marketing. On the other hand, perhaps internal marketing is the most efficacious approach to take. Or, the situation may call for business-to-business marketing. If a media-based approach is chosen, the type of media to be utilized becomes an issue for the implementation plan. The techniques utilized will be dictated by the nature of the marketing initiative.

THE EVALUATION PLAN

While the evaluation process is important for all types of planning processes, it is particularly important in marketing planning. Since the objectives of the marketing process are typically fairly focused, measures of marketing effectiveness are essential and typically easy to perform.

Evaluation techniques focus to two types of analysis: process (or formative) analysis and outcome (or summative) analysis. Both of these have a role to play in the project. Outcome evaluation is particularly important for the marketing planning process. Changes in image or sales volume must be measured, and the success of the project is likely to be calculated in much more precise terms than it is for other types of planning.

Although evaluation techniques are often praised for their bottom-line objectivity, they are also useful in healthcare where it is not possible to place a dollar value on everything. Thus, cost-effectiveness analysis should take into consideration the non-tangible aspects of the service delivery process in its evaluation.

REVISION AND REPLANNING

As noted earlier, it is unlikely that a plan will be completed without being modified for one reason or another. This type of "on the fly" revision is inevitable in a rapidly changing environment. At the end of the planning period, it is important to reaccess the internal characteristics of the organization and the external environment. What developments have subsequently occurred that will affect the plan or the implementation of its provisions? What actions have been taken supportive of the plan that were not anticipated? Have there been developments that affect resource requirements? Have actions on the part of competitors affected the "strategic balance"?

The marketing approach chosen should be reviewed to determine if it is still the best approach in view of possible changes in the environment. The goals and objectives should be revisited to assure that they are still appropriate in the light of any changes in either the internal or external environment.

References

Hillestad, S.G., and Eric N. Berkowitz (1991). *Health Care Marketing Plans*. Gaithersburg, MD: Aspen Publishers.

Additional Resources

Bashe, Gil, and Nancy Hicks (2000). *Branding Health Services*. Gaithersburg, MD: Aspen.

Berkowitz, Eric N. (1996). *Essentials of Health Care Marketing*. Gaithersburg, MD: Aspen Publishers.

Berkowitz, Eric N., Pol, Louis G., and Richard K. Thomas (1997). *Healthcare Market Research*. Burr Ridge, IL: Irwin Professional Publishing.

Kotler, Philip, and Gary Armstrong (2000). *Marketing: An Introduction*. Upper Saddle River, NJ: Prentice-Hall.

Rogers, Stuart C., and Richard H. Thompson, Jr. (1992). *The Medical Marketing Plan*. Burr Ridge, IL: Irwin Professional Publishers.

Rynne, Terrence J. (1995). *Healthcare Marketing in Transition*. Burr Ridge, IL: Irwin Professional Publishing.

Siegel, Michael, and M. Doner (1998). *Marketing Public Health*. Gaithersburg, MD: Aspen.

Wayne, James A. (1998). *Strategic Marketing of Your Long-Term Care Facility: A How-To Approach*. Springfield, IL: Charles C. Thomas Publishers.

10

Business Planning

INTRODUCTION

Business planning is a well-established activity in other industries but is relatively new process for health service providers. Business planning was introduced to healthcare organizations in the 1980s when the industry was being transformed into its "modern" form. Due to increased competition and a more volatile environment, healthcare organizations needed to behave more like businesses, and this meant adopting business practices long common in other industries. Prior to this time, business planning activities had been restricted to more "retail" oriented healthcare entities (e.g., pharmaceutical companies, insurance companies).

The adoption of business planning techniques was also given impetus by the entrance of entrepreneurs from other industries into healthcare during this same period. These newcomers may not have known much about healthcare, but they knew a lot about business. Old line healthcare administrators found themselves at a disadvantage vis-a-vis these new competitors, and they had to adopt business planning principles in order to continue to compete.

Business planning can be defined simply as follows: *The systematic development of a plan for meeting a business objective.* The business plan establishes the outline for developing a project or business in terms of its potential for generating profit. The plan describes the what, when, who, where, why and how of the business. If the plan is for a new business or service line, it should describe the process to be followed in establishing the business or service. If it involves an existing business, it reviews the organization's history and the manner in which the business will be developed in the future.

The Nature of Business Planning

While the business plan by definition has a specific purpose, it is increasingly seen as a tool for analysis and management. How better to assess the "health" of one's business than to work through the business planning process? How better to understand issues related to the management of the operation than through examining it within the context of the business plan? The business planning process introduces the discipline and logical thought necessary for moving the business forward, in addition to laying out the roadmap map for effective business development.

The business plan should be framed within the context of the organization's strategic plan. The objectives of the business plan should support the objectives of the strategic plan and be in keeping with the mission and goals of the organization. It should also be coordinated with any other types of planning being carried out by the organization.

The business plan can be distinguished from strategic plans and marketing plans in one important way. The business plan is inherently conservative, even if it deals with an innovative service or product. While the strategic plan should be visionary and the marketing plan creative, these traits are generally not encouraged in a business plan. Its bottom-line orientation calls for a conservative approach.

Business planning is also distinguished from strategic planning in that the objective of the plan is typically foreordained. With strategic planning, the planning team may be starting out with a blank slate and, through the interaction of those involved, a planning agenda is developed. In most cases, there are few preconceived notions concerning the strategic direction the organization will take. On the other hand, the business plan is generally formulated to support a business concept that has already been conceived and now needs to be operationalized.

This implies that the business plan is relatively rigid compared to some other plans. However, plans can only go so far in anticipating unexpected developments, uncontrollable circumstances, and other complexities of the market. Like all plans, the business plan should be sensitive to potential developments that may require mid-course corrections. It should have the flexibility to adapt to changing circumstances without losing sight of the business objective.

Business planning is seldom applied in the community-wide planning process, as the nature of community-wide planning does not lend itself to this approach. However, healthcare organizations within the community should be encouraged to adopt business planning principles in their efforts to contribute to the objectives of the community-wide plan.

When Should a Business Plan Be Developed?

It is difficult to imagine any healthcare organization operating in today's environment without a business plan of some type in place. Regardless of the competitive situation or the stage of development of the organization, a healthcare organization should have a business plan to guide its actions. The plan defines the organization in relation to its environment and its competitors. It establishes general planning objectives and provides a context in which business decision making can occur.

Any time there is a need to analyze an existing business and determine its future direction, a business plan is necessary. A plan should also be developed whenever a decision is being made that will impact the business. This may involve the addition of a new service, the introduction of a new product, staff changes, and a variety of other actions.

Certainly any effort at initiating a new venture requires a business plan. This is especially true if the venture is a startup and has no history to guide it. Even if the new venture is being launched within an existing framework, a business plan for the new component is necessary.

Business plans typically are developed for either an internal or an external audience. Quite often business plans for existing organizations are developed to guide the overall direction of the organization or for the benefit of some subunit. If a new service or product is envisioned by the organization, a business plan may be developed to justify the initiation of this new line.

Increasingly, healthcare organizations are seeking outside funding for business development. This funding may be derived from traditional investment sources, venture capitalists, or even foundations. They may also be seeking funds from major donors. In every case, it is important to have a well-conceived business plan to present to a funding source.

Why Healthcare Is Different

Every discussion of planning so far has noted the uniqueness of healthcare. Business planning may be the situation in which healthcare is the most unique, and it is unique in a variety of ways. The mission of the healthcare organization is likely to be quite different from that of organizations in other industries undergoing business planning activities. The mission may emphasize the charity or service orientation of the organization, rather than a bottom-line concern with profits. The mission is also likely to be more diffuse than that for organizations in other industries. A mission of "improving the health status of the community" is a lot different than the bottom line-oriented missions of most corporations in other industries.

The objectives of the healthcare organization are also likely to be much more diverse that those of its counterparts in other industries. The hospital, with its myriad of functions and interests, is the epitome of the multipurpose organization. A business plan for an organization this complex must be able to consider a wide range of perspectives, especially when few of these components were established with an eye to the bottom line.

The constituencies of healthcare organizations are typically quite different from those of other industries. Although a growing number of healthcare organizations must be accountable to stockholders, most are more directly accountable to other types of constituencies. A public hospital may have to cater to politicians, consumer interest groups, vested interests in the medical community, and other entities. A church-affiliated hospital not only has a board of directors to which it reports, but it may be accountable to the denomination's leadership as well.

Healthcare organizations are also different in the sense that they are "required" in one way or another to provide comprehensive services. In other industries, an unprofitable product line can simply be eliminated. Hospitals and some other healthcare organizations, however, may feel they cannot compete on equal terms unless they are comprehensive in their service offerings. For a hospital to drop an unprofitable obstetrical program may have negative implications for other aspects of the operation. Indeed, state regulations may mandate the operation of the unit and eliminating it may not be an option.

Ultimately, the healthcare industry is still primarily not-for-profit it its orientation. The main objective is to provide a service needed by the community or to fill a gap in the organization's complement of services. If a business line is profitable, that is a plus. There is no other industry where an organization would knowingly enter into a business venture that has no prospect of being profitable.

This situation reflects, among other things, the intangible aspects related to the provision of health services. In many cases, the intent is not to make a profit on the specific business but to use a service line to support other aspects of the operation. Perhaps the best example involves the establishment of a network of urgent care clinics that will be marginally profitable at best, with the notion that 20 percent of the patients will be referred to the organization's specialists and 20 percent of these will end up being admitted to the organization's inpatient facility. The indirect benefits, in this case, are considered to be more important than any profits that would derive directly from the operation of the urgent care centers.

Expertise Required

Although some of the expertise necessary for developing a business plan will be available in house to large healthcare organizations, many smaller ventures will not have the required capabilities. While much of the data collection process is similar to that for other types of planning, business planning requires much more detail on the financial aspects of the operation. This means that the planners must know the right questions to ask and then know how to interpret the information that is generated.

Business planning is also different in the sense that, once financial data are collected, this information must be converted into pro formas and other financial statements that depict the likely future direction of the business initiative. This requires a certain level of skill that may not be readily available in all organizations. There are many sources of assistance in developing financial statements, and outside expertise may be required for the development of an effective plan.

ORGANIZING FOR BUSINESS PLANNING

The business plan is perhaps the most technical of the plans that are featured in this book. At the same time, it is probably the most straightforward. The components of the plan are highly standardized and much of the process can be reduced to a formula. In fact, computer software has been developed to support business planning more so than other types of planning.

The business plan should be a tool for setting the direction of the company over the next several years and indicate the action steps and processes needed to guide the company through this period. With a well thought out plan, the organization can better anticipate future crisis situations and deal with them proactively.

Planning for Planning

Planning for planning is somewhat different for the business plan than for most other types of planning. In general, the organizational phase involves identifying and enlisting the various parties appropriate for and necessary to the development of a plan. In the case of a business plan, the ultimate goal will have been established prior to initiation of the planning process. Whereas the strategic planner may ask "What do we want the organization to look like five years from now?", the business planner will ask "What do we need to do to introduce the new service?" The anticipated end point is predetermined, and the planning process serves to demonstrate the feasibility of reaching that goal and provide the means for completing the steps necessary for its achievement.

Today, it has become common in hospitals to expect managers in various departments to justify their requests for staff, programs, equipment or other resources in terms of business considerations. This is sometimes carried to the absurd point of making a business case for the purchase of a desktop computer. For the most part, however, business planning is left to the organization's business planners (although they are likely to carry some other title), and relatively few of the organization's staff will have regular involvement in the business planning process. Key individuals may be involved as necessary, especially in that any activity being planned is likely to overlap or interface with activities in other departments. And, certainly, appropriate experts from within or without the organization will be utilized as appropriate.

Initial Information Gathering

Initial information gathering should begin with a review of any available organizational materials. These would include publications produced by the organization such as annual reports, press releases, and marketing materials. It may even be appropriate to review the "resumes" of management and key clinical and technical personnel. Other potential sources of information include any reports filed with regulatory agencies, grant proposals, and certificate-of-need applications. Certain internal documents, such as executive committee minutes, planning retreat summaries, and evaluation studies may also be useful. Of course, detailed financial statements for several previous years should be reviewed.

The *major issues* should be identified, particularly as they relate to the business side of the organization. In the case of a business plan, the information sought through this initial research will center around the project being contemplated. This will involve an analysis of the *organizational structure* for the existing or proposed program. This involves a review of the division of labor, the chain of command, and the internal communications channels.

The *key players* in the organization should be identified through this process and, when appropriate, any influentials external to the organization as well. Some key players are obvious, such as those in formal positions of authority. Other key participants may be those who are positioned to have access to critical information. The business plan particularly requires the identification of management capabilities and other personnel resources, since these will be critically reviewed by those considering the proposal.

This stage of the process should also identify the key constituents of the organization. Constituents may include patient groups, referring physicians, employee benefits managers, insurance plan representatives, politicians and any number of other categories of constituents. If it is a publicly-held company, the board of directors and its shareholders represent constituents of some importance.

The initial information-gathering process for the business plan is not likely to be as comprehensive as it is for most other types of plans. The plan by definition is much more focused and there is no need, for example, to identify the issues affecting the organization above and beyond those that relate to the planning effort.

Profiling the Organization

This initial information gathering should allow the planner to develop a sense of what the organization is and which business it is in. The products or services of the organization need to be clearly defined for the business plan, since these will be the focus of the plan. The resources available for carrying out the business plan must be identified in more detail and earlier in the process than for, say, strategic plan development. Similarly, the customers for these products or services must be identified in order to tailor the plan to their needs.

The stating of assumptions at the outset and throughout the planning process is important in business planning. Any number of assumptions might be made with regard to the market, consumer behavior, the competition, and many other aspects of the environment or the organization. In particular, assumptions must be made that justify the financial statements that are developed. Assumptions should be stated with regard to the potential consequences of the business development initiative.

The nature of the assumptions made at the outset reflects the extent to which a product or service is already in the market and already has some level of awareness and utilization. In addition, the extent to which related business activities are already underway will affect the assumptions that are made.

BASELINE DATA COLLECTION

As with other types of planning, both an internal and external analysis is likely to be performed.

The Internal Audit

The "internal audit" as described in Chapter 7 is used in business planning to collect most of the necessary data on the organization. The intent of the internal audit is to determine who does what within the organization, when and where they do it, how they do it, and even why and how well they do it.

The internal audit will require access to a wide range of internal data describing operations, staffing, finances, physical plant, policies and procedures, information systems, and any other relevant aspect of the organization and its operation. The internal audit may even require the use of primary research methods to obtain certain information.

A more thorough assessment of the organization is likely to be performed for the business plan than for other types of plans. This is not only important for the sake of the planning effort, but, to the extent that outside funding sources are to be involved, a thorough assessment is critical. Considerable emphasis is placed on the current management of the organization and detailed data on its capabilities, experiences and traits are likely to be required. This should include information on the combination of skills and experience, degree of integrity, industry contacts, and previous experiencing working together on the part of management. (It has been purported, in fact, that investors base 60 percent of their decision to fund a project on the characteristics of the management team that is to be involved.)

If the project represents a startup operation or a new product line for an existing organization, the management team may not be in place. In such cases, assurances as to the level of management skills will be required. External funding entities will probably want to see letters of commitment, in fact.

The business plan also goes further in examining the human resources available to the organization and the characteristics of the employee pool. The availability of the appropriate staff to carry out the business plan will be a consideration, as is access to additional personnel if a new initiative is being considered. Access to consultants and specialists in key areas may be a factor as well.

The legal status of the organization needs to be specified, along with the ownership structure. Whether the organization is for-profit or not-for-profit will often make a difference in the process. For for-profit organizations, its legal status (e.g., partnership, corporation) will be a consideration for potential investors. At the same time, the ownership structure will provide information on the resources available to the organization on the one hand and on potentially contentious stakeholders on the other. For this reason, one of the first questions asked by external funding sources typically has to do with the organization's owners.

The business plan obviously goes much further than other types of plans in compiling financial data on the organization. Detailed statistics on the organization's past financial experience and its current financial status will be required. This will include balance sheets, profit and loss statements, and cash flow statements. Any unusual situations related to the organization's finances should be clearly explained.

Detailed information on sources of revenue will be required on the organization, and for most organizations this will be fairly straightforward. For a hospital, however, specifying distinct sources of revenue is much more complex. In some cases, personal financial statements and tax returns may be required of the owners.

Any existing contracts with clients should be identified and the prospects for continued relationships determined. The extent to which these contracts can be leveraged into new business for the proposed project will often be a consideration. For example, if the proposed business line is in direct response to requests from existing customers, converting them to the new service may be almost automatic.

Fortunately, a great deal of the information required for the business plan is likely to be readily available, since much of what is required involves standard business reporting. Many of these reports will have been routinely generated. Contemporary accounting software can generally accommodate the additional requirements of the business plan.

External Audit

The external audit in the business planning process involves the same steps described in earlier chapters for assessing the organization's environment. The process starts with an analysis of the macro-environment and progresses through the various levels down to the micro-environment. Broad social trends are reviewed and developments within the economy are analyzed for their implications for healthcare. Health industry trends are reviewed, with attention paid to developments in the regulatory and reimbursement arenas.

In the case of business planning, a great deal of emphasis is likely to be placed on the industry analysis. An overview of the industry (or more likely the industry segment) will be required. For example, if a hospital is considering entering the long-term care market, background information on both the hospital industry and the long-term care industry will probably be required. The overview should consider trends in the industry, including its stage in the industry life cycle. (See Box 10-1 on industry life cycle analysis.)

This overview should also pay particular attention to reimbursement trends and technological developments. Changes in reimbursement patterns could mean the difference between the success or failure of a business enterprise. Technological advances can quickly make a product or service obsolete.

This industry overview should also consider competitors within the industry. Other organizations that are in direct competition with this particular product or service should be identified, as well as those that are offering different but competing products.

With regard to the market in which the organization plans to compete, a market share analysis should be conducted. For an existing service, the organization's current market share should be determined, along with past trends in market share. To the extent this share can be disaggregated into components (e.g., demographic categories, payor types), the more useful the data will be. The analysis should consider the extent to which the organization might be able to capture additional market share.

For a new product or service, much of the emphasis will be placed on potential market share that can be captured. Consideration should be given to whether the project will involve capturing market share from existing players or if new markets are going to be tapped through this business venture.

In business planning, it is essential that the planning team get out into the market and talk to existing customers, potential customers, and industry experts. It will also be worthwhile to talk to healthcare colleagues offering similar programs in other markets. Third-party payors and potential referral agents should be contacted as appropriate. It is also worthwhile to attend trade shows, conferences, and professional association meetings to develop a better appreciation of what is transpiring in the market. Although the planning team may think it "knows the market", there are always going to be new developments that must be identified and evaluated.

The current and anticipated positioning of the organization with regard to the market is an important consideration. More precisely, what is the business positioning of the proposed product or service? Whether the proposed business line represents an innovative service, an improved or less expensive version of an existing service, or a convenient alternative to what is currently in the market makes a big difference in the business planning process.

Obviously, the identification of potential customers for the proposed business line is an important consideration. The size of the market should be determined and the capturable market share indicated. The extent to which existing relationships can be capitalized on should be determined.

BOX 10-1
Industry and Product Life Cycles

Regardless of the type of planning being initiated, an understanding of the stage of the industry or product life cycle is critical. For strategic planning initiatives, for example, the life cycle stage that characterizes the relevant segment of the industry should be considered. If the organization is primarily involved in providing inpatient services, for example, an appreciation of the point in the industry life cycle where inpatient services can be placed is required. If a business plan is being developed for a specific procedure, the point in the life cycle where this product resides must be determined.

The position in the industry or product life cycle has numerous implications for planning activities. It is likely to influence the packaging of service and products, promotional techniques, approaches to competitors and relationships with other organizations.

The first stage in the life cycle for an industry or product is the introduction or market development stage. At this point, a new product or perhaps an entirely new industry is emerging. Because the industry or product is likely to be innovative, most of the effort is directed toward creating awareness and cultivating "early adopters" in the market. At this stage, there are relatively few competitors, and products and services are not standardized. Entry into the market is relatively easy because there are few established players.

The second stage is the growth phase. At this point, the industry has become established, and the product or service has been accepted by the market. Expansion is rapid as new customers are attracted and additional competitors enter the arena. Products or services become increasingly standardized, although enhancements may continue to contribute to product evolution. Marketing planning at this stage emphasizes differentiation of the organization, product, or service.

During the third stage, the industry or product achieves maturity. At this point, most of the potential customers have been captured and growth begins to tail off. Because few new customers are available, competition for existing customers increases. Product features and pricing are highly standardized, and little differentiation remains between competitors. The

(continued)

number of competitors decreases as consolidation occurs among the various players in the market, and it becomes increasingly difficult for new players to enter the market. Marketing activities emphasize retaining existing customers and/or capturing competitors' customers.

At the final stage in the life cycle, the industry or product experiences a period of decline. The number of customers decreases as consumers substitute new products or services. There is typically a "shakeout" among industry players as the dominant competitors squeeze out the less entrenched and other competitors adopt a different strategic direction. Competition among the remaining players for existing customers becomes even more heated. Because no innovations are being introduced and the customer base cannot be expanded, there is increasing emphasis among the remaining competitors on reducing costs in order to maintain profitability. The graphic below depicts the life cycle progression, including examples from the health industry.

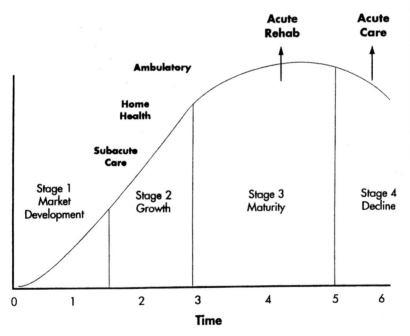

Figure 10-1. Product of life cycle (Developed by Fowler Healthcare affiliates, Inc.)

State-of-the-Business Report

At this stage of the process, it is usually worthwhile to present a state-of-the-business report. The nature of the report will depend on a variety of factors, including whether the plan is for a stand-alone facility or for a component of an existing organization, whether a new operation is being contemplated or the modification of an existing program, and whether the target is existing customers or new ones.

The state-of-the-business report should include the following sections summarizing the data collection up to this point:

- ✓ Overall industry/industry component trends
- ✓ Market area delineation
- ✓ Market area population profile
- ✓ Market area population health characteristics
- ✓ Current position of the organization or service
- ✓ Competitive situation
- ✓ Financial "health" of the organization
- ✓ Likely future developments

This status report should include the strengths, weaknesses, opportunities and threats identified during the analysis. This is an opportunity to frankly describe the state of the market and the organization's position in it. With the business plan, in fact, this is likely to represent a go/no go decision point. Assuming that the project will continue, this should be the launching point for subsequent plan development.

Project Planning

Project planning is an inherent component of the business planning process. In effect, the business plan is a project plan. More so that other plans, the business plan includes a month-by-month and year-by-year outline of the business development process. This will be involve input on staffing, expected expenses, and anticipated revenues for the time period being planned for.

DEVELOPING THE BUSINESS PLAN

The effort up to this point provides the foundation for the actual development of the plan. If the initial work is properly carried out, the planning process should flow smoothly, at least from a technical perspective. (See Figure 10-1 for a depiction of the business planning process.)

Specifying Goals

The goal or goals that are established for the business plan should reflect the information that was provided in the state-of-the-business report. As in other planning

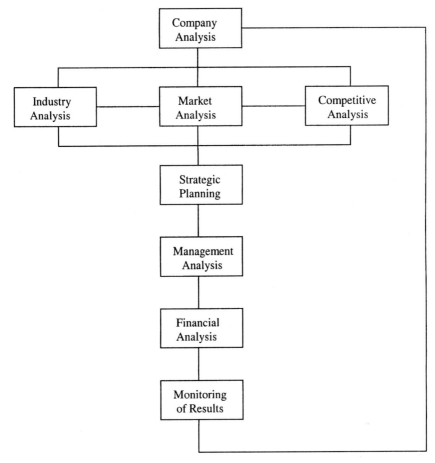

Figure 10-1. Business Planning Process. (*Source:* R.L. Leza, and J.F. Placencia (1988). *Develop Your Business Plan.* Grants Pass, OR: The Oasis Press)

activities, the goal should meet certain criteria before it is accepted. Chief among these is the goal's support of the organization's strategic plan and its compatibility with the organization's mission statement.

The number of goals to be established depends on the complexity and size of the organization and the nature of the issues at hand. However, with business planning there is likely to be a specific goal that reflects the focused nature of the project.

This phase of planning is somewhat different for business planning in the sense that, from the outset, the goal was likely to be clearly defined. This is in contrast to some other types of planning in which the goal may not be determined until well into the planning process. The emphasis in business planning is specifying how the organization is going to achieve predetermined goals.

Establishing Objectives

For every goal a number of objectives may be specified. Four or five objectives are fairly common, although many more than that becomes unwieldy. Objectives are stated in such terms as: The hospital will hire a manager for the pain management unit within three months (in support of the stated goal of establishing a pain management product line). Or, alternatively, the project will reach a breakeven point in 36 months.

Processing Financial Data

The business plan differs from other plans in that it is not enough to collect and analyze appropriate data; it must be further massaged to develop the information needed for fleshing out the plan. Obtaining past financial records is only one step. These figures must be converted into projections, with projected data being especially important in the case of a new organization. Since there would be no organizational history, projections have to be developed based on various assumptions. While one set of assumptions will guide the planning process, another set of assumptions will be developed for the financial analysis.

A complete set of financial statements should be prepared to support the proposed project. Typically these will be extended five years into the future. These documents should include balance sheets, profit and loss statements, and pro formas. They should also include projections of staffing, capital investment and any other activities that will impact the progress of the business venture. (Sample pro forma statements are included in Appendix III.)

To a great extent, the business plan represents an implementation plan per se, so that aspect of the planning process will not be discussed here. It should also be noted that the business plan will require a marketing plan as part of its overall development process.

PRESENTING THE BUSINESS PLAN

While other types of plans can follow a variety of formats, the business plan typically requires a standardized approach. For that reason, an outline of the business plan is presented in this chapter. The length of the business plan and the level of detail depend on the nature of the project and the anticipated audience. A generalized plan may suffice in some cases, but considerable detail will typically be required. In most cases, it is probably appropriate to develop two versions of the plan. One of these contains all of the detail required and provided for will ultimately be review *en toto* by a handful of individuals. A summary version of the business plan should also be developed that can be more widely circulated.

The following components should be included in the business plan.

✓ *Overview/Summary Statement on the Organization*
Present status
Strategic opportunities
Company thrust
Business strategies
Resource requirements
Expected benefits
Net cash requirements
Performance measures and milestones

✓ *Description of the Business or Department*
Philosophy
Goal(s)
Corporate overview
  Corporate history
  Products/Services
  Current customers
  Technology position
  Cost comparisons
  Operational resources
  Strengths/weaknesses
  Bases for competition
  Key success factors
  Competitive position

✓ *Industry Analysis*
Overview
Definition
Key growth factors
Industry life cycle
Competitors
Competing products
Financial measures

✓ *Market Analysis*
Overview of market/strategic opportunities
Market segmentation
Changes in demand/trends

Position in the market
Major customers/concentrations
Potential customers
Location(s)
Distribution capabilities
Pricing trends
Existing promotions/advertising
Competition
Promotional strategy
  (e.g., differentiation)
Market share and sales

✓ *Strategic Planning Status*
Overview of the plan
Plan assumptions
Long-term goals
Realistic assessment of strengths/weaknesses
Key performance indicators
Milestone schedule
Red flags
Company strengths to exploit
Weaknesses to overcome
Market opportunities to exploit
Risk analysis (See Figure 10-2.)

✓ *Organization Assessment*
Ownership structure
Management
Personnel
Consultants/specialists
Legal structure
Requirements in terms of permits, CON, regulatory agencies, licensure

✓ *Financial Data*
Sources of investment funds
Capital equipment
Real estate/insurance
Balance sheet
Profit and loss statement

Element	Ratings		
	Low	Medium	High
Industry	X		
Market			X
Competitive position		X	
Strategy		X	
Assumptions	X		
Financial performance	X		
Management performance		X	
Level of future performance	X		
Others			
Overall risk		X	

Figure 10-2. Risk Analysis (*Sourcee:* R.L. Leza, and J.F. Placencia [1988]. *Develop Your Business Plan*. Grants Pass, OR: The Oasis Press.)

Break-even analysis
Personal financial statements/tax
    returns
✓ *Conclusions*
✓ *Appendices*
Resumes

Pictures of facilities, equipment,
    other pertinent tangible
    factors
Existing contracts, relationships
Market studies
Pertinent published materials

THE OPERATIONAL PLAN

An important component of the business plan is the operational plan. Unlike the rest of the document, this component is primarily for internal use. The management team will use this for coordinating the efforts of corporate players in reaching the objectives set out in the business plan.

The operational plan incorporates components of the project plan and the implementation matrix discussed in other planning contexts. As such, it provides an indication of how the project will be carried out over the five-year planning period. The plan is "operational" in the sense that its lays out the actual process of operating the facility, service or program and not simply for its establishment.

Additional Resources

Abrams, R.M. (1998). *The Successful Business Plan: Secrets and Strategies.* Grants Pass, OR: The Oasis Press (software available).

Jian Tools for Sales (2003). *BizPlan Builder.* Computer Software. Jian Tools for Sales, Mountain View, CA.

11

Research Methods for Health Services Planning

INTRODUCTION

The significant role played by research in the planning process should be obvious from even a casual review of the preceding chapters. Much of the time and effort involved in planning can be attributed to the research activities that lead up to and support the planning function. Every type of planning requires some degree of research support. Even traditional types of organizational planning that are essentially introspective require some spadework. For more externally oriented planning initiatives, extensive research activity is inevitably required. Without the appropriate knowledge base, the planning team will have little foundation for developing the plan.

The type and amount of research undertaken during the planning process is dictated by a number of factors, including the kind of planned being formulated, the nature of the organization, the available resources, and the intended use of the findings. A critical skill for the planner is the ability to determine the type and scope of research appropriate for a particular planning initiative.

In an ideal world, the research necessary to support planning would be an ongoing function within the organization. It is not practical to initiate discrete research projects from scratch to support every planning initiative. By the time most organizations can mount a data collection process, the planning period is likely to be over. With ongoing monitoring systems in place, the ability to track changes in physician referral patterns, trends in admissions, or emerging market niches, for example, is certainly enhanced.

Because of the various aspects of planning that could come into play, this chapter can only serve as an introduction to the research activities that support planning. The resources listed at the end of the chapter will provide some additional guidance.

PLANNING RESEARCH: WHO'S RESPONSIBILITY?

Early in the planning process a decision must be made concerning the project's research requirements. Even the most basic type of planning research is likely to require certain skills, substantive knowledge, and familiarity with multiple methodologies and perspectives. In cases where the community or the organization does not have an on-going planning effort, the requisite skills may be lacking. While a community may have certain research skills resident within various organizations, these resources may not be readily available to the planning team. There may, in fact, be resistance to any particular organization having a dominant role in this important function.

A major decision, thus, involves the assignment of responsibility for the research function. The range of research options available to communities and organizations includes: performing all planning research in-house using internal resources; totally outsourcing the research process; and utilizing a combination of internal and external resources. The last named may involve performing some research functions in house while outsourcing others. Another "compromise" approach might involve bringing in an outside consultant to coordinate the use of internal resources for the planning research. The option chosen will depend to a great extent on the overall approach taken to the planning process. If the planning itself is being outsourced, the research activities would probably be carried out under that auspices. If the planning is being done totally in house, it might be more practical to use internal resources. The corporate culture of the organization will also be a factor influencing the approach taken.

There are numerous advantages to bringing an outside expert into the research process, regardless of the level of internal capabilities available. An outside resource is likely to introduce a broader perspective than that held by those closely involved with the organization, in addition to having had experience with similar organizations. The outside consultant may have expertise in specialized techniques that are required for the project or may already have expensive resources (e.g., geographic information systems) that would otherwise have to be acquired. From a political perspective, the outsider may bring a measure of objectivity and neutrality that might not be available internally.

There are disadvantages to using outside experts as well. They can be very expensive and a certain level of sophistication is required in order to negotiate a reasonable contract. (Note that there are no small costs involved in carrying out research activities in house, particularly if no dedicated function is already in place.) There may be situations in which such sensitive data is involved that outside access may be undesirable. Further, an outsider is an outsider, and there may be aspects of the community or organization that are difficult to understand without having an insider's perspective. Ultimately, every organization will have to weigh the pluses and minuses of using outside resources for planning research.

THE APPROACH TO PLANNING RESEARCH

Planning research involves a number of distinct components that generally follow a certain sequence. With each component the intent is to collect data that can be converted into information that can, in turn, serve as the basis for identifying solutions. Raw numbers are of limited use until they are converted into meaningful information. Information is only beneficial if it can contribute to decision making.

Within this general framework, the following functions served by the planning research process can be identified:

Describing

The first responsibility of the health services planner is to describe the community or the market under consideration. Description here refers to the development of a (usually) comprehensive profile of the target area being studied. It may be a population, a patient grouping, or any number of other appropriate targets for the analysis. The planner must develop an informed description of the chosen subject, taking into consideration the relevant dimensions of that subject.

Identifying

Typically the description of a community or market is followed by the identification of distinct patterns or noteworthy attributes related to the target community or organization. These phenomena may involve unserved or underserved populations, a service niche that is not being addressed, a lack of certain equipment, or a variety of other conditions. Identifying patterns and attributes takes description a step further and extracts from the numerous possibilities within the typical market the meaningful options (and threats) within that context.

Comparing

An important step in the processing of data collected during research is the comparison of findings to relevant benchmarks. Depending on the plan, this may involve comparing one population to another, one health indicator to another, or one hospital to another. Analysis of the health indicators for a community may involve comparisons with historical figures, with other comparable communities, with national averages, or with established benchmarks. Similarly, an analysis of the data collected on a community hospital may involve comparisons to the hospital's past performance, a competitor's performance, JCAHO guidelines, or a benchmark set in the hospital's business plan. Through comparative analysis, the planner can begin to determine what the research findings *mean*.

Comparative analysis can be extended further in the research process when different options present themselves. A community may need to compare potential sites for a public health clinic. A healthcare organization may need to compare one market to another or one business opportunity to another. There are seldom going to be clear-cut choices in terms of appropriate services to be offered. The planner must be able to comparatively analyze the options, employing both quantitative and qualitative techniques.

Evaluating

It is seldom enough to describe a community or organization or to simply identify noteworthy patterns. The status of the community or organization must be evaluated based on relevant criteria. The comparative analysis above provides a basis for evaluating existing services, personnel or market opportunities. The analyst's ability to assess whether a situation is favorable or unfavorable is critical for the planning activities that follow.

Ultimately, the planner must determine if a situation is "good" or "bad". If it is found, for example, that the community reports 5 hospital beds per 1,000 population, this figure must be evaluated. If the national standard is 4 beds / 1,000, it could be concluded that, all things being equal, the community has overcapacity in terms of beds. If, on the other hand, the community is a regional medical center and draws patients from surrounding counties that lack hospitals, a different "read" could be made on the statistics. This is where the skills of the planner start coming into play.

Monitoring

Planning research activities typically involve the monitoring of various phenomena. This may mean monitoring population trends in a potential target area, tracking changes in patient satisfaction, or measuring the impact of marketing initiatives on the consumer image of the organization. Especially to the extent that planning is an on-going function, monitoring in some form is likely to be one of the responsibilities.

Interpreting

At a time when few sources of health data existed, decision makers were happy with any information they could get access to. Today, with access to data less of an issue, the emphasis is on the ability to interpret the massive amounts of data that have become available within the industry. The ability to analyze and interpret the data that have been collected (i.e., convert data into information) is what distinguishes a planner from a technician.

Recommending

The next step beyond interpreting the data involves recommending actions suggested by the planning research. This may involve a go/no go decision or a choice among a number of different options. Increasingly, planning analysts are being asked to go beyond simply turning the numbers over to someone else for decision making. The planning team is likely to expect the one answer they are looking for and not a lot of confusing options. The growing emphasis on generating recommendations reflects the shift from a technically-oriented planning approach to a management-oriented approach.

TYPES OF RESEARCH

The research component of the planning process is likely to involve a variety of methodologies, the choice of which are determined by the type of organization and the type of plan involved. In formulating the research design to support the planning effort, three general categories of research should be considered based on the type of information required. These three categories of research are *exploratory, descriptive*, and *causal*.

The goal of exploratory research is the discerning of the general nature of the problem or opportunity under study and identifying the associated factors of importance. Exploratory research is characterized by a high degree of flexibility, and usually relies heavily on literature reviews, small-scale surveys, informal interviews and discussions, and a subjective evaluation of the data. Exploratory designs are typically used for initial information gathering in the early stages of a planning initiative. The objective here is to gain insights into the planning context and gather information, even if anecdotal, that may inform further planning research.

Descriptive research involves the development of a factual portrait of the various components of the community or organization that are being examined. Market profiles, community assessments, and resource inventories are examples of the products of descriptive research. Any source of information can be used in a descriptive study, although most studies of this nature rely heavily on secondary data sources and survey research. Carefully designed descriptive studies represent the backbone of planning research, and they provide the basis for any subsequent research that is performed. The bulk of the effort in planning-oriented data collection is geared toward descriptive studies, with no pretense of explaining the "why" of any of the observed findings.

Causal (or inferential) research attempts to specify the nature of the functional relationship between two or more variables in the situation under study. For example, a study of the relationship between place of medical training and physician referral patterns would probably involve an analysis of cause-and-effect relationships. A study on the market response to a promotional campaign would seek to isolate and identify the ways in which increased advertising, for example, fostered a rise in outpatient visits. Causal research designs typically infer relationships, since a direct causal relationship usually cannot be conclusively demonstrated.

Little of the planning-oriented research conducted in healthcare in the past could be characterized as casual research. Although causal research has contributed to an understanding of the motivation for consumer behavior in other industries, health services planning has a long way to go to arrive at this level of sophistication.

STEPS IN THE RESEARCH DESIGN PROCESS

The planning research process can be conceptualized as a multistage endeavor. The exact number of stages varies from planning analyst to planning analyst and from problem to problem, but all research designs include certain basic elements. The process leads from the initial inquiry (e.g., is the management of eating disorders a service worth pursuing?) to the ultimate decision made by the organization (e.g., a pilot eating disorders program should be initiated). No two experts agree completely on the steps involved in the research process, and research that supports health services planning has unique characteristics that distinguish it from the process in other industries. The steps below represent the general order of activities in the research plan, although there is nothing sacred about the order in which they occur. The steps in the design process sometimes interact and often occur simultaneously, and they should be modified as appropriate to suit the particular planning exercise.

Initial Information Gathering

In planning research the first step typically involves developing a generalized understanding of the community or organization for which planning is occurring. For community-wide planning, a general knowledge of the community is clearly required. If a strategic planning initiative is being undertaken for an organization, a reasonable knowledge of the nature of the organization needs to be developed. For a marketing planning initiative, information on the product or service is required, as well as information on the market area. If it is a business planning initiative, a reasonable understanding of the financial operation of the organization is necessary.

A review of the existing literature is an obvious place to start the research process. "Literature" is used here in a very broad sense. In traditional research this typically refers to the professional journals in which the field's conventional wisdom is codified. Unfortunately, health services planning has yet to develop a body of professional journals comparable to those in other industries. (In fact, the term "health planning" was virtually absent from the industry literature during the 1980s and early 1990s.) The literature for health services planning will include not only traditional journals but newsletters, government reports, technical papers, professional meeting presentations, annual reports, and the publications of professional associations.

Today, planners can gain access to the Internet for literature reviews and other sources of relevant information. Most bibliographic databases can be accessed through the Internet and any number of other sources—some of them quite serendipitous—can be uncovered by accessing the World Wide Web. Another type of electronic "literature review" involves the growing volume of e-mail exchanges among networks of health professionals. An increasing amount of health-related data is becoming available via the World Wide Web and the Internet is becoming a standard research tool. (See Box 11-1 for a discussion of health data on the Internet.)

Identifying Issues

Issue definition is an important step in the planning research process. Unless the issues are properly defined, the information produced by the research process is unlikely to have much value. In planning research, the "problem" is likely to be defined in terms of a process or the specific issues related to a process. The scope of the research is thus much broader and diffuse than it is in many other types of research projects.

Isolating the relevant issues becomes an important early task in the research process. Planning initiatives are typically triggered by a crisis or a concern of some type. The "iceberg" effect often can often be found, in that the apparent issue is simply the tip of the iceberg and suggests that there are other, perhaps more serious, underlying concerns. It is also often the case that the problem posed by the party initiating the process may be quite different from the "real" problem. This is part of the art of planning research, with the planner being able to examine the situation and determine the nature of the underlying issues. A more precise statement of the issues may imply a very different research problem from the initial statement.

BOX 11-1
Health Data and the Internet

As the world has now discovered, the World Wide Web is becoming a global information repository that can be easily accessed via the Internet. At the time of this writing, there was thought to be more health-related data available via the Internet than on any other topic. Not only are there more sites dealing with more aspects of health, but some of the most extensive sites have been established by healthcare organizations.

Despite the spate of health-related data available via the Internet, most of it has been of limited usefulness to the health professional until recently. The overwhelming majority of health sites offer data geared to healthcare consumers. The ready "market" has been for consumer data, and there was no shortage of consumer-oriented organizations eager to establish a presence on the Web. Today, healthcare consumers can find a doctor, diagnose a condition, or order prescription drugs and nutritional supplements via the Internet.

By the mid-1990s the information needs of health professionals were beginning to be recognized. In response to this need, various organizations responded by offering data via the Internet. This involved making data files available to be viewed, browsed and downloaded. More advanced sites may actually allow the user to manipulate the data in some basic ways. Even commercial data vendors are searching for ways to make data more accessible via the Internet.

The federal government has led the charge to make raw data available on the Web. Agencies such as the Census Bureau, the Centers for Disease Control and Prevention, the National Center for Health Statistics, and the Center for Medicare and Medicaid Services have expended significant effort toward posting their data files on the Web. Not only do these data files represent improvements over the cumbersome output formats (e.g., print, magnetic tape) that these agencies historically used, but Web-based files can be posted much more expeditiously than the data can be published in print form. Plus, many of these sites offer data for downloading at no charge, data that often had to be purchased from various agencies in the past. Some of these data sets would never be published in print form, making, for example, data available for levels of geography that would be much to cumbersome to publish in hard copy in any case. As print versions of data reports are steadily eliminated by the federal government and other data generators, the importance of Internet distribution will increase.

The initial response of health data users has been enthusiastic. At last it has become possible to obtain data on a variety of topics from a "single source". However, as one gets serious about using Web-based data files from any of these sources, this enthusiasm can be quickly dampened. The following issues face health professionals who see the World Wide Web as a valuable source of data:

Ease of Access

While the sites that are posting data files are generally easy to access, the user can quickly run into roadblocks when searching for data. (As is always the case, if one knows exactly where to look it is less of a problem.) Sites maintained by the Census Bureau or the Centers for Disease Control, for example, are extensive and complex. Further, the provision of data files for use or download may not be the primary function of these organizations and their Web sites. Thus, the data user may have to wade through a number of screens before the issue of data is even broached. Even then, the data files are likely to be numerous and, in the absence of any standard categories, searching the site becomes problematic.

Ease of Use

One of the advantages of electronically formatted data files should be their ease of use. By being posted in what is typically a "spreadsheet" format, the user should be able to easily navigate through these files and manipulate the data in them in a number of ways. Unfortunately, many of these files simply replicate the print version in electronic format. As such, they are not searchable, and their use as spreadsheets is therefore limited. In fact, there are some advantages that print versions actually offer over those in an electronic format.

File Size and Structure

In many cases, Web-based files represent too much of a good thing. Since the amount of data that can be included in an electronic file is essentially unlimited, there is a tendency to post such large files that it becomes difficult to manage them. There also appears to be a tendency to place "unedited" files out on the Web. For example, a federal database may be made available

(continued)

for downloading that contains mostly internal variables that are of no use to the user. Thus, processing an otherwise useless file may require more effort than it is worth in some cases.

Documentation

Any data file is going to require an extensive amount of documentation in terms of sources of data, calculation methodologies, explanation of variable names, etc. The electronic format offers the advantage of unlimited space for the presentation of documentation. However, the rush to post data files on the Web has caused many to overlook an important intermediate step: developing standard documentation formats. Even within a single government agency, the data files posted may include a variety of different formats with different approaches to documentation.

Downloading Issues

One of the advantages of Web-based data files should be the ability to download them for use in another environment. While this advantage generally exists with regard to these data files, there are issues related to downloading that represent barriers to efficient use of these resources. Many of the files are in formats that require specialized software for downloading and reading. While these "utilities" may be readily available and often free via download, they are not necessarily intuitively obvious to the beginner trying to access

Developing the Research Plan

As in any research process, a carefully thought out research plan must be developed. The initial information gathering stage should provide a guide to the types of data that will be required. The nature of the planning initiative will also dictate certain research requirements. Thus, a community-wide plan will typically require a broader range of data than an organization-level plan; a strategic plan will involve a broader research scope than a technology plan; research on the competitive situation will be more important for a business plan than for a community-wide plan; and so forth.

The nature of the planning initiative will determine the objectives of the research plan, and various action steps will specify the effort required. The categories of data to be considered, the means of collecting the relevant data, the indicators to be utilized, and the analytical techniques to be employed, among other attributes, are included in the research plan.

these data files. Some of these downloading applications do not work on all computers and downloading the utilities themselves requires a certain level of technical expertise. Further, some of the files are huge, and appropriate software may be required for decompressing these files.

Quality Issues

As with other Internet sources of data, it is easier and quicker to post health-related data on the Web than it is to verify their accuracy and usefulness. Data files that are posted may include provisional data or be otherwise incomplete. If they include data collected from different states, for example, the data may vary in methodology or time period. This may not be obvious to the user, although this is an issue with print data files as well.

The use of the Internet as a vehicle for making data files available for viewing and downloading represents a giant step forward in health data distribution. In fact, the Web may come to truly be a single source for health-related data. Today, however, there are significant issues associated with the data files that are being made available via this environment. There are obvious barriers to efficient use that will be obvious to users but not so obvious ones that could be disastrous. While hard copy data files will continue to be useful, the presence of the Internet is likely to steadily expand the importance of electronic access to data files.

The research plan specifies the sequence in which various research efforts are to be carried out, the responsible party(s), the resources required, and the timeframes involved. The plan should also specify the "products" that are expected from the research effort.

Specifying the Analytical Approach

Data are useful only after they have been analyzed. Data analysis involves converting a series of observations, however obtained, into descriptive statements and/or inferences about relationships. The types of analyses chosen reflects such factors as the nature of the sampling process, the measurement instrument utilized, and the data collection method.

Since most planning research is essentially descriptive, the analytical methods utilized may not be as complex as in more basic research. Nevertheless, it is important to visualize the types of output that the research is expected to generate and specify the analytical approaches that provide the desired outcome.

A variety of different analytical approaches can be utilized, with the choice being dictated to a great extent by the type of plan. Virtually all plans will involve a demographic analysis, but the use of epidemiological analysis, for example, may be more appropriate for community-wide planning than for organization-level planning. Examples of useful analytical techniques are presented later in this chapter.

Research Resource Allocation

Once the research plan has been developed, the planner must estimate resource requirements. The requirements can be quantified in terms of time, money and personnel. If the research is to be conducted in house, resources can be broken down into direct expenses (e.g., to hire additional interviewers) and "in-kind" contributions such as staff time, office space, and supplies. Time refers to both the time needed to complete the project and the time commitment required of personnel. The financial requirement is the monetary representation of personnel time, computer time, and materials requirements. In addition, the opportunity costs incurred by those participating in planning-oriented research must be calculated to the extent possible.

If an outside consultant or resource is to implement the process, the determination of costs must be calculated differently. The consultant will typically present a proposal that includes cost estimates for performing the requisite research. The planning team will work with the consultant to determine the nature of the process and the division of labor between internal staff and consulting staff.

Project management tools like the program evaluation review technique (PERT) and the critical path method (CPM) offer useful aids for estimating the resources needed for a project and for clarifying the planning and control process. PERT involves dividing the total research project into its smallest components activities, determining the sequence in which these activities must be performed, attaching a time estimate for each activity, and presenting them in the form of a flow chart that allows a visual inspection of the overall process. The time estimates allow planners to determine the critical path through the chart.

Data Collection

Data collection involves the actual process of acquiring the raw data that will be converted into the information needed for the planning analysis. The data collection process can take a variety of forms, but will typically involve both primary data acquisition and the compilation of secondary data. Secondary data are virtually always collected first because they are likely to be readily available without much in the way of additional expense. Primary research is likely to be used when certain types of data cannot be acquired through secondary research.

Planners obviously have a variety of techniques to utilize for data collection. In considering the alternatives available for any project, the advantages and disadvantages of each approach should be considered. In using any one of these approaches, there are special concerns which the researcher must address and be cognizant of to ensure that the data collected will be reliable and valid.

As noted above, the typical research project will involve both primary data and secondary data. For example, in collecting data to support planning for a proposed new health service, an analyst may (1) examine hospital records for information relating to the past introductions of similar services (secondary data); (2) conduct a set of interviews to determine current consumer attitudes about the service (primary survey research); and (3) conduct a pilot study in which consumer reception of the proposed service is measured (primary experimental research).

Since an unlimited amount of data on an infinite number of topics can be collected, the planner must ensure that any data collected are relevant to the issues at hand. In particular, care must be taken to assure that the data collected is "actionable". Some things may be interesting to know, but, if they do not contribute to the process, they may not be necessary. Specifically, the planner should list the questions that need to be answered by the end of the study and structure the data collection process accordingly. The potential benefit of any information should be determined prior to collection.

Methods for conducting primary research are discussed later in this chapter. Sources of secondary data are described in Chapter 12.

Data Analysis

Data analysis involves the processing, manipulation and analysis of the data collected through the means specified in the research plan. A variety of techniques for statistical analysis can be applied, although the descriptive nature of most planning research mitigates against the use of sophisticated analyses. Basic statistics will typically suffice for most planning analyses.

On another level, however, there are a number of analytical approaches that could be utilized that contribute to the interpretation of the data. For example, the health services planner should probably be familiar with the techniques utilized in demographic analyses, the methods developed by epidemiologists, and approaches to evaluation analysis. Several of these techniques are described later in this chapter.

Drawing Conclusions

The main objective in analyzing the data that have been collected is the generation of conclusions related to the planning issues. The conclusions drawn will rely heavily on the analysis step described above. Properly chosen analytical techniques should generate useful findings.

Conclusions may be drawn at various levels in keeping with the tiered approach (described in the discussion of the environmental assessment). There are likely to be conclusions drawn concerning trends at the national level, the state level, and for the local market. These may relate to findings concerning market share, utilization trends, or changing market characteristics.

These conclusions should provide the basis for subsequent planning activities. Some of them, in fact, become a part of the assumptions that have been stated and restated throughout this process.

Formulating Recommendations

The formulation of recommendations is a relatively new role for the researcher, but one that is likely to grow in significance. Historically, planning research has been seen as a technical support function. The researcher's role was to turn over numbers to administrators and they would make the appropriate decisions.

As planning issues have become more complex and research methods more sophisticated, planners are increasingly asked to offer recommendations. Rather than providing the decision maker with three objectively compared options for review, the analyst is likely to be asked to indicate the best choice among the three given the results of the various analyses.

PRIMARY DATA COLLECTION METHODS

Virtually every planning study is going to require the collection of primary data. There are always going to be situations when the desired information is simply not available. This is particularly the case in an industry undergoing the rapid and dramatic changes that characterize healthcare today.

The major advantage of primary data is that the information is collected for the particular problem or issue under investigation, making the data more directly relevant and current than most secondary data. Another major advantage is that primary data collection allows the organization to maintain the proprietary nature of the information collected. Conducting primary research also gives the planner control over the types of information elicited, rather than having to rely on questions asked by another party perhaps with quite different intentions.

Primary data collection, however, has some disadvantages. The collection of primary data can entail significant costs and require an extended period of time to complete. The administration of primary research also requires some fairly sophisticated skills that may not be available within the organization.

When initiating primary research activities, the "right" data collection method depends on a number of factors. There are many alternative methods to choose from in conducting such research (Creswell, 1994). Several commonly used methods—both quantitative and qualitative—for collecting primary data are described below. (Box 11-2 compares qualitative and quantitative approaches to research.)

BOX 11-2
Bringing Back Qualitative Data

For much of the last half of the 20th century, the importance of quantitative data eclipsed that of qualitative data in healthcare as it did in other fields. Researchers and administrators became enamored with survey research in particular. Because there was a substantial body of knowledge related to survey research, it was relatively easy to conduct virtually any kind of study that involved interviews of patients, their families and friends, healthcare professionals, and physicians. Indeed, there were even those who argued against any use of qualitative data, claiming that such information was "soft" and the qualitative research process lacked scientific rigor.

By the end of the century, however, the use of qualitative data had become increasingly common, even in the healthcare industry. It became standard practice for healthcare providers to conduct focus groups and other interviews. The use of observation for data collection and content analysis for examining health-related data were increasingly used to supplement quantitative approaches. New software designed for the analysis of qualitative data facilitated the use of qualitative data.

This renewed interest in qualitative research reflects to a certain extent the growing willingness of researchers to concede the shortcomings of strictly quantitative research in healthcare. There are numerous subjective dimensions to the experience of illness and the operation of the delivery system. Further, many aspects of healthcare simply cannot be understood without the use of qualitative methods.

As healthcare enters the 21st century, researchers and planners recognize the value of both qualitative and quantitative methods, and the importance of using these methods in tandem is being increasingly appreciated. Surveys in healthcare are no longer limited to closed-ended questions that restrict responses. Open-ended questions are frequently employed and the answers subjected to qualitative analytical techniques. In data-driven healthcare organizations, continuous collection, monitoring and analysis of both types of data is becoming standard procedure.

The research required to support the planning process should involve both quantitative and qualitative techniques. Planners must strive to coordinate the two types of data collection and analysis in order to successfully implement the research component of the planning process.

Observation

Observational research involves techniques in which the actions and/or attributes of those being studied are observed either by another individual or through a mechanical recording device such as a video camera. Information is not so much elicited from the subjects as it is observed. Data collection by means of observation is performed according to specified rules based on stated objectives.

Before observation can be used in planning research, three minimum conditions must be met. First, the data must be accessible via observation. Motivations, attitudes, opinions, and other "internal" conditions cannot be readily observed. On the other hand, behavior in a waiting room, for example, can be observed and recorded. Second, the behavior must be repetitive, frequent or otherwise predictable, since the primary objective is to identify patterns. Finally, an event must be of relatively short duration. Thus, we are usually restricted to observing activities that can be completed in a relatively short time span, such as clinic visits or segments of activities with a longer time span.

Observational methods are typically used in planning research when data cannot be obtained through interviews or from secondary sources. This approach is particularly useful when a process is being analyzed. For example, a hospital might place a trained observer in its patient waiting area to observe the admitting process. Observers might track individual emergency patients from their initial encounter in the admitting area through their examination in the emergency room. Some organizations may even use a "professional shopper" program to improve the organization's ability to perform this type of observational research. By actually going through the admissions process, for example, simulated patients may obtain more information about the process than any other method would yield.

Observational techniques are characterized as either participatory or nonparticipatory. In participatory observation, the researcher becomes part of the group or activity that is being observed. Participant observation allows the observer to analyze the group, situation or process as an "insider". Also, by becoming part of the group, the impact of the observation process on behavior hopefully is minimized. However, the participant observer typically cannot take notes or otherwise record the observations that are being made. Thus, the observer must rely on memory for the recording of observations at a later date. The greatest concern, of course, relates to the possibility of the observer's mere presence altering the behavior of those being observed.

Non-participant observation involves a situation in which the researcher is detached from the individuals, situations or processes that are being observed. In some cases the observer may view the subjects from afar or, in more controlled environments, through the one-way mirror of an observation booth. The advantage of this approach is that the process typically does not affect the phenomena being observed, since the subjects do not know they are being observed.

One disadvantage of observational research is that the researcher is not in a position to control the variables under study, either physically or statistically.

Further, observational data are difficult to quantify. There are likely to be a small number of observations, and the open-endedness of the information collected typically does not lend itself to quantitative analysis.

Although observational data are useful in observing what people do, they cannot address *why* people behave in the way they do. Thus, it is often necessary to supplement observational research with personal interviews or some other form of data collection to determine the motivations underlying of the observed behavior.

Indepth Interviews

Complicated questions, or questions that do not lend themselves to simple dichotomous responses, often require personal interviews. Indepth interviews typically involve one respondent and one interviewer. The indepth interview is of value when the respondent must be probed regarding his or her answers. The interview does not necessarily follow a defined set of questions that must be asked in a predetermined order, but probes and questions as necessary to elicit the required information.

Indepth interviews are sometimes referred to as "key informant" interviews. They typically last 30 to 45 minutes, but can last several hours. There is latitude within the interview to ask ad hoc questions, follow up on responses that appear worthy of further exploration, and generally elicit the best information possible within this research framework.

Indepth interviews appear to be the most useful in situations where more superficial data collection techniques will not work. These include situations in which extensive probing is required, where the subject matter may be very complicated, confidential or sensitive, or the group influence (e.g., in the focus group setting) may be a distraction.

Ostensibly, indepth interviews can be conducted with anyone presumed to have knowledge of a particular topic. However, in healthcare indepth interviews are usually carried out with key informants who: possess a particular set of knowledge (e.g., technical innovators); have a broad perspective for the issues (e.g., hospital administrators); are in a position to be familiar with the perspectives of a large number of people (e.g., human resources manager); or are likely to hold influential opinions (e.g., hospital medical staff members).

It is difficult to imagine undertaking any planning initiative within a healthcare organization without including indepth interviews with key informants. One of the initial tasks is to identify the problems or opportunities being faced by an organization. Indepth interviews provide an excellent setting for this type of problem/opportunity identification. In fact, such interviews are typically used as a basis for constructing the survey forms that are used in subsequent quantitative research.

Personal interviews have some limitations. This method requires skilled interviewers, and even then there is potential for bias on the part of interviewers or misrepresentation on the part of respondents. There is also the danger of "experts" going off on a tangent. A physician-respondent on a "soapbox" may be difficult to rein in.

Group Interviews

In recent years one of the most popular qualitative research techniques in healthcare has been the group interview. Group interviews can be relatively structured, as in the case of *focus groups*, or more informal, as in the case of *naturally occurring groups*. Focus groups consist of a group of people who are assembled to discuss a particular topic of interest under the direction of a professional moderator. The objective is to have people express their feelings or views on a range of interests. Naturally occurring groups in healthcare might include all persons working the same shift in a particular department or the families and friends of patients admitted to a hospital.

Focus groups can be used for several purposes. For example, information from focus groups might be used in the construction of a survey instrument. A second frequent use of the focus group is in needs assessment. For example, a hospital might want to better understand the type of programs or services they could provide that would be valuable to referral physicians.

Focus groups are often used to test ideas for new programs or services. For example, an orthopedic medicine group might conduct focus groups among parents of youth between the ages of six and eighteen years to assess the feasibility of establishing a pediatric sports medicine program.

Another valuable use of focus groups is in examining the underlying meaning of survey results. Often, in conducting a quantitative survey, the organization examines the response and finds, for example, that fifty percent of the emergency room patients thought the service was unsatisfactory. A focus group among emergency room users might help reveal the reasons behind the quantitative findings.

As with any research methodology there are advantages and disadvantages to focus groups. The advantages of focus groups include:

✓ The synergy created by the group environment
✓ The ability to probe for additional information or follow unexpected directions
✓ Relatively low costs
✓ Short data collection and analysis time spans
✓ The richness of the data collected
✓ Direct input from consumers or patients

While the advantages of a focus group are several, it is also important to recognize the limitations which exist for this technique. Some of these include:

✓ Lack of control of variables
✓ Inability to use quantitative analytical techniques

✓ The challenge of analyzing subjective data
✓ Group variations due to small "samples"
✓ Potential moderator bias
✓ An inability to generalize the results

The focus group method would never be used as the primary tool for planning research. It does serve, however, to provide useful insights that can contribute to a formulation of the issues and the development of subsequent research activities. As such, it is a useful supplement to the other research techniques employed.

Survey Research

Many, if not most, planning projects will involve some survey research. Survey research can take one of three common forms: mail-out surveys, personal interviews, and telephone interviews. Computerized interviews and fax-based surveys are also becoming common. Each of these forms of survey research is described below.

Mail Surveys

Mail surveys are a common method of administering sample surveys. Mail surveys involve the development of a survey instrument, the identification of an appropriate sample of respondents, and the mailing of survey forms to the sample. Returned survey forms are analyzed according to predetermined analytical techniques.

Mail surveys have the advantage of being a relatively inexpensive way to collect data. Typically, administration costs involve the reproduction of the survey form and the postage to send and return it. Mail surveys provide anonymity to the respondent and eliminate potential interviewer bias. Mail is also an efficient way to contact individuals who are dispersed over a large geographical area. For this reason, mail surveys are often used in healthcare to collect patient satisfaction data.

While mail surveys have these advantages, there are several disadvantages to this data collection method. Response rates to mail-out surveys are often low. The instruments are self administered, leaving survey items open to interpretation on the part of the respondent. "Turnaround" time may be lengthy, and the short timeframes characterizing much marketing planning, for example, may preclude the use of this method.

Personal Interviews

A second method of surveying individuals involves personal (or face-to-face) interviews. An individual interview is a valuable way to collect data when the respondent must be probed regarding his or her answers. Complicated questions or questions that require explication on the part of the interviewer can best be handled in a face-to-face situation. In contrast to the indepth interview, these interviews are relatively short, involve a larger number of respondents, and require that those interviewed be representative of the population being studied. Personal interviews typically require a lower level of interviewing skills and less substantive knowledge of the topic than indepth interviews.

In planning research, the focus is often on specific audiences. For this reason, on-site interviews are often conducted. The waiting rooms of clinics, emergency departments and other healthcare facilities offer such an opportunity. This survey approach has become popular in recent years since it has the advantage of face-to-face interviewing without the expense of the door-to-door canvassing involved in community surveys.

There was a day when "community surveys" were routinely conducted, but they are much less common today. With the community survey, a sample of households is selected and an interviewer or a team of interviewers contacts individuals in their homes for the interviews. Today, the costs involved in community surveys have become nearly prohibitive. Further, the perceived danger involved in sending interviewers into various neighborhoods has made many research organizations reluctant to use this approach. At the same time, it is difficult to find respondents at home during much of the day, and potential respondents are increasingly reluctant to open their doors to strangers.

In terms of cost, the personal interview is the most expensive of the survey approaches. Trained interviewers are required, and all travel costs for interviewers must be considered in the budget. Another drawback beside the cost is the potential for interviewer bias. Untrained interviewers may condition responses by their reactions to answers or by their mannerisms, or they may fail to accurately follow the wording of a survey.

Telephone Interviews

The third common survey technique involves the telephone interview. While there have been increasing complaints from consumers about the intrusive nature of telephone surveys, this methodology still offers many advantages. Telephone interviews represent a quick way to acquire information. Using multiple interviewers in a telephone interview bank, considerable data can be acquired in a short time-frame. If the interviewers have some "hook", a high response rate can generally be obtained. Telephone interviewing allows for a reasonable degree of probing by the interviewer. On the other hand, while it is often difficult for a respondent to terminate a personal interview, terminating a telephone interview is easy.

There is an inherent sampling bias with telephone interviews in that they require the respondent to have a telephone. While telephone ownership is high in this country, certain areas or populations may have significantly lower telephone ownership than the national average and many individuals are eliminating the use of land lines in favor of cellular service. Low-income populations and racial and ethnic minority groups, in particular, have lower than average levels of telephone installation.

Increasingly, people are requesting unlisted telephone numbers, making the phone directory, always a questionable sampling frame, even less useful. One method to address this problem uses computerized programs to perform a random digit dialing sequence working from the prefixes utilized in an area and generating the last four digits randomly. Still another approach involves randomly selecting numbers listed in the telephone directory or other directories and systematically adding or subtracting one from the last digit. (See Dillman [1978] for the definitive reference on the effective administration of mail and telephone surveys.)

Computer-assisted telephone interviewing (CATI) has become increasingly common among survey researchers, and inexpensive software has made this technology available to most interviewers. A CATI system involves a survey workstation in which the telephone interviewer enters answers to survey items directly into the questionnaire programmed into the system. The responses are automatically entered into the computer and typically directly into the database to be utilized for analysis. The intelligence built into the software application can "flag" out-of-range answers, adjust subsequent questions based on earlier answers, and automatically lead the interviewer through a series of branching questions.

Computerized Interviews

Computer-based interviews have become increasingly popular as software has become more user friendly, and the general public has become more comfortable with computers. In computerized interviewing, the computer presents the survey items to the respondent on the screen in very much the same form it would take on a printed interview questionnaire.

On-site computerized interviewing is being utilized in more and more health-care settings. The most frequent use to date is for collecting patient satisfaction data. After a clinic visit, for example, a respondent may be asked to sit down at a computer station and "fill out" the questionnaire displayed on the screen. The more user-friendly systems allow the user to touch the appropriate response on the screen. Others may instruct the interviewee to strike certain keys on a keyboard.

This on-site approach to data collection has the advantage of capturing the information at a time when it is top of mind. It allows researchers to obtain responses from virtually every patient rather than relying on a sample. The provision of information is easy for the respondent, and the computer-assisted system often has the ability to modify itself during the course of the interview, edit the responses, and even perform analysis. Computerized interviewing saves time and resources and eliminates much of the paper involved in survey research. The results of the surveys can typically be obtained in hours if not minutes.

The disadvantages of this approach are that the survey must be relatively short, survey items must be very simple and completely clear, and patients must be willing to cooperate, especially if they suffer from computer-phobia. There is always the fear the patients may resent being asked to go to this extra trouble, especially if they are not feeling well or they have just paid a large fee. In addition, some analysts feel that patient satisfaction responses are not valid unless they have had some time to "age"; they would contend that surveys conducted, for example, two weeks after the visit are more valid than those conducted at the time of the visit.

It has become increasingly common to administer surveys through the use of facsimile machines. While this is not a particularly useful approach for data collection from patients or the general public, it is proving to be a reasonably efficacious method for conducting surveys with certain target audiences. A "faxed" questionnaire seems to carry more significance with certain hard-to-reach groups of respondents than a mailed one. It is more likely to get into the hands of the respondent than a mail questionnaire or even a telephone call. It is also easier to return the responses via fax than through the mail. Hard-to-reach respondent groups such as physicians or employee benefits managers seem to be particularly appropriate for this approach.

Some researchers have begun to administer surveys via the Internet, and the growing level of Internet penetration among the general public has made this medium increasingly popular. Assuming that the target population is "wired", data collection via the Internet is convenient and inexpensive. To date, this approach works best in the case of an existing network of customers, an advisory board, or other groupings that may already be linked by electronic mail, rather than for general consumers. As penetration rates increase and consumers become more familiar with this data collection approach, the use of the Internet for survey research will undoubtedly increase.

ANALYTICAL TECHNIQUES

As data have become more widely available in healthcare, some of the emphasis has shifted from data collection to data analysis. Unanalyzed data is essentially useless and must be processed and interpreted to turn it into information. There are a number of analytical methods that are available for this purpose, and some of the more important ones are described below. Space allows only an introduction to these analytical techniques, but ample detail is available elsewhere.

Demographic Analysis

The use of descriptive demographic data is clearly a cornerstone of planning research in healthcare as in any other industry. The researcher must be conversant with the numerous variables considered under the heading of demographics, be able to access them, and be able to apply them to research in an intelligent way.

The need for demographics, however, does not end with basic descriptive demographics. Market analysts must be familiar the three demographic processes that contribute to change in both population size and composition. These processes are fertility, mortality and migration. Each of these has an associated body of statistical techniques that the analyst should be familiar with. These three processes account for much of the dynamics that characterize healthcare markets.

There are also a number of more advanced demographic techniques that should be considered. The planning analyst should be familiar with procedures for *cohort analysis*, since this is so important to an understanding of future changes in health services demand. The analyst should also be familiar with *standardization* techniques, since these are important in comparing markets. *Contextual analysis* is becoming increasingly important as an approach for understanding health behavior.

It is also appropriate to consider population estimates, projections and forecasts under the heading of demographic analysis. The analyst must be familiar with the techniques used to generate such "synthetic" data, since these are important in any planning research. Further, the underlying techniques also are important since the time may come when the analyst is called upon to generate custom estimates or projections. (See Box 11-3 for a discussion of estimates, projections and forecasts.)

Epidemiological Analysis

Epidemiology is the medical specialty concerned with the distribution of disease within the population. As definitions of health and illness have evolved, epidemiology has taken on a broader meaning that includes virtually any factor that is related to the incidence of disease. In recent years, the subdiscipline of social epidemiology has emerged to address the increasingly important relationship between social conditions and health status (Dever, 1991).

Epidemiology has developed its own set of analytical techniques, many of which have relevance for healthcare planning research. Some of the techniques discussed elsewhere were developed by epidemiologists. The procedures for calculating incidence and prevalence rates came out of this field, and many of the indicators utilized in fertility and mortality analyses came out of this tradition. Such advanced analytical techniques as life table analysis and survival analysis can be attributed to epidemiologists.

Epidemiological analysis is particularly useful in profiling a service area or population, particularly from the perspective of public health. The growing interest in population-based healthcare and the revival of concern in public health over the resurgence of communicable diseases will assure that epidemiological methods remain important in health planning research.

BOX 11-3
Estimates, Projections and Forecasts

Almost all analyses conducted by health services planners, of necessity, involve the use of estimates, projections and/or forecasts. In many cases, actual data do not exist related to the service area or healthcare activity under study, requiring the generation of demand or utilization estimates. The inherently futuristic nature of planning calls for the frequent use of projections and forecasts. Also referred to as "synthetic" data, each of these types of data calculations has different characteristics and different uses. Other sources may be consulted to obtain information on the details of these processes.

Estimates involve the calculation of statistics for a current or past time period. Estimates of population are common, but estimates could also be made of the incidence of a health condition or the amount of health service utilization. Estimates typically involve the extrapolation or interpolation of actual data (e.g., census data) for two or more known time periods. The starting point for most planning analyses may be the current population, the patient pool, or even the level of demand. Quite often, these figures must be estimated. A variety of techniques are used to generate estimates and many commercial data vendors have built substantial businesses preparing estimates of population and/or health services demand.

Projections involve estimates of population or some other quantifiable phenomenon for some future period. Planning ideally focuses on future

Spatial Analysis

Spatial analysis is a concept developed by geographers that focuses on the spatial relationships among phenomena within the environment. This approach goes beyond the simple mapping of data (which is certainly important for descriptive purposes) to the calculation of statistics based on the distribution of cases on the map (Plane and Rogerson, 1994). The spatial approach improves on non-spatial representation because it takes into account the proximity or isolation of the phenomena under study.

Geographic information systems (GIS) have been developed that can assist planners in the performance of spatial analyses. GIS software can be used to describe and analyze the geographic distribution, for example, of diseases or persons at risk for developing certain health conditions. It can be used to target population segments and select sites for treatment programs or facilities. The software allows the data to be visualized and facilitates analyses of geographic and

conditions, so some method must be employed to develop a picture of the future. Projections by their nature reflect past trends and carry them forward into the future. Analysts generating projections may simply extrapolate a trend into the future or may apply adjustments based on known or potential developments in the area for which the projection is being made. As with estimates, a number of different methods are used to generate projections and, again, commercial data vendors are heavily involved in synthetically producing projections of future populations or other phenomena of interest to health planners.

Forecasts resemble projections in that they offer an estimation of conditions for some future point in time. Forecasts, depending on the methodology used, may or may not rely heavily on historical trends. The distinguishing characteristic of forecasts is that they attempt to take likely future developments into consideration. For this reason, there is more of a subjective dimension to the formulation of forecasts relative to projections. The forecaster is likely to try to anticipate future developments that will affect the size of the population or the level of demand, perhaps quite independent of any prior developments. Econometric models are often used to generate forecasts rather than projections because of their tendency to incorporate a number of variables that are thought to reflect future developments. The lack of relevance of past trends for future developments in healthcare has encouraged an increasing number of analysts to generate forecasts.

longitudinal variation. This approach has a lot in common with epidemiological techniques, since one of the main applications of GIS systems is in the study of epidemiological phenomena. Recent concerns over the threat of bioterrorism have further raised the interest in spatial analysis as applied, for example, to the geographic dispersion of a biological pathogen.

Spatial analysis can be utilized to generate a variety of map types. The choice depends on the issues under study and the type of analysis being performed. GIS software typically has the ability to link two or more mapped variables and perform statistical analysis. Indeed, accessibility analyses on available health services, made possible by GIS software, have become a standard technique in planning studies. GIS software includes the ability to "geocode" data to a specific latitude and longitude. This means that, for displaying phenomena on maps, the exact location can be plotted.

Although spatial analysis is becoming increasingly important with the introduction of low-cost, user-friendly geographic information systems, this method requires a certain level of specialized skills. Medical geographers and others who have experience in spatial analysis in healthcare are rare and it is likely to be a while before this method is widespread in the healthcare arena.

Evaluation Analysis

Evaluation analysis has a long history outside of healthcare, but is beginning to find a growing number of health-related applications. Evaluation techniques can be utilized in a number of ways in healthcare. They can be utilized to evaluate a particular program or service (both retroactively and prospectively). They can be utilized to evaluate various marketing activities. And to a lesser extent they can be utilized to evaluate a market. The most effective use of evaluation in healthcare is probably related to feasibility studies and business planning. Various evaluation techniques (e.g., cost-benefit analysis) can be used for the planning of new programs.

In their broadest application evaluation practices are designed to: 1) provide a basis for decision making and policy formulation; 2) assess and evaluate progress; 3) monitor and manage programs; and 4) generate information for improving programs. As such, evaluation analysis can serve as a valuable component for virtually any planning study.

Evaluation techniques focus on two types of analysis: process (or formative) analysis and outcome (or summative) analysis. The former evaluates systems, procedures, communications, and other factors that contribute to the efficient operation of a program. Outcome evaluation, on the other hand, focuses more on end results. Process evaluation essentially measures efficiency, while outcome evaluation measures effectiveness.

Although evaluation techniques are often praised for their bottom-line objectivity, they are also useful in healthcare where it is not possible to place a dollar value on everything. Thus, cost-effectiveness analysis can take into consideration the non-tangible aspects of the service delivery process in its evaluation.

SWOT Analysis

The SWOT analysis has become an increasingly common technique for assessing the position of a healthcare organization within its market. It can also be utilized to assess the overall characteristics of a community's health system. The SWOT analysis involves an examination of the *strengths, weaknesses, opportunities* and *threats* relative to the community or the organization.

In the case of community-wide planning, it would be normal to identify the strengths of the community's healthcare system overall, as well as particularly effective or well-developed programs or facilities. Weaknesses within the community's healthcare system would be identified in the same manner. Opportunities may take the form of service niches that could be addressed, new sources of insured patients, or potential collaborative projects. Threats may take the form of system under-capacity or overcapacity, declining reimbursement for "public" patients, or overly aggressive competition among the players. In the case of the organization, the SWOT analysis will take into consideration the findings from both internal and external audits.

The SWOT analysis should include input from the quantitative research that is being conducted as well as from the interviews that are administered. Because the strengths, weaknesses, opportunities and threats that are identified will guide further development of the plan, it is important that consensus be reached on these attributes before proceeding with the planning process.

Gap Analysis

A "gap analysis," as the name implies, assesses the gap between the needs of a population and the existing resources for meeting those needs. Thus, this form of analysis involves assessing the needs of the population, identifying the services or other resources available to meet those needs, and then determining what the unmet needs (or the gaps in services) are. In the case of organization-level planning, the process may involve specifying some ideal state (e.g., a 25 percent market share) and determining the gap between this target and the current reality. Thus, gap analysis can be utilized to assess the gap between where an organization is and where it wants to be.

The gap analysis is frequently used in performing community assessments. The community's healthcare needs are compared to the services available, and unmet needs are subsequently identified. These needs may be expressed in terms of some global rating or linked to specific programs (e.g., there are ample specialists in the community but a shortage of primary care physicians). This same approach can be applied by private sector organizations and this technique, under various guises, serves as the starting point for much strategic decision making.

A supply and demand analysis is an example of a gap analysis utilized in healthcare. An example of such an analysis involves the community's physician supply. In the typical case, the level of physician need for a particular community or population is determined, preferably in terms of specialty categories. The next step is to determine the existing supply of physicians located in the community or otherwise serving the target area. It then becomes a simple matter of comparing the demand for physicians with the current supply to complete the analysis. The analysis should identify the extent to which surpluses or shortages of physicians exist on a specialty-by-specialty basis. The conclusions of the analysis serve as a guide for planning physician services. Gaps can be identified in terms of personnel, as in the example above, facilities, services, equipment, funding, and a variety of other types of resources.

"What-If" Analysis

The "what-if" analysis has become an increasingly important analytical technique as the ability to model processes using computers has become more widespread.

This approach involves a simulation technique in which the components of a particular model are adjusted to determine the likely impact throughout the model. Thus, "what-if" we manipulate the hospital admission? How will that impact revenues or occupancy rates?

What-if models can range from quite simplistic to highly complex. Fortunately, many what-if scenarios can be modeled using a spreadsheet on a personal computer. A market analyst might be asked, for example, to estimate the impact of offering a service at varying fee levels. A what-if scenario could be modeled using a spreadsheet or financial analysis software to determine the impact of different fee schedules. Obviously, a great deal of information is needed for what-if analyses, and the analyst must fully understand the process being modeled for this to work. However, a well constructed what-if model can be very useful to the planning analyst.

References

Creswell, John W. (1994). *Research Design: Qualitative and Quantitative Approaches*. Thousand Oaks, CA: Sage.

Dever, G.E.A. (1991). *Community Health Assessment*. Gaithersburg, MD: Aspen.

Dillman, D.A. (1978). *Mail and Telephone Survey: The Total Design*. New York: Wiley & Sons.

Plane, D.A., and P.A. Rogerson (1994). *The Geographical Analysis of Population*. New York: John Wiley.

Additional Resources

Aday, Lu Ann (1989). *Designing and Conducting Health Surveys*. San Francisco: Jossey-Bass.

Berkowitz, Eric N., Pol, Louis G., and Richard K. Thomas (1997). *Healthcare Market Research*. Burr Ridge, IL: Irwin Professional Publishing.

12

Information Sources and Data Management

The health services planner seeking data to support the planning process is presented with something of a paradox. The healthcare industry generates a wealth of data, but large portions of this bounty are inaccessible to planners. Unlike other industries, healthcare has never developed national clearinghouses for bringing industry data into a central repository. When data are available, they often suffer from a lack of standardized reporting format, thus limiting the comparability of much of the data from site to site or from time period to time period. Since health-related information is often internally generated by private healthcare organizations, potentially useful health data sets may be unpublished, proprietary, and/or difficult to interpret.

In recent years the demand for health-related data has grown dramatically. Historically, interest in health data was limited to organizations involved directly in patient care, a few for-profit components of the system (e.g., insurance, pharmaceuticals), and certain government agencies. Today, a wide variety of other organizations both inside and outside of healthcare now require health-related data for an expanding number of uses. Insurers, employers, benefits managers, policy makers, consultants, and a variety of other interests increasingly seek health-related data for their planning needs. Healthcare providers who made minimal use of available data just a few years ago, now aggressively seek a wider range of data for a growing list of applications within the organization.

265

Data on the external environment have become increasingly important as strategic, business, and marketing planning have become more common in healthcare. Despite this, healthcare still lags behind other industries in the collection and dissemination of market-related data. The local orientation and autonomous nature of many healthcare organizations has impeded data sharing. Much important information lies buried in government reports, organization databases, and proprietary research documents that are inaccessible to most of the healthcare community. Increasingly, the health planner's ability to access, manipulate, and interpret these data means the difference between the success and failure of a planning initiative.

Because of demands for improvement in the quality, quantity, and specificity of the data used for planning purposes, the amount and variety of health-related data have been greatly expanded. Organizations in both the public and private sectors have begun generating new data sets. More importantly, efforts are underway on the part of various entities, particularly within the federal government, to make existing data more accessible and affordable for the healthcare community. The ability to "post" data on-line in electronic format has contributed substantially to this effort.

The primary purpose of this chapter is to outline the categories of data required for various planning initiatives, describe the ways in which they are generated, and indicate sites where they might be accessed. In view of the growing number of types and sources of health-related data, this chapter cannot present an exhaustive discussion of this topic. It should, however, direct the reader to the most important sources of data for health planning. While many of the information sources discussed in this chapter have been introduced in specific contexts earlier in the book, important characteristics of these sources—such as frequency of release, geographic specificity, and methodological limitations—are presented here.

A number of the data sets described here are not traditionally considered health-related data. However, much of what affects the health industry does not result directly from health-related events, and there has been an increase in the demand for data thought in the past to be unrelated to health care (e.g., data on such topics as employment, housing, and crime). Therefore, this discussion has been expanded to include data sets that reflect the more general environment affecting health care-related activities.

DATA DIMENSIONS

The data being considered for use in planning activities can be categorized along a number of different dimensions. By categorizing data along these dimensions, some order is introduced into the data management process. Some of the most important dimensions are addressed in the sections below.

Community vs. Organizational Data

As noted throughout this text, the compilation of health data can be approached at two different levels, the community level and the organizational level. The former involves the analysis of community-wide health data, whether the "community" is the nation, a state, a county or a planning district. This macro-level approach has historically been associated with public sector planning activity. Community-level data focus on top-of-the-organization statistics as opposed to detailed internal data for organizations. The emphasis is more likely to be on overall patterns of health service delivery and on dominant practice patterns than on the details of the operation of various organizations. Thus, community-level data will provide the planner information on such phenomena as patient flow into and out of the service area, levels of overcapacity or under-capacity affecting the area's health facilities, and the adequacy of various types of biomedical equipment within the service area.

At the organization level, data analysis focuses on the characteristics and concerns of specific corporate entities such as hospitals, physician groups, and health plans. The organization-level approach is more typical of the private sector in health care. The emphasis is likely to be on the details of the organization's operation vis-à-vis the activities of competitors and other healthcare organizations within the market area. There is interest in the overall pattern of system operation only to the extent that it affects the particular organization. The specialty physician practice, for example, is primarily interested in the details of competing specialty practices (e.g., patient volume, market share, procedures performed) rather than more general data on the health service area.

Internal vs. External Data

Community-wide and organization planners alike will require the use of data on both the internal environment and the external environment. While it has been natural for health care organizations to turn first to internal information sources, data on the external environment have become increasingly important. Data related to the external environment are sometimes difficult to locate and access but, relative to internal data, are more available to the public. The health care organization's ability to access, manipulate, and interpret external data sets is increasingly the difference between success and failure.

Internally generated data represent a ready source of information at the organization level. Healthcare organizations routinely generate a large volume of data as a by-product of their normal operations. These include data related to patient characteristics, utilization patterns, referral streams, financial transactions, personnel and other types of information that almost always have a demographic dimension. To the extent that these data can be extracted from internal data management systems, they serve as a rich source of information on the organization and its operation. (This chapter will, however, focus on sources of external data, since internal data will be specific to each organization.)

Data on the internal characteristics of the organization typically includes information on patient characteristics, utilization trends, staffing levels, and financial trends, among others. Internal data are usually compiled through an *internal audit*. The internal audit typically includes analysis of the organization's structure, processes, customers and resources. The internal audit may compile data produced through standard reports generated by the organization's data management systems (e.g., patient activity reports). Additional "runs" may be required of the data systems, however, in order to obtain "ad hoc" data. Few data management systems within healthcare organizations were set up with the generation of data for planning in mind and many are too inflexible to produce custom data sets. In these cases, the internal audit is likely to require some primary research. (More detail on the internal audit is provided in Chapter 7.)

Most of the data collection effort on the part of health planners will be directed toward external data. As healthcare providers, in particular, have become more market driven and the emphasis has shifted to strategic planning, business planning, and marketing planning, the interest in external data of all types has grown. And, of course, the primary concern of the community-wide planner is external data since virtually all of the relevant data is "external" to the planning entity.

Strategic, business, and marketing planning are primarily external in their orientation. These types of planning must address the external environment in which they are to operate. They need to take into consideration national, state and local trends in healthcare delivery, financing and regulation. They need to be aware of developments in the local market that will affect their initiatives. They particularly need to have an understanding of the characteristics of other healthcare organizations within the market area, especially those who may compete with them. Much of this chapter is devoted to an understanding of the types and sources of external data.

Primary vs. Secondary Data

Another useful distinction is made between primary data and secondary data. Primary data collection involves the use of surveys, focus groups, observational methods and other techniques for the stated purpose of obtaining information on a specific topic. Secondary data refers to data gathered for some other purpose besides planning, marketing, or business development but that is nevertheless of value in the formulation of strategy and policy.

This chapter focuses on secondary sources of data rather than primary research. Primary research requires a much more detailed treatment than can be afforded in this framework and is better addressed in a research methodology context. Also, primary research activities are usually focused narrowly on specific issues facing an organization at a particular time under certain conditions. While the value of primary research has become well established within health care as evidenced by the growing number of patient satisfaction surveys and focus groups being conducted, these activities usually generate proprietary data that are not likely to be disseminated outside the sponsoring organization. Most of the data compiled for planning-specific research will ultimately be drawn from secondary sources.

Geographic Level

Another dimension of health data that should be noted is the geographic dimension. Health planners are likely to operate at different levels of geography depending on the type of plan and the type of organization involved. The Centers for Disease Control and Prevention, for example, may think in terms of national-level data and examine morbidity trends for the entire U.S. population. Similarly, a pharmaceutical company with a national market may also examine data at that level. Realistically, though, healthcare is primarily a local concern, and most organizations require data at a level much lower than the national level.

Community-wide planners are likely to require data for a fairly restricted service area (e.g., a county or group of counties), but they need it a relatively high level of granularity in order to make distinctions between various parts of the community. Thus, they may collect data at the census tract level, which is the smallest unit of geography for which extensive data are likely to be available. State health planners, on the other hand, are more likely to be concerned about county-level data. These are essentially the administrative building blocks for the state, and sub-county data are likely to involve more detail than state-based planners require.

The type of organization and the nature of the service area will determine the level of geography at which the organization-level planner functions. A large specialty group is likely to draw patients from a wide geographic area covering several counties; in this case, the county is probably the best unit for data collection. A family practitioner in a solo practice is likely to serve a fairly circumscribed service area within a particular county. In this case, the ZIP code may be the level at which data should be collected and analyzed.

The choice of geographic unit for the analysis is important not only because of its implications for the service area under study, but because different types of data are available for different geographies. For many types of information, the county may offer the most extensive range of data and, generally, the smaller the unit of geography, the less data are available. While use of the ZIP code or census tract as the unit of geography may allow for more precise delineation of the service area, access to certain types of data becomes more limited. Thus, there is likely to be a tradeoff related to the specification of the service area and the types of data that are available.

Temporal Dimension

One other dimension of data that needs to be taken into consideration is the temporal dimension. Health professionals typically think in terms of current data—that is, data that relate to the present timeframe or, at least, to the immediate past (e.g., last year's hospital admissions). The nature of healthcare focuses the practitioner on the present and, hence, the interest in information management systems that can provide "real time" access to data.

From a planning perspective, current data are important but, in some ways, are less important than future data and even historical data. The value of current data rests with its ability to provide a baseline against which past and future figures can be compared. Planners routinely collect historical data on the community or the organization. To a great extent, the planning process relies on the ability to extrapolate past trends into the future. Thus, historical patterns of population growth, hospital admissions, and disease prevalence can provide the basis for predicting future trends. While it could be argued that, since healthcare has changed so dramatically over the past two or three decades, the past is not a good predictor of the future. While there is considerable merit in this position, it would be reckless to not consider the trends that led up to the current situation for the community or the organization.

"Future" data refers to data that describe conditions at some point in the future. By definition, planning is future oriented, and effective planning requires insights into the future of the healthcare environment. Since actual data do not exist on the future, efforts must be made to generate projections of future conditions relevant to the community or the healthcare organization. Increasing emphasis is being placed on the production of "synthetic" estimates of future populations, service demands and utilization patterns. The growing interest in predictive modeling among health plans and other care managers is encouraging the development of techniques for predicting future trends.

DATA GENERATION METHODS

The methods for data collection discussed in this chapter are divided into four general categories: censuses, registration systems, surveys, and synthetically produced data. Censuses, registries, and surveys are the more traditional methods of generating data supportive of health planning activities, although synthetically produced statistics such as population estimates and projections have become standard tools for most planning analyses.

Censuses

A census of the population involves a complete count of the persons residing in a specific place at a specific time. The U.S. Census Bureau (within the Department of Commerce) conducts an enumeration of population and housing every ten years (the decennial census) and the 2000 enumeration was the twenty-second decennial census. A lesser-known enumeration of business units, or an "economic census," is conducted every five years.

Although a census theoretically includes a complete count of the population, it is increasingly difficult to strictly apply this term to the decennial census conducted in the U.S. While the U.S. census ostensibly counts every resident, it falls short of a true census in two aspects. First, every decade a certain portion of the population is missed in the enumeration, resulting in some level of "undercount". While the undercount is typically less than three percent, its mere existence creates myriad problems. This undercount tends to be concentrated among certain segments of the population, resulting in a situation in which members of some groups have a greater chance of being enumerated than members of others. This has significant practical implications, since the results of each census are used as the basis for redistributing Congressional seats and allocating government funds. Because of the undercount, the publication of initial census figures every ten years produces a spate of lawsuits related to the accuracy of the census itself and, with the 2000 census, it led to Congressional intervention into the determination of the "official" count.

The second factor diminishing the enumeration's value as a census is the fact that a large portion of the data on population and housing characteristics is obtained from a sample of the nation's households. Only a fraction of the population and housing questions are asked of all U.S. households. The remainder are asked of approximately one out of every six households. While the use of sampling significantly reduces the cost of conducting the census, it generates figures that some might incorrectly assume to represent complete counts. Users of census data should become knowledgeable about the validity of the figures, especially when small geographic units are being studied.

The infrequent administration of the census is another source of problems. In a society where rapid change is common, collecting data at ten-year intervals has its shortcomings. As time elapses after the census year, the usefulness of the data is diminished. Nevertheless, commercial data vendors and other organizations that generate population estimates and projections continue to use these "dated" data as their baseline for calculations. This practice opens the door for potential miscalculations for which the magnitude might not be known. (The Census Bureau has instituted the American Community Survey, a national survey that involves a large sample of U.S. populations. This survey is expected to eventually replace the decennial census and is discussed under surveys below.)

The census collects data on the number of persons residing in each living unit (e.g., house, duplex, apartment, or dormitory) and the characteristics of those individuals. Information is gathered on such characteristics as age, race, ethnicity, marital status, income, occupation, education, employment status, and industry of employment. There are also questions about the dwelling unit in which the respondent lives, eliciting information on the type of dwelling unit (e.g., apartment or duplex), ownership status, value of owned house, monthly rent, age of dwelling unit, and a number of other housing characteristics.

Health-related items are noticeably absent from the census, since very few have been mandated for collection through legislative action. Other government agencies, as will be shown later, have a much more significant role in the collection of health-related data than does the Census Bureau.

The value of the census to health planners clearly rests with its demographic data. These data have direct application to the performance of market analyses and indirect applications as input into models for generating prevalence and demand estimates. Although the census is only conducted every 10 years, the Bureau maintains the capacity for generating population estimates and projections on an on-going basis. These federally generated intercensal figures may not be as detailed as some commercially produced ones—e.g., they are only calculated down to the county level—but they are broken down in terms of age, race, income, and other important variables.

Census data are tabulated by the Census Bureau for virtually every formally designated geographic unit in the United States, and this is a clear advantage of census data over some other type of data. Statistics generated by the census are disseminated for states, counties, zip codes, metropolitan areas, and cities. Data are also published for specially designated areas created by the Census Bureau, including census tracts, block groups, and blocks.

Census data may be accessed through a variety of sources. Many libraries are designated as depositories of U.S. government publications and maintain most or all of the census reports in print, microfiche or CD format among their holdings. The U.S. Government Printing Office also makes these publications available to the public at a reasonable cost. Census data sets in electronic format are sold by the Census Bureau and by other organizations that repackage the census data. The Bureau offers free and relatively user-friendly on-line access to its data sets and most census data can be accessed through the American Factfinder feature of the Bureau's Web site (www.census.gov.) With each successive census, the number of printed reports is reduced, with the intent of eventually restricting census output to electronic formats, thereby making use of on-line data increasingly important.

The modern economic census was initiated in 1954 and is conducted every five years (currently in years ending in 2 and 7). The census covers businesses engaged in retail trade, wholesale trade, service activities, mineral industries, transportation, construction, manufacturing, and agriculture, as well as government services. The information collected through the economic census includes data on sales, employment, and payroll, along with other, more specialized data. These data are available for a variety of geographic units, including states, metropolitan areas, counties, and places with 2,500 or more residents.

While it may appear that these data are unrelated to health issues, the economic census actual compiles a lot of data on healthcare "businesses". All businesses are assigned a code using the North American Industry Classification System (NAICS). Aggregated data on businesses within the NAICS categories that involve health-related activities (e.g., physician practices, pharmacies, medical laboratories) are available from this source. There is no other all-inclusive source that will indicate the number of hospitals, pharmacists, and chiropractors, for example, that are located in a particular area. As with the population and housing data, the Bureau is increasingly distributing data from the economic census in electronic form.

Registration Systems

A second method of data collection that produces information useful for health planners is represented by registration systems. A registration system involves the systematic compilation, recording, and reporting of a broad range of events, institutions, and individuals. The implied characteristics of a registry include the regular and timely recording of the phenomenon in question. Most of the registration systems relevant to this discussion are sponsored by some branch of government, although other types of registration systems will be discussed below as well.

The best-known registration activities in the United States are those related to "vital events", including births, deaths, marriages, and divorces. However, other registries can prove valuable, especially when examining changes in the level and types of health services required by a population. These include registration systems sponsored by the Centers for Disease Control and Prevention (CDC), the Social Security Administration (SSA), Medicare, and the Center for Medicare and Medicaid Services (CMS), among others.

A variation on registries that is finding increasing use in health-related research is the "administrative record". Administrative records systems are not necessarily intended to be registries of all enrollees or members of an organization or group but a record of transactions involving these individuals. Thus, the list of all Medicare enrollees would constitute a registry, but the data generated by virtue of Medicare enrollees' encounters with the healthcare system would be under the heading of administrative records (since not all Medicare enrollees would use services during a given time period). Data sets made available by the federal government on Medicare activity, for example, involve administrative records that are useful for a number of purposes. Some examples of registries are described below.

Vital Statistics

The tracking of vital statistics in the United States involves data collection on births, deaths, marriages and divorces and, in some jurisdictions, induced abortions. The collection of data on vital events is initially the responsibility of the local health authority. Health departments at the county (or county equivalent) level are charged with filing certificates for births and deaths. These data are forwarded to the vital statistics registry within the respective state governments. The appropriate state agency compiles the data for use by the state and transmits the files to the National Center for Health Statistics (NCHS). NCHS has the responsibility of compiling and publishing vital statistics for the nation and its various political subdivisions. (See Box 12-1 for a description of the National Center for Health Statistics.)

BOX 12-1
The National Center for Health Statistics

The National Center for Health Statistics (NCHS) is considered by many to be the Census Bureau of health care. As a division of the Centers for Disease Control and Prevention (CDC), NCHS performs a number of invaluable functions related to health and healthcare. For over 40 years the Center has carried out the tasks of data collection and analysis, data dissemination, and the development of methodologies for research on health issues. The NCHS also coordinates the various state centers for health statistics.

Part of the Center's responsibilities includes the compilation, analysis, and publication of vital statistics for the United States and each relevant subarea. This is a massive task, but the results provide the basis for the calculation of fertility and mortality rates. These statistics, in turn, provide the basis for estimates and projections made by other organizations. The compilation and analysis of data on morbidity is another important function, and the Center has been responsible for the development of much of the epidemiological data available, for example, on chronic disease and AIDS.

In addition to the data compiled from various registration sources, the Center is the foremost administrator of healthcare surveys in the nation. Its sample surveys are generally large scale endeavors that fall into two categories: community-based surveys and facility-based surveys. Perhaps the Center's most important survey is the National Health Interview Survey (NHIS), in which data are collected annually from approximately 49,000 households. The NHIS is the nation's primary source of data on the incidence/prevalence of health conditions, health status, the number of injuries and disabilities characterizing the population, health services utilization, and a variety of other health-related topics. Surveys that involve a sample from the community include the Medical Expenditure Panel Survey

Standard birth certificates capture data on the time and date of birth, place of occurrence, mother's residence, birth weight, pregnancy complications, mother's pregnancy history, mother and father's age and race (ethnicity in selected states), and mother's education and marital status. Data elements available from the standard death certificate include age, race (ethnicity in selected states), sex, place of residence, usual occupation, and industry of the decedent, along with the location where the death took place. In addition, data are collected on the immediate and contributing causes of death and on other significant health conditions.

(MEPS), the National Health and Nutrition Examination Survey (NHANES), and the National Survey of Family Growth (NSFG). Another survey, the National Maternal and Infant Health Survey (NMIHS), involves a sampling of certificates of birth, fetal death, and infant death.

One NCHS survey is arguably the most important source of information on the increasingly important topic of ambulatory care. The National Ambulatory Medical Care Survey (NAMCS) samples the patient records of 2,500 office-based physicians to obtain data on diagnosis, treatment, and medications prescribed, along with information on the characteristics of both physicians and patients. Important facility-based surveys include the National Hospital Discharge Survey and the National Nursing Home Survey.

The data collected through NCHS studies are disseminated in a variety of ways. Much of the information is distributed as printed material. The Center's publications include annual books such as *Health, United States* (the "official" government compendium of statistics on the nation's health), and publications such as *Vital and Health Statistics*. Data from NCHS surveys are also available in tape, diskette, and CD formats. The NCHS sponsors conferences and workshops offering not only the findings from the Center's research but training in its research methodologies. NCHS-generated data sets are being made increasingly available via the Internet and can be accessed at www.cdc.gov/nchs.

From the perspective of a health data user, there are other resources that the Center can offer. By contacting the appropriate NCHS division, it is possible to obtain detailed statistics, many unpublished, on all of the topics for which the Center compiles data. Center staff are also available to help with methodological issues and provide that "one number" that the health data analyst might require. In short, the NCHS is a service-oriented agency that provides a number of invaluable functions for those who require data on health and healthcare. Much of the information required for the U.S. system to adapt to the changing healthcare environment, in fact, will be generated by the National Center for Health Statistics.

Birth and death statistics are regularly reported in federal government publications and, now, via the Internet (http://www.fedstats.gov). The compiled statistics are typically presented based on both the place of occurrence of the event (e.g., the location of the hospital) and the place of residence of the affected individual. Considerable detail is provided in federal reports for a wide range of geographic units including states, MSAs, counties, and urban places. Data for other geographic areas may be available through state or local government agencies. Yearly summary reports are produced and published by the National Center for Health Statistics, though monthly summaries are also available through the monthly vital statistics reports. NCHS is offering a growing number of reports and data sets in electronic format and via the Internet.

Vital statistics reports are also made available by most state governments and most local health departments. Although basic data will always be reported by these agencies, the format, detail and coverage varies from state to state and county to county.

CDC Disease Surveillance

The Centers for Disease Control and Prevention (CDC) have been involved in disease surveillance activities since the establishment of the Communicable Disease Center in 1946. Surveillance activities now include programs in human reproduction, environmental health, chronic disease, risk reduction, occupational safety and health, and infectious diseases. One purpose of the surveillance system is to provide weekly provisional information on the occurrence of diseases defined as "notifiable" by the Council of State and Territorial Epidemiologists (CSTE). To this end, the CDC maintains a number of registries on various disease categories.

Notifiable disease reports are received by the CDC from 52 U.S. jurisdictions (Washington, D.C., and New York City report separately) and five territories. The number of diseases and conditions reported is quite large. The list of monitored diseases includes, among others, anthrax, botulism, cholera, diphtheria, food-borne disease, leprosy, mumps, and toxic shock. Statistics on notifiable diseases are published weekly by the CDC in *Morbidity and Mortality Weekly Report* (MMWR) and compiled in an annual report published by the agency. The CDC is now providing a growing amount of information via the Internet.

Because of the historical focus of the CDC on communicable diseases, chronic diseases are generally not officially tracked as part of the public health agenda. This situation creates a serious void in ability to monitor the chronic conditions that now account for the bulk of morbidity within the U.S. population. Although our knowledge of these conditions has been advanced through survey research on the part of the National Center for Health Statistics, information derived from sample surveys limits our understanding of the epidemiology of chronic conditions and, thus, the system's ability to monitor their prevalence. As a result, the CDC and other agencies are currently exploring possibilities for improving capabilities for identifying and monitoring chronic conditions.

Health Personnel

Registries constitute the main source of data on many categories of health personnel. Most health professionals must be registered with the state in which they practice. In addition, most belong to professional associations whose rosters become *de facto* registries. Like other registries, the registration of healthcare personnel involves the regular and timely recording of persons entering a given profession.

The federal government is the primary source of registry data on health personnel at the national level. The Department of Health and Human Services is responsible for collecting and disseminating data on the status of health personnel in the United States. These requirements have led to the establishment of registries for various categories of health professionals. The Department also generates projections of the future personnel pool for selected categories of professionals. In addition, the listing of health professional shortage areas maintained by the Health Resources and Services Administration within DHHS is often of use to health planners. This database tracks the counties, communities, and special populations (e.g., Indian reservations) that report less than the recommended number of primary care physicians. In addition, the Center for Medicare and Medicaid Services maintains detailed registries of many types of health professionals that receive reimbursement under federally sponsored health programs.

Other examples of sources of health personnel data include the AMA physician master file; medical, osteopathic, dental, and nursing school enrollment data; the American Academy of Physician Assistants master file; the American Dental Association dental practice survey; the Inventory of Pharmacists; and licensure information from the National Council of State Boards of Nursing and various accrediting bodies and professional associations serving the allied health profession (e.g., laboratory technicians, dietitians, physical therapists).

State governments often represent more direct sources of information on health personnel than federal agencies, since the various states have the primary responsibility for the licensing and monitoring of virtually all health professions. As part of their administrative activities, they necessarily establish registries for specific categories of health personnel. The databases created at the state level for physicians, nurses, physician assistants and other categories of health personnel are typically up to date. However, the detail provided and the usefulness of the data collected for planning, marketing, and business development purposes varies widely from state to state.

While data on professional licensure are often available to the public, mere registration in a jurisdiction does not necessarily indicate employment in healthcare. Further, these databases are likely to include only the barest of data required to carry out the mandated functions of the licensing agency. Specialty boards and other organizations also maintain registries on their members or certification recipients. While this information is often available in printed directories, the availability of the actual databases varies.

Many local organizations have begun to develop and maintain personnel databases for their particular service areas. Since most healthcare markets are local, national databases are of limited usefulness. Business coalitions have led the way in support of database development in many local markets.

Commercial data vendors maintain databases of physicians and other personnel, and some of these are comparable to the more traditional databases maintained by the professional organizations and government agencies. Data vendors may identify emerging professions or "marginal" practitioners that do not have an association base or are not tracked by the government. Other vendors repackage data from government organizations or association sources, and resell the data in modified form.

Health Facilities

The federal government is the major source of nationwide data on health facilities. The National Master Facility Inventory (NMFI) is a comprehensive file of inpatient facilities maintained by the National Center for Health Statistics. The institutions included in this NCHS data collection effort are hospitals, nursing homes and related facilities, and other custodial or remedial care facilities. The NMFI is kept current by periodically adding the names and addresses of newly established facilities licensed by state boards and other agencies. Annual surveys are used to update information concerning existing facilities.

The facilities databases established by NCHS include data on facility size, personnel, admissions, discharges, services offered, type of ownership, and type of certification. These data are available through various published reports, with much of this information obtained initially from professional associations and processed by the NCHS or some other federal agency. CMS makes available a set of data files on health facilities and other providers of care. Its "Provider of Services" files include every provider that has filed claims with Medicare.

Arguably, the nation's most complete hospital registry is maintained by the American Hospital Association (AHA). Data are compiled annually on the availability of services, utilization patterns, financial information, hospital management, and personnel (American Hospital Association, 2003). The database is continuously updated through an on-going survey of the nation's hospitals. These data are available for a variety of geographic units (including regions, divisions, states, counties, and cities). They are available via published reports, CD-ROM, and the Internet. Some of the information is reprinted in secondary sources such as the *County and City Data Book* and *Health, United States*. Certain commercial data vendors have also established hospital databases. Solucient, one of the nation's largest health data vendors, produces an annual profile of hospitals based on its database.

Since most health facilities are licensed by the state, information is usually available from the state agency charged with that responsibility. Many states now require that hospitals submit utilization data to a designated state agency. These data may be made available to the public. The Agency for Healthcare Research and Quality (AHRQ) has begun compiling data from the various states. Increasingly, local organizations such as planning and regulatory agencies and business coalitions maintain facilities databases. For facilities other than hospitals, some private data vendors have begun collecting and disseminating data. There are now vendors selling data on health maintenance organizations, urgent care centers, freestanding surgery centers, and a variety of other types of facilities.

Mental Health Facilities

An inventory of mental health organizations is maintained by the Center for Mental Health Services (within the U.S. Department of Health and Human Services) and is updated every two years. The agency publishes periodic reports on the status of mental health services in the United States, although the format varies from edition to edition. Additional information can be obtained from the Center's Web site (http://www.samhsa.gov/cmhs/htm).

Since many mental health services are administered by state governments, the respective state agencies represent a source of mental health statistics, although the data provided vary in terms of accessibility, content, and format. While rather detailed statistics have become available on ambulatory care services for physical illness, this is not the case for mental illness. Some limited data on mental health outpatient activity may be available through reports filed by community mental health centers.

Surveys

A sample survey involves the administration of an interview form to a portion of a target population that has been systematically selected. The sample is designed so that the respondents are representative of the population being examined. This allows conclusions to be drawn concerning the total population based on the data collected from the sample.

The federal government is the major sponsor of survey research related to healthcare. Primarily through the National Center for Health Statistics, the federal government maintains a number of on-going surveys that deal with hospital utilization, ambulatory care utilization, nursing home and home health utilization, medical care expenditures, and other relevant topics. The National Institutes of Health and the Centers for Disease Control and Prevention also conduct surveys, although more episodically, that generate data of interest to health demographers. Some of the more useful sample surveys for health demographers are discussed in Box 12-2.

There are also a few surveys sponsored by commercial data vendors that contain data useful for health planning. These organizations sponsor nationwide surveys every year or two that may include as many 100,000 households. Through these surveys, data are collected on health status, health behavior, and healthcare preferences. Certain market research firms collect health-related data as part of their consumer surveys and public opinion pollsters may also collect data on health and healthcare. Some of the data collected in this manner is considered proprietary and is generally not available except to the vendor's clients. Other vendors make data available for purchase to the general public.

BOX 12-2
Federal Sources of Survey Data

The combined agencies of the federal government represent the nation's largest data collection force. Led by the National Center for Health Statistics (NCHS), federal agencies conduct a variety of surveys on health-related issues. The sections below describe a sample of these federal survey activities that have particular relevance for healthcare planning.

The *National Health Interview Survey* (NHIS) is an ongoing national survey of the noninstitutionalized civilian population in the United States. Each year, a multistage probability sample of 49,000 households is selected. The data gathered are quite detailed and include demographic information on age, race, sex, marital status, occupation, and income. Information is compiled on physician visits, hospital stays, restricted-activity days, long-term activity limitation, health status, and chronic conditions. Recently, questions regarding AIDS knowledge and attitudes have been added to the survey. Food nutrition knowledge, smoking and other tobacco use, cancer, and polio are also subjects sometimes addressed.

The *National Health and Nutrition Examination Survey* (NHANES) is conducted by the National Center for Health Statistics. This survey has been designed to collect information about the health and diet of people in the United States. NHANES is unique in that it combines a home interview with health tests that are done in a mobile examination center. Tens of thousands interviews are conducted annually and, during a 12-month period, examinations are performed on some 5,000 of the interviews. The survey collects information on physical health status, dental health and nutrition. Data are used to determine cholesterol levels, trends in obesity and other health characteristics of the population.

The *National Hospital Discharge Survey* (NHDS) is a continuous nationwide survey of inpatient utilization of short stay hospitals. All hospitals with six or more beds reporting an average length of stay of less than 30 days are included in the sampling frame. A multistage probability sampling frame is used to select hospitals from the National Master facility Inventory and discharge records from each of the hospitals. The resulting sample has ranged from 192,000 to 235,000 discharge records. Information is collected on the demographic, clinical, and financial characteristics of patients discharged from short-stay hospitals.

The *National Ambulatory Medical Care Survey* (NAMCS) is a nationwide survey designed to provide information about the provision and utilization of ambulatory health services. The sampling frame is office visits made by ambulatory patients to physicians engaged in office practice. A multistage probability sampling frame is used to select physicians from the master files maintained by the American Medical Association and the American Osteopathic Association. A sample of the patient records maintained by these physicians is then examined for a randomly assigned one-week period. Recent samples contain about 35,000 records. Data regarding the age, race, ethnicity, and sex of the patient are gathered, along with the reason for the visit, expected source(s) of payment, principle diagnosis, diagnostic services provided, and disposition of visit.

The *National Nursing Home Survey* (NNHS) is a periodically-conducted national survey of nursing and related care homes, their residents, their discharges, and their staffs. Last administered in 1999, data are collected using a two-stage probability design. Once facilities are selected, residents and employees of each facility are sampled. Six separate questionnaires were used to gather data in the most recent survey. The first addresses characteristics of the facility and involves an interview with the administrator or a designee. The second focuses on cost data and is completed by the facility's accountant or bookkeeper. Information on the current and discharged residents is obtained by interviewing the staff person most familiar with the medical records of the residents. Additional resident data is gathered using telephone surveys of the resident's families. Full-time and part-time employees, including nurses, complete a nursing staff questionnaire. This data set includes approximately 1,400 facilities, 5,100 discharges, 3,000 residents, and 14,000 staff records.

The *National Home and Hospice Care Survey* (NHHCS), last conducted in 2000, involves the collection of data from a sample of 1,200 home health agencies and hospices. Patient questionnaires are administered for the various agencies and information is collected on the demographic and health characteristics of the patients served by these agencies.

The *National Survey of Family Growth* (NSFG), last administered in 1995, involved a survey of approximately 10,000 women ages 15–44 years (U.S. Department of Health and Human Services 1997b). This survey collects data on factors affecting birth and pregnancy rates, adoption, and maternal and infant health. Specific characteristics that are examined include sexual activity, contraception and sterilization practices, infertility, pregnancy loss, low birth-weight, and the use of medical care for family planning and infertility.

(continued)

The *Medical Expenditure Panel Survey* (MEPS) was initiated in 1996 as a replacement for previous surveys focusing on expenditures for health services. Co-sponsored by the Agency for Healthcare Research and Quality (AHRQ) and the National Center for Health Statistics (NCHS), MEPS is designed to generate data on the types of health services Americans use, the frequency with which they use them, how much is paid for these services, and who pays for them. In addition, MEPS provides information on health insurance coverage.

The *Behavioral Risk Factor Surveillance System* (BRFSS), sponsored by the Centers for Disease Control and Prevention (CDC), was initiated in 1995 to collect information on the health behavior and lifestyles of the U.S. population. Over 90,000 persons respond to the survey annually. The survey includes data collection on factors that affect health such as smoking, alcohol and drug use, seat-belt use, and obesity, as well as other factors that might contribute to one's health risk profile.

In the area of behavioral health, the Center for Mental Health Services (CMHS) conducts an annual survey of mental health organizations and general hospitals that provide mental health services. These surveys collect data on the characteristics of all providers of behavioral health services and on the characteristics of the patients served. Other related surveys include samples of patients admitted to various treatment programs.

The *Current Population Survey* (CPS) is the Census Bureau's mechanism for gathering detailed demographic data between the decennial censuses. Since 1960, the sample size has ranged from 33,500 to 65,500 households per year. Data are collected on many of the items included in the census of population and housing (e.g., age, race, and education). Questions are included on some health issues and on fertility issues that have implications for healthcare. Of particular interest to the healthcare industry are the data on health insurance coverage for the U.S. population. These data were the basis for recent estimates of the size the population that lacks health insurance.

This sample does not exhaust the list of government sources of data relevant to health planning, but only provides a sampler. Publications of the federal National Technical Information Service (NTIS) provide a good starting point for finding other relevant databases and, of course, the NCHS Web site (www.cdc.gov/nchs) provides links to most of these surveys.

Public opinion polls are often overlooked as sources of certain types of data. Methodologically sound opinion polls are constantly being conducted by research organizations of various types. While the sample sizes are relatively small, opinion polls can provide insights into developing national trends. For example, the shift in the perception of home healthcare as an inferior alternative to hospital care to the notion of the home as the preferred setting for care was first identified through opinion polls.

Synthetic Data

Synthetic data refers to figures that are generated in the absence of actual data by using statistical models. Synthetic data are created by merging existing demographic data with assumptions about population change to produce estimates, projections, and forecasts. These data are particularly valuable given that census and survey activities are restricted because of budgeting and time considerations. Since there is a large and growing demand for information for years between the administration of the census, the production of synthetic data has become a major business. Since no actual data are available for future points in time, any such data must be produced through synthetic means.

The demand for synthetic data is being met by both government agencies and commercial data vendors today. Within the federal government, population estimates for states, MSAs, and counties are prepared each year as a joint effort of the Census Bureau and the state agency designated under the Federal-State Program for Local Population Estimates (FSCPE). The purpose of the program is to standardize data and procedures so that the highest quality estimates can be generated.

Overall, the Census Bureau produces 30 different series of population projections for each year. The Bureau provides relatively detailed population estimates for the current year and projections as far as 50 years into the future down to the county level. Most states also generate population estimates and projections that are available through state agencies.

A number of commercial data vendors have emerged in recent years to supplement the efforts of government agencies in this regard. Data generated by these vendors have the advantage of being available down to small units of geography (e.g., the census block) and they are often provided in greater detail (e.g., sex and age breakdowns) than government-produced figures. They also offer the flexibility to generate estimates and projections for "custom" geographies (e.g., a market area) that government statistics do not have the ability to do. The drawback, of course, is that some precision is lost as one develops calculations for lower levels of geography and for population components. However, the ease of accessibility and timeliness of these vendor-generated figures have made them a mainstay for health services planners.

There is an ongoing debate over the quality of the synthetic data available. Users are demanding the most current data possible and, in an effort to serve the market, the question of quality has sometimes become a secondary concern. Users of synthetic data should develop knowledge of the methodologies utilized by various vendors and of the quality of the data used for baseline purposes.

An important category of synthetic data for our purposes involves estimates and projections of health services demand. Since there are limited sources of actual data on the use of health services and projections of future demand are often required, a variety of approaches have been developed for synthetically generating demand estimates and projections. The general approach involves applying known utilization rates to current or projected population figures. To the extent possible, these figures are adjusted for, at a minimum, the age and sex composition of the target population. Utilization rates generated by the National Center for Health Statistics are the basis for most such calculations, and the demographic data are likely to be obtained from a variety of different sources.

Commercial data vendors have led the way in the development of demand estimates and projections. Some vendors have developed calculations for the full range of inpatient and outpatient services, although these are often available only to established customers. Other vendors can provide selected data on, for example, the demand for a particular service line.

A somewhat different type of synthetic data is generated by the Bureau of Labor Statistics (within the U.S. Department of Labor). The Bureau maintains data on all occupational categories within the economy, including healthcare occupations. As part of the Bureau's responsibilities, it produces projections on the size of various occupational categories in the United States for 10 to 15 years into the future. Six projection models are generated, each containing a number of variables involving different scenarios reflecting changes in the total labor force, the aggregate economy, industry demand, and industry employment, among other factors.

Three sets of employment projections are created based upon differing sets of assumptions. Of interest here are the various categories of health-related occupations (e.g., dentists, physicians and surgeons, and therapists by specialty) and supportive occupations (e.g., dental and medical assistants, as well as nurse's aides). In recent years, health professions have been prominent among the occupations with the greatest projected growth. Projections for occupational categories are available from the Department of Labor through regularly published reports and, increasingly, via the Internet. (Additional information on health professions can be obtained by accessing http://www.hrsa.dhhs.gov/bhpr.)

SOURCES OF DATA FOR HEALTH PLANNING

There are numerous sources of data for health planning available today and the number of sources continues to grow. The sections below group these sources into four main categories: government agencies, professional associations, private organizations, and commercial data vendors. Although the sources presented in each section refer to the agencies and publications responsible for the specific data set being discussed, numerous compendia exist that users should find quite useful. (Box 12-3 describes the more important of these compendia.)

Government Agencies

Governments at all levels are involved in the generation, compilation, manipulation and/or dissemination of health-related data. The federal government, through the decennial census and related activities, is the world's largest processor of demographic data. Other federal agencies are major managers of data for the related topics of fertility, morbidity, mortality and migration statistics.

The federal government is a major generator of health-related databases. Through the National Center for Health Statistics, the Centers for Disease Control and Prevention, the National Institutes for Health, and other organizations, a large share of the nation's health data is generated. The Bureau of Health Resources (Department of Health and Human Services) maintains a master file of much of the health data compiled by the federal government entitled the *Area Resource File* (ARF). Other federal sources outside of health-related agencies, such as the Bureau of Labor Statistics (e.g., health occupations) and the Department of Agriculture (e.g., nutritional data), create databases of supporting data. The number and variety of databases generated by federal agencies is impressive, but the variety of agencies involves means that databases vary in coverage, content, format, cost, frequency and accessibility.

State and local governments are also major sources of health-related data. In fact, a survey of health data users indicated that various state agencies were their primary source of data for planning, marketing, and business development (Thomas 1996). State governments generate a certain amount of demographic data, with each state having a state data center for demographic projections. Vital statistics data can often be obtained in the most timely fashion at the state level, in fact. States vary, however, in the types and quality of data they generate. University data centers may also be involved in the processing of demographic data. Local governments may generate demographic data for use in various planning functions. City or county governments may produce population projections, while county health departments are responsible for the collection and dissemination of vital statistics data.

Professional Associations

Various associations within the health industry represent another source of health-related data. Chief among these are the American Medical Association (and related medical specialty organizations) and the American Hospital Association. There are also other organizations of personnel (e.g., American Dental Association) and facilities (e.g., National Association for Home Care) that maintain databases on

---

BOX 12-3
Compendia of Health Data

There is currently no national clearinghouse for data on health and health-care in the U.S. This makes identifying and acquiring needed data a challenge for health planners. There are, however, a few "compendia" of health data that might prove useful for many purposes. While no one of these publications provides all of the data a planner is likely to need, they offer a reasonable starting point. Not only do they compile specific data on certain topics, but they can often direct the reader to the origin of the data and other useful resources.

The best known of the compendia of health-related data is entitled *Health, United States*. This work is published annually by the National Center for Health Statistics and includes data gathered from NCHS and many other sources. The publication includes data on health status, health behavior, health services utilization, healthcare resources, healthcare expenditures, and insurance coverage. These data are available mostly at the national level, although some state and regional data are available.

A companion publication, *Mental Health, United States*, is published less frequently than *Health, United States* but represents the primary source of data on behavioral health care. The statistics are based on data collected by the Center for Mental Health Services.

Another more specialized compendium is also published by the Center for Medicare and Medicaid Services (CMS). Simply referred to as *Data*

---

their members and on activities related to the organization's membership. These databases are typically developed for internal use, but are increasingly being made available to the outside parties.

A number of organizations have been formed in recent years that focus specifically on health data, while others have established formal sections that deal with health data within their broader context. The National Association of Health Data Organizations (NAHDO), for example, brings together disparate parties from the public and private sector who have an interest in health data. The National Association of County and City Health Officials (NACCHO) has become very active in terms of access to health data for local planning purposes. The Health Information and Management Systems Society (HIMSS) is one of the largest organizations that is addressing this issue as a collateral consideration to data management systems issues.

Compendium (with the publication year presented as part of the title), this book brings together data on Medicaid and Medicare. The data presented are drawn primarily from CMS files, although data from sources outside the agency are also included. The information compiled by CMS is presented only at the national level, with some data reported at the state level. No data are presented for sub-state levels of geography.

Since demographic data are so important to health planners, it is worthwhile to mention some compendia that focus on this type of data. The *County and City Data Book* is published every two years by the Census Bureau and includes over 200 separate items for each county and 134 items for each city of 25,000 or more persons. Data of interest to healthcare analysts include population statistics, vital records, and hospital, physician, and nursing home statistics, as well as certain insurance data.

The *State and Metropolitan Area Data Book* is published by the Census Bureau every four years and contains 128 data items for each state, 298 variables for each MSA, and 87 variables for each MSA's central city. *County Business Patterns*, prepared by the Bureau of the Census, provides a comprehensive count of the various health care businesses operating in each U.S. county.

The *Statistical Abstract of the United States* is published every year by the Census Bureau. The *Abstract* contains detailed data for the nation as a whole for 31 different subject categories (e.g., vital statistics, nutrition), as well as data for states and metropolitan areas. Most states publish a statistical abstract that includes comparable data for that state and its counties and cities.

In recent years, many professional associations have made an increasing amount of information on their members available to the research and business communities. Not only do such organizations have an interest in exchanging information with related groups, but they also have recognized the revenue generation potential of such databases. Some of these databases include only basic information, while others offer a wealth of detail.

Private Organizations

Many private organizations (mostly not-for-profit) collect and/or disseminate health-related data. Voluntary health care associations often compile, repackage and/or disseminate such data. The American Cancer Society, for example, distributes morbidity and mortality data as it relates to its areas of interest. Some organizations, like Planned Parenthood, may commission special studies on fertility or related issues and subsequently publish this information.

Many organizations repackage data collected elsewhere (e.g., from the Census Bureau or the National Center for Health Statistics) and present it within a specialized context. The Population Reference Bureau, a private not-for-profit organization, distributes population statistics in various forms, for example. Some, like the American Association of Retired Persons (AARP), not only compile and disseminate secondary data but are actively involved in primary data collection, as well as the sponsorship of numerous studies that include some form of data collection.

Commercial Data Vendors

Commercial data vendors represent a fourth category of providers of health-related databases. These organizations have emerged to fill perceived gaps in the availability of various categories of health data. These include commercial data vendors that establish and maintain their own proprietary databases, as well as those that reprocess and/or repackage existing data. For example, SMG Marketing maintains databases on nursing homes, urgent care centers, and other types of facilities and makes this information available in a variety of forms. Also included in this group are the major demographic data vendors (e.g., ESRI Business Information, Claritas) who do not necessarily create health-related databases but incorporate health-specific databases into their business database systems.

Because of the demand for health-related data, several commercial data vendors have added health data to their inventories, and a few health-specific data vendors have emerged. These vendors not only repackage existing data into more palatable form, but some also are developing their own proprietary databases. At least three vendors are conducting major nationwide health consumer surveys.

Because of the increasing demand for health-related data, improvement in the quality, coverage, timeliness and availability of such data has become a priority with many organizations. The federal government has taken a lead in the public sector through its efforts to make its extensive health-related databases and registries available to the research and business communities. Through its various programs, the federal government is supporting projects that involve the application of contemporary computer technology to the processing, manipulation and dissemination of health-related data, an area in which health care lags far behind other industries. Commercial data vendors continue to develop proprietary databases and to repackage and distribute databases produced by government and/or association sources.

The Internet is already becoming a force with regard to health data. Although the focus at the time of this writing has been on consumer-oriented health information on the World Wide Web, data for use by health professionals is not far behind. Bibliographical and text files are already becoming available, and some healthcare organizations are transferring patient data over the Internet. In the future, there is every reason to believe that data for health services planning, marketing, and business development will be widely available on the World Wide Web. (See Chapter 11 for a discussion of health data on the Internet.)

HEALTH DATA MANAGEMENT

The expansion in the availability of health data has generated a problem of a different sort for those involved in health planning. This involves the challenge of managing and ultimately exploiting the growing mountain of data on health and healthcare.

Early attempts at managing health data were primitive by any measure and focused almost entirely on such practical dimensions as patient billing. The mainframe environment characterizing hospitals and other large health care organizations created a slow, inflexible process. Data management was controlled by information systems technicians who were essentially isolated from the operation of the organization. If healthcare professionals were to harness the power of the growing volume of data and exploit it for planning, marketing, and business development purposes, a better technical solution was necessary.

During the early 1980s it was realized by some that the ability to manage this growing volume of data was going to be critical. Most other industries had already addressed this issue and had developed fairly sophisticated means of processing and analyzing industry data. Because of its peculiar characteristics, the healthcare industry lagged well behind other sectors of the economy in terms of information management.

The introduction of the microcomputer opened the door for more efficient data management. Bringing the power of the mainframe to the desktop, personal computers quickly transformed the data management environment. The transformation involved more than technical capabilities, however, as it allowed the control of data management to shift back to the administrators and health professionals that ultimately utilized the data.

In the mid-1980s, as the health data industry expanded, computerized applications for managing this growing wealth of data emerged. Several companies introduced "desktop" marketing and planning systems designed to run on microcomputers. Many were patterned after those developed in other industries, but most of these could not survive the transition. Others developed healthcare-specific desktop systems and two major vendors emerged to serve primarily the hospital market. Today, health data management is increasing being handled via the Internet.

The introduction of desktop market analysis systems made possible the transformation of marketing research from a slow, plodding process of questionable accuracy to a scientific, accurate, and expeditious activity. Proprietary desktop analysis systems offered a number of advances over previous approaches to market analysis. Now, most of these capabilities can be provided on line. Internet-based data management systems can produce standardized or custom reports, tables, graphics, and maps pertinent to any application. They have the capability to import data sets in a variety of formats and to incorporate them easily into existing applications.

Although some technical details have yet to be resolved with regard to Web-delivered data, it appears that the distribution of health-related data via the World Wide Web is gaining momentum. While the mainframe environment emphasized the centralization of data management, the burgeoning personal computer environment has served to fragment data within an organization. The Internet offers a framework for integrating data from disparate sources, and various federal agencies have committed to making their data accessible via the Internet.

Another important consideration with regard to the management and analysis of data for health planning is the growing importance of geographic information systems (GIS). Spatial analysis, in its various forms, has always been an inherent aspect of the community assessment process. At the same time, epidemiological fieldwork includes spatial analysis as a basic analytical technique. The introduction of high performance, low-cost GIS applications has contributed greatly to the use of spatial analysis in health-related research. The power of mainframe-based spatial analysis has been brought to the desktop by applications such as MapInfo and ArcView, and even unsophisticated computer users can now generate complex maps. The opportunity for advanced spatial analysis is available to those that require it. Further advances in GIS applications are likely to make these systems even more important for health demographers in the future.

The ability to process, manipulate and disseminate health-related data has improved tremendously due to the advances that have occurred in computer technology. New developments in the areas of data warehousing, data standardization and large-scale database management capabilities continue to improve the prospects for those requiring health data. Advanced techniques, such as artificial intelligence, fuzzy logic and neural networks, are now being applied in the health care arena, and "predictive modeling" is coming into use by many healthcare organizations.

Ultimately, all of these developments reflect the changes that are occurring in the manner in which health data are being utilized. The demand for better data management and analysis capabilities is being driven by the new approach to health planning demanded by the changing environment. While being able to simply describe a situation in terms of data was a major breakthrough in the past, the new healthcare environment is calling for a much more proactive approach to the use of data. It is no longer sufficient to be able to describe a market area, for example, but the data must be used proactively for decision support and strategic planning.

References

American Hospital Association (2003). *Hospital Statistics* (2003 Edition). Chicago: American Hospital Association.

Additional Resources

American Hospital Association (2003). *AHA Guide to the Health Care Field* (2003 Edition). Chicago: American Hospital Association.

American Medical Association (2002). *Socioeconomic Characteristics of Medical Practice, 2002*. Chicago: American Medical Association.

American Medical Association (2002). *Physician Characteristics and Distribution in the U.S., 2002*. Chicago: American Medical Association.

Bureau of Health Professions, U.S. Department of Health and Human Services. Web site: http://bhpr.hrsa.gov.

Census Bureau, U.S. Department of Commerce, Washington, DC. Web site: http://www.census.gov. (See in particular "American Factfinder:").

Census Bureau (2002). *County Business Patterns, 2002*. Washington, DC: U.S. Government Printing Office.

Census Bureau, U.S. Department of Commerce, Washington, DC. Information on the North American Industry Code System. Web site: http://www.census.gov/epcd/www/naics.html.

Center for Mental Health Studies, U.S. Department of Health and Human Services, Washington, DC. Web site: http://www.samhsa.gov/cmhs/htm.

Centers for Disease Control and Prevention, U.S. Department of Health and Human Services, Atlanta, GA. Web site: http://www.cdc.gov.

Centers for Disease Control and Prevention (Weekly). *Morbidity and Mortality Weekly Review*. Atlanta: Centers for Disease Control and Prevention.

FedStats on-line resource. Web site: www.fedstats.gov.

Health Resources and Services Administration, U.S. Department of Health and Human Services, Washington, DC. Web site: http://www.hrsa.dhhs.gov.

Bureau of Primary Health Care, U.S. Department of Health and Human Services, Washington, DC. Web site: http://bphc.hrsa.gov/

National Center for Health Statistics, U.S. Department of Health and Human Services, Hyattsville, MD. Web site: http://www.cdc.gov/nchs

National Center for Health Statistics (2002). *Health United States, 2002*. Washington, DC: U.S. Government Printing Office.

Wellner, Alison S. (1998). *Best of Health: Demographics of Health Care Consumers*. Ithaca, NY: New Strategist Publications.

13

The Future of Health Services Planning

INTRODUCTION

With the dawning of the 21st century, health services planning appears to be entering a new era. By the mid-1990s articles dealing with the issue of health planning began to reappear in the healthcare and health policy literature. New journals geared to academicians with planning interests were established, and newsletters devoted to planning-related topics appeared in the private sector. Papers featuring planning themes were appearing more frequently on the programs of professional meetings and planning issues were openly being discussed by various parties in public forums. "Population-based health care" became one of the "buzz-words" of the late 1990s, and both public and private sector organizations began to cautiously adopt this approach.

Today, health professionals in both settings are increasingly planning-like activities even though they may go by some other name. Integrated delivery systems are being formed, private and public entities are coming together to address community issues, and community-wide attempts to collect and share health-related data are being initiated. After almost two decades in the closet, the "p" word is once again being said aloud.

The reasons for this renewed interest in health planning are complex and reflect the changing nature of the healthcare system itself. The factors encouraging

293

this new emphasis on planning include (1) the movement toward local, community-based approaches to health issues, (2) the perceived failure of "market" approaches, (3) identified deficiencies in public health, (4) the "excesses" that have characterized the private sector, (5) the costs of providing health services under current conditions, and (6) the perceived ineffectiveness of the health care system overall.

The healthcare environment has clearly changed in many ways over the past 20 years, and virtually all of the developments that have occurred make a planning approach in healthcare increasingly important. The paradoxical nature of just a few of the developments reflects the growing need for planning. Who would have ever thought that hospital administrators would be desperately trying to empty beds, providers would be avoiding sick people, clinicians and administrators would be aggressively trying to limit utilization of services, non-clinical personnel would be making "clinical" decisions, and no one would be using the word "patient" anymore? These developments clearly indicate a healthcare world turned on end, and the paradoxes they represent have gone a long way toward fostering renewed interest in health services planning.

The most prominent development in healthcare over the past several years, however, has been the paradigm shift from an emphasis on "medical care" to an emphasis on "healthcare". The implications of this shift are staggering, to the extent even of redefining such basic concepts as "health" and "illness". This shift involves an expansion of the notion of health into a qualitatively different concept and the broadening of the notion of healthcare to include a wide range of services and behaviors never before considered under this heading.

The emergence of this new health care paradigm has been paralleled by shifts in the type of responses offered by the delivery system in the face of a health problem. The traditional approach could be considered to involve an "episodic response." Subsequently, this approach was broadened to take the form of "care management." Today, care management has been expanded to become "patient management". Patient management is now being displaced by an even broader paradigm that involves "population management". Once one moves to a population management paradigm, the need to plan for the provision of health services becomes even more pronounced.

Ultimately, this paradigm shift (and virtually every other trend that is occurring in healthcare) demands the development of a planning mentality. Whether it is the shift to managed care, the new interest in demand management, the growing focus on the continuum of care, or any number of other developments, the ability to formulate and implement plans is becoming increasingly critical.

THE NEW COMMUNITY HEALTH PLANNING

While the renewed interest in health planning might be viewed by some as a revitalization of the comprehensive health planning of the 1960s and 1970s, it is not appropriate to think of contemporary health planning in the same light. Just as the medical care model of the 1960s and 1970s does not represent an appropriate metaphor for today's healthcare environment, the traditional approach to health planning has little place in today's healthcare world.

In considering a more contemporary approach to planning, it might be worthwhile to review some of the reasons offered for the failure of comprehensive health planning. These range from underfunding to a paucity of planning skills to a lack of a constituency for planning. While these may have been the proximate "causes of death" for community health planning, the underlying cause can probably be linked to the assumptions on which traditional health planning was founded. These assumptions include the following:

✓ Health care is primarily concerned with the treatment of disease.
✓ Sick people are the focus of any system of healthcare.
✓ Community health status represents the sum of individual health statuses.
✓ Utilization is a reasonable indicator of actual healthcare needs.
✓ Utilization can be controlled through restrictions on facilities and services.
✓ Health care can be addressed in isolation from other systems in society.
✓ Healthcare is measured in terms of quantity rather than quality.
✓ The existing delivery system is appropriate but requires that some constraints be applied.

Of course, no one could be faulted for accepting these assumptions thirty years ago. They did, after all, represent the conventional wisdom among health professionals. However, these assumptions are now being replaced by others (many of them in direct opposition) that reflect the new healthcare mindset. This new mindset calls for an approach that emphasizes the greatest good for the greatest number and for a comprehensive approach that emphasizes health maintenance and promotion. This approach sees outcomes in terms of improvement in the health status of the community, not in terms of short-sighted objectives such as reducing the number of hospital beds.

Shifting Emphases

This changing approach to community health planning is illustrated by a number of "shifts" that are occurring within healthcare, shifts that can be expected to contribute to a milieu more conducive to planning. These include shifts in the system's conceptual framework, in the scope of healthcare, and in the actual delivery of services. Some of the more important shifts in evidence are outlined below.

1. *From disease control to health management.* The traditional approach to health planning mirrored the healthcare system of the day with its emphasis on treatment and cure. It operated under the assumption that the healthcare system was not activated until an illness or injury occurred. The new health

planning focuses on well people rather than sick ones, reflecting the notion that it is easier to keep someone healthy than it is to cure them after they are sick.

2. *From healthcare in isolation to integrated health delivery.* Traditional health planning did not interface with other types of planning, there was no coordination with other institutions or systems in society, and non-clinical issues were felt to have no bearing on health status and health behavior. The more holistic approach of the new health planning involves interfaces with all relevant institutions and emphasizes an "integrated" approach to healthcare delivery.

3. *From a reactive stance to a proactive stance.* The approach to traditional health planning typically represented a reaction to developments that had already occurred in the healthcare arena. Much of the effort was intended to redress wrongs and correct defects in the system. The new health planning, while not ignoring past and present issues, attempts to proactively address anticipated future developments.

4. *From bureaucratic process to democratic process.* Traditional planning, regardless of the intent, was essentially bureaucratic in nature. Federal sponsorship, in fact, guaranteed that standardized approaches would be emphasized and that top-down policy setting would occur. The historical approach could not accommodate the uniqueness of individual communities and mandated a standardized approach to planning that did not fit all communities. The fact that the new planning has it origin at the grassroots engenders a bottom-up approach to planning. This more "democratic" perspective allows for the consideration of variations in local conditions.

5. *From a formalistic orientation to a pragmatic orientation.* Because of federal sponsorship, the traditional approach exhibited a formal/legal dimension that in many ways handcuffed those involved in planning activities. Rigid guidelines were passed down that were often grudgingly accepted but then ignored in the implementation. The new health planning emphasizes a pragmatic approach that is tailored to the needs of the particular community or organization.

6. *From maintaining control to providing direction.* Traditional planning took a legalistic approach in an effort to regulate the operation of the system. Regulations often became the technique of choice for controlling the system. This created an inflexibility that, of necessity, led to a focus on very narrow goals. The new approach emphasizes the development of a framework for system development rather than trying to control its various components.

7. *From nominally comprehensive to broadly comprehensive.* Ostensibly, "comprehensive" health planning took all aspects of the healthcare delivery system into consideration and, in all fairness, probably did include what was considered the totality of the system at the time. In general, non-clinical aspects of healthcare were not taken into consideration and,

importantly, the patient/consumer dimension was not a consideration. The new planning approach incorporates a much broader notion of health and healthcare in an effort to be truly comprehensive in its orientation.

8. *From a public only approach to public/private cooperation.* Traditional community health planning was something that government agencies carried out and, to many, had little to do with the real world of patient care. While private sector healthcare organizations may have tried to influence or even control the process, most felt like it was not about them. The new planning approach is about everyone. Widespread participation is being called for, and the success of these efforts will depend on the extent to which an interface between community-wide and organization-level planning and between public sector and private sector organizations can be effected.

9. *From a narrow constituency to a broad constituency.* Despite mandated calls for community involvement in the traditional planning process, any meaningful intercourse inevitably involved a handful of vested interests. It was believed that the operation of the process would directly affect only a few parties and, as implemented, this was probably true. The new planning recognizes a much wider range of interests, and even planning at the organization level is increasingly taking the perspectives of various groups outside the organization into consideration.

10. *From a utilization-based approach to a need-based approach.* The analysis of the health system in the past focused on utilization. Utilization levels were considered a proxy for both demand and need. The new health planning, theoretically at least, begins with a realistic view of the true prevalence of health problems and predicates planning decisions on that basis. In this view, utilization patterns should represent a response to the actual healthcare needs of the population rather than a phenomenon existing seemingly independent of other factors.

11. *From narrowly defined outcomes to broadly defined outcomes.* Under the traditional planning paradigm, outcomes were narrowly defined either in terms of the health status of individuals or compliance with bureaucratic mandates (e.g., no more than four hospital beds per 1,000 population). The new approach focuses more on community-wide outcomes such as improved health status and improved access to services.

12. *From impact on facilities/services to impact on population outcomes.* The yardstick in traditional planning for measuring success was the impact that the process had on the inventory of facilities and services. The extent to which these were added or not added to the service complement was the measure of planning effectiveness. There was a clear disconnect between the technical application of planning methodologies and the actual impact the actions had on the community's health status. The ultimate question becomes: What was the impact of the activity on the health status of the population?

While each of these developments has important implications in its own right, taken together they represent a major reorientation for the healthcare arena. This is clearly a situation that demands efficient change management processes, and the planning process provides a framework for addressing change. The need for a revitalized planning approach has been recognized by various parties, and increased support is slowly emerging from a variety of quarters.

Federal agencies like the Health Resources and Services Administration (HRSA) within the Department of Health and Human Services have begun supporting planning initiatives through various programs. If not directly supporting planning activities, other programs are providing funds to improve the healthcare infrastructure to allow for more effective planning, through improvements in information technology and data availability, for example. National foundations like the Robert Wood Johnson Foundation are funding initiatives that involve a community planning component. Professional associations like the American Hospital Association have developed software applications to support community planning. While these developments still represent relatively isolated events, they do provide evidence of a discernible surge of interest in health planning.

THE NEW ORGANIZATIONAL HEALTH PLANNING

Planning at the organization level does not seem to be undergoing the same degree of change as community-wide planning. However, organization-level planning does appear to be gaining momentum. Planning has become an increasingly important function within all types of healthcare organizations, although the term "planning" may not always be used. It is becoming increasingly difficult to find any health professional, in fact, who has not been involved in some type of planning activity.

Many of the developments in healthcare that have encouraged community-wide planning are also contributing to the interest in planning within healthcare organizations. Pressure to contain costs, be accountable, demonstrate effective outcomes, and efficiently manage data are as important for private sector healthcare organizations as they are for public health entities. In fact, in many ways they are more important given the increasingly competitive healthcare environment.

On the other hand, there are some important differences in what is happening at the two different levels of planning. At the organization level, for example, the implications of not planning are often immediate and disastrous. This reflects the fact that a rapidly evolving healthcare environment demands the ability to expeditiously make decisions in response to market developments. Another difference evinced by organization-level planning is the focus on the consumer. The fact that organization-level planning has become market driven means that the behavior patterns and attitudes of consumers take on new meaning within the planning context. The costs involved in a wrong decision are certainly another consideration facing planners at the organization level.

One final difference that might be noted between community-wide and organization-level planning is the involvement of large, national corporations in the healthcare "space" occupied by many organizations. These organizations, which are often for-profit, are likely to have experience in various types of planning that a local organization might not have. The ability to plan from a national perspective sets organization-level planning apart from more community-based health planning initiatives.

Two major trends related to the industry life cycle are also influencing the course of organization-level planning. One involves the maturing and even decline in some cases of certain components of the healthcare system. The other involves the emergence of new growth areas within the industry.

Many components of the healthcare industry have progressed through the stages of the industry life cycle to the point of maturity and beyond. Perhaps the most outstanding example of this phenomenon relates to traditional inpatient care. As is typical of a mature industry entering the decline phase, organizations that provide hospital services find that few new patients or population groups are demanding the service, most of the desirable patient groups have been captured, and relationships between providers and consumers are typically well established. There are few new major breakthroughs in treatment, the major players are becoming consolidated, and profit margins are becoming leaner. Since there are few new customers, the emphasis is on retaining existing customers and extracting as much from them as possible.

Providers of hospital-based care and most other services must adopt a planning approach consistent with their stage in the life cycle. The needs of organizations that are mature or in decline are much different from those experiencing growth. The planning approach must be tailored to the organization's position within the life cycle and its particular market. Planning for an approach that emphasizes "maintenance" is much different from planning for one that emphasizes expansion.

A parallel phenomenon reflects the emergence of new growth markets within healthcare. Healthcare might be likened to an air mattress to the extent that a reduction of services in one area is invariably offset by an expansion in services in another. As certain segments of the industry have declined in importance, other segments have emerged. New services and products, as well as the repackaging of existing services and products, are frequent developments within the industry. Further, new organizational structures and innovative relationships are continually evolving.

Developments of this type in healthcare today are almost too numerous to mention. Some are fairly specific and include therapeutic techniques like laser surgery and other forms of microsurgery, new drug offerings like Viagra, and the various nutritional regimens that are being promoted. Others may involve emerging systems of care such as the various alternative therapy techniques that are being made available. Some of these may even involve repackaging existing services in a more contemporary guise. This would include the repackaging of sub-acute care, rehabilitation services, and home healthcare as "post acute care". In many cases, this means converting a mature or declining service into a new business line.

Organizations attempting to plan for these types of developments obviously face a different situation from those planning for a mature or declining service line. While the issues may be different, the fact remains that the situation demands a planning orientation. Planning, in fact, is particularly important for a program or service that is undergoing rapid expansion.

Although the changes in planning at the organization level have not been as radical as they appear to be in the community planning arena, there is one area in which this shift appears to be more dramatic. This involves the long-overdue change in the mindset of health professionals. Health professionals have been perhaps the most resistant of any group of professionals to the notion of planning. Yet, today, there is a growing conviction that planning should be an integral function of any healthcare organization. Indeed, many health professionals laboring in the trenches today blame a lack of planning for many of the challenges they face—from nursing shortages to fragmentation of services to the increase in uninsured patients.

Clearly the shift in focus from internally oriented types of planning to more externally oriented approaches has progressed significantly. The emphasis appears to be increasingly on strategic planning, marketing planning and business planning, while less attention is devoted to facilities planning and operational planning. This trend is likely to continue as healthcare organizations become less tied to bricks-and-mortar and more dependent on relationships with other organizations.

RESOURCE AVAILABILITY

The improved availability of planning resources has contributed to the increased effectiveness of the planning efforts of health planners at both the community and organization levels. In retrospect, it is amazing that planning with any degree of effectiveness was even possible during the "golden age" of comprehensive health planning. Few people, inside or outside of healthcare, had much planning expertise. There was very limited data available with which to work, and virtually no applicable technology. Today, a number of developments are contributing to a more positive planning environment. Some of the major advances in planning support are described below.

Planning Expertise

At the inception of the comprehensive health planning act in the 1960s, planning as an art and science was not well developed. There were few individuals with the skill to develop a planning process and few models to emulate. Planning was only becoming established in other industries and, even here, these experiences did not translate well into the healthcare arena.

Today, planning methodologies, particularly at the organization level, have become highly developed. While other industries have progressed to a new level of sophistication, healthcare organizations are still struggling with the basics. Nevertheless, numerous tools are now available, and there is considerable expertise to draw upon. While much of this expertise has not been developed in a formal planning context, skills in research, analysis, project planning, marketing and so forth provide a base on which to develop planning capabilities.

Data Resources

Traditional health planning emerged in a data-poor environment. This is not to say that healthcare organizations were not generating data, they were. However, the data that were generated tended to be proprietary for the most part and inaccessible to planners or the general public. There was little in the way of national databases, and federal and state governments were decades away from making their data readily available.

Today, not only do we have access to many more databases than we have had in the past, but we have detailed data on utilization and costs heretofore unavailable. Although gaps still exist with regard to certain types of data, the availability of most types of data has increased dramatically. Organizations in both the public and private sectors have begun generating new data sets. Moreover, efforts are underway by various entities, particularly the federal government, to make existing data more accessible and affordable for the healthcare community.

Technology Resources

Traditional health planning emerged in an environment with virtually no technological support. These early initiatives predated the widespread use of computers by nearly twenty years. Without computers there could be no database management systems and no geographic information systems. (In fact, until the 1980s, maps were still typically colored by hand by health professionals.)

If only the basic technological capabilities available today are considered, this alone would carry planning to a new era. Widespread access to computer technology that brings the power of the mainframe to the desktop has expanded the capabilities of even a novice planner. Inexpensive, user-friendly geographic information system software has made the creation of sophisticated maps relatively easy. These basic technological capabilities are now being supplemented with data warehousing and other data integration capabilities, on-line analytical capabilities, advanced GIS capabilities, and a wide range of software development resources that have carried this process light years beyond even the beginning of the 1990s.

Financial Acumen

The approach to the financial component in healthcare in traditional health planning was superficial at best. Only now are we beginning to gain an understanding of the costs of providing care and to develop adequate financial analysis capabilities. Driven primarily by the changing reimbursement environment, healthcare organizations have been forced to develop a much more indepth understanding of costs than at any time in the past. The notion that it was impossible to truly cost out healthcare has been discarded, and sophisticated approaches to cost accounting are being developed.

THE CONVERGENCE OF COMMUNITY AND ORGANIZATIONAL PLANNING

One trend that is likely to influence the future of health planning is the convergence of community-level and organization-level planning. It has already been observed that public health agencies are being expected to apply a more private sector orientation to their tasks and that private sector organizations are adopting techniques from public health to address the needs of their enrolled populations. While these activities do not constitute the actual convergence of these two distinct approaches, they do suggest the existence of much more commonality than in the past.

Some of the areas of commonality that are emerging include an interest in community assessment and the health status of the total population (rather than only patients), a more proactive approach to addressing the needs of the medically indigent, and a growing emphasis on health promotion and health education. The "community" is increasingly being defined as the "customer" by both public and private organizations. To the extent that planning is occurring, at both levels it appears to be adopting an "outside-in" approach.

This convergence is also evidenced by the establishment of public/private initiatives to address a variety of health issues, including many, such as housing, drug abuse, and violence that have historically been considered outside the healthcare arena. This has extended to the sharing of health-related data, and there are now numerous attempts to establish community health information networks underway.

THE NEW HEALTH PLANNER

These developments in planning call for a new type of health planner and a new skill set. This does not mean simply adding contemporary quantitative techniques to traditional approaches but involves the adaptation of a different mindset from that of the traditional planning approach of the 1960s and 1970s. The planning concept at that time involved a narrowly technical approach that emphasized the mechanical and quantitative aspects of planning. It was also an approach that isolated planning from implementation.

This is not to say that the skills that were important in the early days of health planning are no longer important, they are. These skills must be supplemented by different types of skills that are more appropriate for the new planning paradigm. The traditional planning approach—indeed all planning activities—require analytical skills, an attention to detail, precision, timeliness and follow-through.

The new planning paradigm calls for a higher order of skills to supplement these basic technical skills. The planning process is becoming much more system oriented and involves a much wider range of stakeholders than the traditional approach. Health services planners—in both the public and private sectors—must be able to think much more conceptually, possess qualitative as well as quantitative skills, and be able to work successfully in multiple settings. The new planner must be politically astute, be able to demonstrate leadership, carry out negotiations, and facilitate the planning process.

Unlike the lock-step planning environment of the past, the new planner must be able to live with ambiguity and demonstrate flexibility and creativity. It is one thing to perform calculations to determine if there is an oversupply of hospital beds; it is quite another to develop a plan for the creative reuse of an abandoned hospital building. This calls for broad experiences on the part of the planner and a grounding in the real world. After all, health services planning is increasingly business planning.

Skills are also required in technical areas such as information management and financial analysis. With regard to the former, a grounding in technology is not so important—the technology rapidly changes—but an appreciation of information management issues is critical. Every plan in the future is going to have a financial component, so a working knowledge of financial analysis, third-party reimbursement, and managed care negotiations will become increasingly important.

Communications skills will become more important than ever. The planner-as-facilitator will be required to make a case in written and oral form. As the role of the planner expands and the emphasis becomes more qualitative, the importance of communications skills increases.

The highly circumscribed role of the planner under the traditional planning paradigm is giving way to a much broader role that is essentially without boundaries. It can be argued, in fact, that by virtue of being a planner, no aspect of the system or organization is off limits. The technical support function of the planner is being replaced by one of facilitator. This is being expanded by increased demands for decision making on the part of the planning team. The responsibilities will be further expanded as planners are increasingly urged to take part in the implementation process.

Additional Resources

Garrett, Martha (ed.) (1999). *Health Futures: A Handbook for Health Professionals*. Geneva: World Health Organization.

Landrum, L. B. (n.d.). *Health planning is alive and well*. Retrieved February 1, 2003, from http://www.ahpanet.org/policy.html.

Wing, K. (2000). Health care reform in the year 2000: the view from the front of the classroom. *American Journal of Law and Medicine, 26*(2–3), 277 (18 p).

Glossary

Access   The ability of individuals or groups to obtain health services. Access may be it influenced by service availability, as well as access to transportation, insurance and other factors.

Accessibility analysis   An analytical technique that determines the extent to which plan enrollees or members of the general population have geographical access to providers or other health services. Access in this analysis typically is measured in terms of geographic distance or drive time.

Activities of daily living (ADL)   The tasks that individuals must perform in order to take care of themselves (e.g., dressing, toilet use). The level of disability characterizing an individual is often determined by the number of ADLs the individual can or cannot perform.

Acute condition   A health condition characterized by rapid onset, usually short duration, and a clear-cut disposition (e.g., cure, death), typical of developing countries and younger populations.

Administrative records   Data collected routinely during the course of operations by healthcare organizations or government agencies; certain national registries (e.g., Medicare) are based on administrative records.

Admission The formal placement of an individual into a hospital or other inpatient facility, typically limited to episodes of care involving an overnight stay. The number of admissions is a commonly used measure of hospital utilization.

Adverse selection Situation in which a health plan experiences enrollment of a disproportionate number of individuals with a higher than average risk of utilizing services and thereby filing claims against the plan.

Advertising Promotional activities, typically in the form of media-based promotions, undertaken to influence the demand for a product or service.

Age-specific rates The level of occurrence (per 1,000, 10,000 or 100,000 population) of a phenomenon for specific age cohorts.

Agency for Healthcare Research and Quality (AHRQ) A federally funded research institute that supports studies on the utilization of health services and the efficacy of various treatment modalities.

Alternative therapy An umbrella term that refers to a variety of therapeutic modalities (e.g., homeopathy, acupuncture, nutritional therapy) utilized by patients as alternatives to mainstream allopathic medicine. Increasingly referred to as complementary therapies.

Ambulatory care Any type of treatment that is provided to an "ambulatory" patient that does not require an overnight hospital stay. Also referred to as outpatient care.

Ambulatory Payment Classification (APC) The classification system developed by the Center for Medicare and Medicaid Services for reimbursing services provided to outpatients. It is essentially the ambulatory care version of the Diagnosis Related Group system.

Attitude An individual's cognitive evaluations, feelings, or action tendencies toward some person, object, or idea.

Audit, external An assessment of the external environment of a health system or organization, involving a range of data collection activities on the market area and its population.

Audit, internal An assessment of the internal environment of an organization, involving a thorough analysis of operations, staffing, systems, policies and procedures, customer characteristics and other factors that contribute to a description of the organization.

Average length of stay (ALOS) The number of days on average patients remain in a hospital or other institution, calculated as the number of patient days during a period (usually a year) divided by the number of admissions during that period.

Baby Boomers   The segment of the U.S. population (born between 1946 and 1964) that constitutes the largest cohort in the age distribution and exhibits characteristics that set it apart from older and younger age cohorts.

Bed day   One patient filling one bed for one day. Used as a measure of service utilization.

Break-even analysis   A mathematical determination of the volume of revenue required to cover total costs of a good or service at a given price.

Business coalition   A cooperative formed by businesses in a community in order to jointly negotiate with healthcare providers with the intent of containing healthcare costs.

Capitation   An arrangement whereby providers are paid a predetermined per capita fee for providing a specified range of services to a specified population.

Case analysis   A technique used by epidemiologists to identify the incidence of specific health conditions within a population and track the progression of these conditions over time.

Case-mix   The combination of diagnoses that make up the distribution of cases treated by a particular provider (e.g., the proportion of cases that are obstetrical, cardiac, etc.). Alternatively, the overall characteristics (e.g., age, sex) of a group of enrollees for which a case manager is responsible.

Catchment area   The geographic area from which a healthcare organization draws its patients or enrollees; sometimes formally designated for assigning patients to various providers.

Causal research   Research that attempts to identify cause-and-effect relationships by means of specifying the functional relationships between two or more variables in a research study.

Cause of death   The reason for the death of an individual entered on the standard death certificate and used in mortality analyses.

Census   A data collection technique that involves obtaining data from the entire population.

Census Bureau, U.S.   The federal agency within the U.S. Department of Commerce with responsibility for conducting the decennial census and a variety of other censuses and survey activities.

Census block   The smallest geographic area for which the Census Bureau collects and reports data during the decennial census. A census block is the square or other polygon that is formed by the streets that comprise the four (usually) sides of a block.

Census tract   A geographic area established by the Census Bureau for the collection and reporting of census data.

Center for Medicare and Medicaid Services (CMS)   The federal agency within the U.S. Department of Health and Human Services that manages the Medicare and Medicaid programs.

Centers for Disease Control and Prevention (CDC)   The CDC is the federal agency responsible for monitoring various infectious diseases and tracking the course of any epidemic condition. The CDC is an important source of epidemiological data.

Certificate-of-Need (CON)   In many states, a certificate-of-need application must be filed in order to obtain approval for the establishment of a new health facility or an addition or change in services provided. The states that maintain CON programs vary widely in terms of the types of services provided and the provisions for CON regulations.

Cherry picking   The practice in which a healthcare provider or health plan targets only the most desirable patients or enrollees.

Chronic condition   A health condition characterized by slow onset, lengthy progression, and a usually indefinite disposition, typical of modern, industrial societies and older populations.

Cohort   A segment of the population that is distinguished by a particular attribute—e.g., all people born in the United States between 1946 and 1951 or all American soldiers exposed to Agent Orange in Viet Nam.

Cohort analysis   An analytical technique that monitors the movement of cohorts of individuals over time and the implications of this movement for health services utilization.

Cohort effect   The observed impact that certain experiences and conditions exert on a cohort of individuals as that cohort is monitored over time—e.g., the analysis of the baby boom cohort's adaptation to aging.

Collection, data   Any one of a number of procedures (both primary and secondary) for acquiring the data required for the implementation of a research plan.

Commercial insurer   A category of for-profit insurance plan that typically reimburses providers on a fee-for-service basis.

Community health information network (CHIN)   A system established by a coalition of healthcare providers and/or purchasers for the purpose of collecting, processing, sharing and disseminating patient data collected from the community or plan enrollees.

Community survey   A type of sample survey conducted on the community at large, typically using households within the community as the sampling frame.

Community-based care   The range of health services provided to individuals or families outside formal institutional settings.

Competitive analysis   Research conducted on the characteristics of a healthcare organization's competitors within a market area.

Comprehensive Health Planning Act   The original legislation that established the first formal health planning structure in 1966. This Act was replaced by subsequent health planning acts. All federal support for health planning was eliminated in the early 1980s.

Computer-Assisted Personal Interview (CAPI)   Interview situation in which the interviewer directly enters responses in a laptop or hand-held computer, thereby eliminating the need to transfer data later on.

Computer-Assisted Telephone Interview (CATI)   Interview situation that utilizes a computer software application for question generation and data entry while the interviewer talks to the respondent via telephone.

Consumer   Any individual in the community that is a potential user of an organization's products or services.

Consumer panel   A sample of respondents who agree to provide information to researchers over an extended period of time.

Contextual analysis   A research technique that involves an examination of the context in which the phenomenon under study exists as a factor in interpretation.

Cost shifting   The process through which healthcare providers increase charges to certain categories of customers in order to compensate for the portion of charges that other customers cannot or do not pay.

Cost-benefit analysis   A form of analysis that identifies the benefits (both tangible and intangible) that will be derived from a project and compares the benefits to the costs involved in carrying out the project.

Covered lives   Total individuals that are covered under an insurance plan (as opposed to the number of individuals who participate in the plan)—i.e., plan participants plus any covered dependents.

Crude birth rate (CBR)   A simple measure of the level of fertility of a population based on the number of births per 1,000 population; the birth rate may be misleading since the denominator includes the total population and not just the population at risk.

Crude death rate (CDR)   A simple measure of the level of mortality of a population based on the number of deaths per 1,000 population; the crude death rate may be misleading since there are significant variations in death rate by age. Also referred to as the crude mortality rate.

Current Procedural Terminology (CPT)   A coding system used by physicians to code procedures performed. This code is tied to the fees charged.

Custodial care   Refers to non-medical care provided to individuals, typically in long term care facilities, who cannot take care of themselves. There is no intent to cure, thus the term "custodial". Also referred to as "personal care".

Customer   A patient or other type of client that currently utilizes one or more of the organization's products or services.

Decision support system (DSS)   A computerized application that includes relevant databases, a system for manipulating the data, and a user interface that allows users to generate information to support decision making.

Deinstitutionalization   Process through which institutionalized patients (typically the mentally ill) are discharged from inpatient facilities with the assumption that supportive services and treatment will be provided within the community.

Demand (for health services)   The combined healthcare needs and wants of a population that constitutes the volume and type of health services "demanded" by the population (which may or may not approximate utilization).

Demand management   An approach utilized primarily by managed care plans to proactively limit health services utilization by limiting the demand for services rather than trying to control utilization once demand has been manifested.

Demographics   The numerical, biosocial and sociocultural characteristics of a population that constitute its demographic composition.

Density, population   An indicator of the density or sparseness of the population in a geographic area, usually measured in terms of persons per square mile or, in urban areas, per acre.

Dependency ratio   An index that compares the number of "dependent" individuals within a population to the number of independent individuals that are expected to support them. The very young and very old are typically included among the dependent population.

Descriptive research   Research that describes the population, market, or situation under study, but does not attempt to explain the patterns that are identified.

Desktop marketing system   A microcomputer-based system that interfaces databases useful for marketing and planning and provides applications with which the user can manipulate the data in these databases and generate reports, graphics, maps and other output.

Diagnosis Related Groups (DRGs)   A system of categorizing diagnoses and/or procedures for hospital inpatients into groupings based on relative resource utilization and used as a basis for prospective reimbursement by the Medicare program.

Diagnostic and Statistical Manual of Mental Disorders (DSM)   A coding system patterned on the International Classification of Disease that is utilized for classifying mental disorders.

Differentiation strategy   A business development or marketing approach that attempts to distinguish one organization or product from its competitors in ways significant to consumers or to create the perception that there is difference, even if there is not.

Disability   The level of incapacity within a population as measured by the number of cases of physically and/or mentally handicapped individuals, or by the level of restricted activity (e.g., school-loss days or work-loss days).

Discharge   The official release of a patient after an episode of care at a hospital or other inpatient facility involving at least one night in the hospital. The number of discharges is a frequently used indicator of the utilization level for a hospital.

Disease   A term used in a number of different ways but generally referring to a state of pathology within an individual organism.

Disease management   An approach to patient care that emphasizes the long term, continuous, and often comprehensive management of a patient's disease, rather than an episodic approach to the treatment of the condition.

Diversification   Process through which health care organizations diversify their service offerings beyond their traditional service complement. Hospitals frequently diversify by establishing outpatient facilities to serve different needs. Other healthcare organizations may diversify into unrelated areas (e.g., real estate, assisted living facilities) in order to expand their revenue base.

Durable medical equipment (DME)   Biomedical and assistive equipment that is utilized in the provision of care for institutionalized, homebound and ambulatory patients. Wheelchairs and hospital-type beds are examples of durable medical equipment.

Elasticity   The tendency for the demand for health services to rise or fall in response to non-clinical factors (e.g., insurance coverage, consumer preferences).

Elective procedure   A procedure that is not covered by insurance typically because it is not considered medically necessary (e.g., cosmetic surgery). A consumer may "elect" to have such a procedure performed if he is willing to pay out of pocket for the service.

Encounter Refers to one patient visit to a provider, usually regardless of the number of procedures performed.

Epidemiological analysis An approach to the study of health phenomena that involves the relationship between individuals and their social environment and the distribution of health problems among various segments of the population.

Episodic care The traditional approach to the provision of health services in which each physician visit for each reason is considered a separate episode unrelated to any other episodes of care for that condition. This is in contrast to managed care that focuses on the total and continuous management of the condition or the patient.

Estimate, population A calculated estimation of the population for a particular area or population category for some current or past time period.

Evaluation analysis An analytical technique that involves the assessment of the effectiveness of the processes and outcomes associated with a program or service.

Exploratory research Preliminary (often informal) analysis that examines the general nature of the problem or opportunity under study and provides guidance for the development of more formal descriptive analyses.

Extrapolation A projection technique that graphically, mathematically or statistically identifies a pattern in a number of periods of past utilization, and then extends that pattern into the future to predict utilization.

Family life cycle The stages the "typical" consumer passes through from childhood to death, including stages of marriage, childbearing, "empty nest", and retirement.

Fee-for-service The traditional means of paying for health care in the United States whereby insurers or patients pay a separate fee for each service that a physician, hospital or other provider performs. This is in contrast to managed care in which the provider receives a specified amount of reimbursement for managing a range of services.

Fertility The reproduction experience of a population, most often expressed in terms of total births and/or birth rates.

Flow diagram The visual presentation of a sequential process or logic.

Focus groups Interviews conducted with typically 8 to 10 persons and a trained moderator following an interview guide for the purpose of collecting qualitative data.

Forecast   A prediction of future reality, based on an examination of present or past reality together with judgment regarding how reality might change.

Full-time equivalent (FTE)   The amount of labor that would represent one employee working on a full-time basis. The FTE unit is used to standardize labor force counts where different organizations utilize varying amounts of part-time labor.

Gap analysis   An analytical technique used to assess the gap between needs of a population and the resources required to meet those needs, or between the current status of an organization and the position in which it would like to be.

Gatekeeper   The person or organization that controls a consumer's access to health services. Traditionally, the physician has served as the gatekeeper for the system. Other gatekeepers such as health plan authorization personnel and discharge planners also play an important role in managing utilization in today's healthcare environment.

Geographic information system (GIS)   Computerized application for performing spatial analysis and generating maps reflecting the analysis.

Goal   A generalized statement indicating the desired position of an organization or health system at some point in the future.

Gusher analysis   An analytical technique that identifies particularly promising market opportunities that are immediately available (although they may not have much long-term benefit).

Health   A state of wellness whose definition depends on one s perspective. In the narrowest sense, health has been defined as the absence of disease and disability. In its broadest sense, it has been defined as a state of complete physical, social, mental and spiritual well-being.

Health maintenance organization (HMO)   An organization of healthcare providers that offers a comprehensive range of services to an enrolled population for a fixed, prepaid sum.

Health plan   A generic term that applies to any type of insurance program that provides coverage for health services, including companies that self-insure their employees.

Health Plan Employer Data and Information Set (HEDIS)   An attempt to standardize health plan performance in terms of quality, access, satisfaction, utilization, and finance for use in comparing various health plans; the survey instrument used to gather HEDIS data.

Health Professional Shortage Area (HPSA)   Area designated by the U.S. Public Health Service that has a shortages of specified categories of healthcare providers.

Health promotion Any activity or system that is designed to proactively maintain, improve, or enhance the health status of individuals or populations. Health promotion generally includes both preventive care and lifestyle-related health behavior.

Health service area The geographic area served by a healthcare provider. The federal government designates formal health service areas covering the entire United States for some of its data management activities.

Health status indicator A measure of the relative health condition of a person or population, usually in the form of an index score and generated through self-reports or from statistics produced on the population in question.

Holism An approach to healthcare that involves holistic perspective on the diagnosis and treatment of health problems. This approach involves an emphasis on the whole person rather than a specific disease or organ and takes into consideration non-clinical factors related to the patient.

Incidence The number of new cases of a disease, disability, or other health-related phenomenon recorded during a specified period of time, reported in terms of the number of cases per 100, 1,000, 10,000 or 100,000 population.

Indemnity insurance The traditional form of health insurance in the United States in which the insured pays the cost for each service after it has been provided (assuming it is covered by the benefits package). This is in contrast to a managed care approach that involves prepayment for a package of services that are covered under the health plan.

Indepth interview Research technique involving (usually) one-on-one interviews with key informants that are lengthy and involve indepth probing for information.

Index A composite "score" usually calculated from responses, on a survey or the characteristics of a population that have been identified; the index score can then be compared to other respondents or populations.

Indigent care Health services provided at no cost to individuals who are considered "medically indigent"—i.e., they are not covered under any type of insurance plan. Such patients are not necessarily impoverished but they lack the ability to pay for health services.

Industry life cycle The process that an industry typically follows involving: the emergence of the industry as a new phenomenon, a growth phase, a maturity phase, and a period of decline as the industry's functions are replaced by other industries.

Infant mortality rate (IMR) The number of deaths to infants under one year of age per 1,000 live births during a specific time period (usually one year). Also referred to as the infant death rate.

Information   Data that have been rendered meaningful by means of statistical analysis and interpretation.

In-migration   The flow of new residents into a geographic area.

Inpatient   Technically, any patient that spends at least one night (or 24 hours) in an institution such as a hospital or residential treatment program. Traditionally, most patients requiring any significant type of care were admitted to a hospital as inpatients.

Integrated delivery system (IDS)   Arrangement for integrating physicians, hospitals and other medical services into a network for the provision of coordinated health services to a defined population of enrollees.

Intercept interview   A research technique that "intercepts" potential respondents as they carry out routine activities—e.g., shopping at a mall or waiting in a clinic reception room—and performs interviews at the point of intercept or in a nearby interview area.

International Classification of Disease (ICD)   The standard classification system utilized to categorize the universe of diagnoses and procedures utilized in contemporary medical science.

Interpolation   An estimation technique for calculating estimates between two points in time for which data are available—e.g., if population figures are available for 1980 and 1990, an estimate for 1985 could be made through interpolation.

Interview, computerized   A technique in which a respondent interactively completes a survey form at a computer, either by touching the screen, typing at the keyboard, or through voice activation.

Interview, mail(out)   A research technique that involves mailing out survey forms to respondents, who then return completed forms to the organization that mailed them or to some third party for analysis.

Interview, personal   A research technique that involves face-to-face administration of a survey instrument.

Interview, telephone   A research technique that involves the administration of a survey instrument over the telephone.

Key informant   An interview subject chosen as a key source of information due to his position within the organization, his role as opinion leader, or some other characteristic that makes the informant a critical source of information.

Length of stay   The number of days an individual remains in a hospital or other healthcare facility. The length of stay is an important consideration in utilization management.

Lifestyle The set of attitudes, values, preferences and behavior patterns that distinguish subsets of the population from each other; often used interchangeably with "psychographic characteristics".

Lifestyle analysis An analytical approach that evaluates a population on the basis of the lifestyle characteristics associated with various subsets within the population; often used interchangeably with "psychographic analysis".

Limitation of activity A measure of disability that involves a determination of the ability of an individual to carry out various activities. Usually presented in terms of bed-restricted days, school-loss days, work-loss days, etc.

Living arrangement Used to describe the nature of household relationships as a supplement to marital status. Includes such categories as married without children married with children, living alone, cohabitative relationship, and unrelated individuals living together.

Long term care (LTC) Refers to any type of care for the elderly and/or disabled that involves on-going institutionalized management of the patient whether or not medical care is necessary. Nursing homes are the traditional form of long term care but various other types of long term care facilities have become common.

Maintenance strategy A strategic approach adopted by healthcare organizations when the industry is in the mature phase of the life cycle. Since there is limited expansion occurring, the emphasis is on maintaining existing business and extracting as much benefit from it as possible.

Marital status The official status of individuals in terms of marriage, typically including the categories of never married, married, divorced, widowed and, sometimes, separated.

Managed care A planned and coordinated approach involving positive and negative incentives for both enrollees and providers for "managing" the services received by a population enrolled in a particular health plan.

Market Any geographic area or population grouping that can be conceptualized as a source of potential customers.

Market area The targeted geographic area in which the primary market potential for a healthcare organization is located; often used interchangeably with "service area".

Market research A multi-step process involving the systematic gathering and analysis of market data that assists an organization in developing strategies and making decisions.

Market segment A specific subset of a population that differs from other subsets in terms of their use of health services.

Market share   The proportion of health services utilization that any single provider is able to capture in a given time period.

Marketing mix   The combination of the "four Ps" of marketing–product, price, place and promotion—characterizing the marketing activities of a particular organization or product line.

Marketing plan   An outline of the methods and resources needed to achieve organizational goals with regard to a specific target market.

Marketing research   The process by which the marketer acquires information to be used to identify and define marketing opportunities and problems; generate, refine and evaluate marketing actions; and improve understanding of marketing as a process.

Matrix analysis   An analytical technique that involves simultaneously examining the various possible outcomes that are associated with a combination of factors that are likely to influence an outcome.

Measurement   The assignment of numbers to characteristics of objects, persons, states or events according to pre-specified rules.

Median age   An indicator of the average age of a population, whereby the median age represents that age at which half of the population falls below and half falls above.

Medicaid   The federally sponsored and state-administered government insurance program for the low-income population in the United States. The Center for Medicare and Medicaid Services (CMS) manages the program, with the characteristics of the program varying from state to state.

Medically indigent   Individuals who for whatever reason do not have access to health insurance and or not able to pay for health service out of pocket. The medically indigent may not be poverty-stricken but are "insurance poor."

Medically necessary   A characteristic of a procedure or service provided under an insurance plan that reflects a clear medical need for the procedure or service. This is in contrast to elective procedures (e.g., cosmetic surgery) that nay be performed in the absence of medical necessity.

Medicare   The federally-sponsored insurance program that provides coverage for the elderly population in the United States. All elderly citizens are eligible for basic coverage, with certain additional coverage optional. The Medicare program is administered by the Center for Medicare and Medicaid Services (CMS).

Metropolitan statistical area (MSA)   An official designation for a large concentration of population that includes a central city, a county and its surrounding counties.

Migration The physical movement of individuals or groups from one location to another, typically with the intent of a permanent change of residence.

Minor civil division (MCD)/Census county division (CCD) Sub-county geographical areas established by the Census Bureau as the basis for data collection and reporting when census tracts are not used.

Mission statement A short statement (usually one or two paragraphs) describing an organization's reason for being.

Model A statement (mathematical or otherwise) that specifies the conceptual relationship between two or more variables—e.g., a model may depict the manner in which healthcare decisions are made with a hospital.

Morbidity The level of sickness and disability within a population, usually expressed in terms of incidence and prevalence rates.

Mortality The level of death characterizing a population, usually expressed in terms of the number of deaths and/or death rates.

Mystery shopper A term applied to the use of an individual Pretending to be a customer who utilizes the services of a healthcare organization in an effort to obtain information on procedures, employee behavior, prices or other information that might not be readily available.

National Center for Health Statistics (NCHS) The "census bureau" of health care, the NCHS is the federal agency responsible for the collection, management and dissemination of most national data on health and healthcare

Naturally occurring groups Groups suitable for conducting interviews because of the "natural" setting in which they are found—e.g., the family and friends of a hospitalized patient.

Necessity strategy A strategic approach that involves the introduction of services as a prerequisite for effectively competing in a market, rather than as a direct basis for revenue. Hospitals often feel compelled to offer certain services, although there is little opportunity to achieve significant market share.

Need In this context, need refers to the actual need for health services within a population as measured by the prevalence of clinically identifiable health problems. This is in contrast to wants and desires for health services that might characterize a population. Need should represent the baseline level of health problems affecting a population.

Niche, market A market opportunity, usually narrowly defined in terms of population, geographic location, or service category, that is not being exploited by mainstream providers.

Niche strategy A strategic approach that focuses on identifying and exploiting one or more niche markets within a service area. Rather than offering a full range of hospital services, a hospital may elect to focus on certain segments of the market (e.g., eye surgery, foot surgery).

Notifiable disease   A disease whose presence must be reported to public health officials. Typically an infectious disease, notifiable conditions are generally first reported to local health departments and this information is compiled nationally by the Centers for Disease Control and Prevention (CDC).

Objective   A formally designated achievement to be accomplished in support of a goal that is specific, concise, and time bound.

Observation, non-participatory   A form of observation research in which the observer is detached from the group or activity being observed and those being observed typically are unaware of the research taking place.

Observation, participatory   A form of observation research in which the observer becomes a part of the group or activity being observed in order to collect information as an "insider".

Occupancy rate   The percent of the beds in a hospital or other inpatient facility that are occupied by patients during a particular time period. The occupancy rate is an indicator of the level of utilization of a hospital, with occupancy for licensed beds and operational beds often calculated separately.

Office visit   The standard measure for use of physician services and the typical "encounter" that is recorded to measure utilization of physicians and other services.

Operationalization   Process for representing a concept in the form of a measurable variable. E.g., "social class" is often operationalized for research purposes in terms of "median household income".

Opportunity cost   The potential benefits to be derived from a project that are forfeited by virtue of turning attention to another project.

Out-of-pocket payment   Reimbursement for health services provided by consumers who are not covered by insurance or for whom the particular service is not covered. Certain procedures are never covered by insurance and consumers who require these services must pay out of pocket.

Outcome measurement   A formal process for assessing the effectiveness of treatment and/or patient satisfaction with treatment results.

Out-migration   The flow of residents out of a geographic area.

Outpatient   An individual who receives any type of health service that does not require an overnight stay in a hospital or other inpatient facility. Similar to an ambulatory patient, although homebound patients would be considered outpatients but not ambulatory patients.

Over-the-counter drug (OTC)   A drug that can be purchased from a pharmacy without a prescription written by a physician.

Patient   Any individual who receives "formal" health services from a licensed healthcare provider. This does not include self care since the individual has not been formally diagnosed.

Panel survey   A sample of respondents who have agreed to provide information for a research project over an extended period of time.

Patient origin   The source of patients for a health service based on place of residence (usually identified by zip code).

Payer (or payor)   See Third-Party Payer.

Penetration   The percentage of business captured by a health plan or plans, usually used in reference to managed care. E.g., a managed care penetration rate of 20 percent indicates that managed care plans have enrolled 20 percent of the area's potential health plan enrollees.

Period effect   The effect of the specific events and conditions uniquely occurring at a particular time to a particular cohort within the population.

Plan   A systematic approach to specifying and striving after a future goal, typically involving the matching of existing resources with market opportunities.

Planning   The process for developing a systematic plan for identifying and reaching some future goal.

Plan, business   A systematic approach for reaching a specific business objective at some point in the future.

Plan, human resources   A systematic approach for allocating resources to meet future needs for personnel.

Plan, implementation   A systematic approach for carrying out the activities specified in a strategic plan or other type of plan. The overall plan typically defines what is to be done, while the implementation plan determine how it will be done.

Plan, marketing   A systematic approach for utilizing a marketing initiative to reach some objective of the organization.

Plan, operational   A systematic approach for maintaining operations and reaching some specified operations-related goal in the future.

Plan, strategic   A systematic approach to positioning the organization in the market, utilizing existing resources to exploit market opportunities.

Plan, technology   A systematic approach for evaluating, acquiring and implementing appropriate technology for use at some point in the future.

Population at risk   The total number of persons within a population that are at risk of a particular condition. E.g., the number of persons at risk of childbirth would equal the number of fertile child-bearing age women within the population.

Population-based healthcare   An approach to the provision of health services that focuses on the needs of the total population rather than the needs of individuals. Outcomes are measured in terms of improvement in overall health status rather than by individual clinical successes.

Population pyramid   A stacked bar graph visually depicting the age and sex composition of a specific population.

Preferred provider organization (PPO)   A form of health plan that encourages the use of a specified network of providers in exchange for lower rates for plan enrollees. The PPO typically negotiates discounted rates with providers in the network, with the intent of passing these discounts to consumers in the form of lower premiums.

Prevalence   The total number of cases of a disease or disability within a population at a specific point in time, reported in terms of the number of cases per 100, 1,000, 10,000 or 100,000 population.

Preventive care   Any activity intended to prevent disease and/or improve health status carried out prior to the onset of a health problem. Preventive care includes health education, screening, and various health behaviors (e.g., tooth brushing) that protect the individual from the onset of health conditions.

Price   The dollar amount that a provider charges for a service provided, typically referred to as a "fee" in health care. This is distinguished from "cost" which refers to the provider's cost of providing the service.

Pricing strategy   A strategic approach that attempts to capture customers and market share by offering a price advantage to consumers.

Primary care   The provision of basic, routine health services including preventive services. The physicians typically involved in primary care are general and family practitioners, general internists, obstetricians, and pediatricians, although other types of providers (e.g., behavioral health therapists) may be thought to provide "primary" care.

Primary data   Information collected specifically to address a particular research issue.

Product life cycle   The process that a product or service might follow as it evolves—i.e., involving the emergence of the product or service as a new phenomenon, a growth phase, a maturity phase, and a period of decline as the product or service is replaced by other products or services.

Product line   See Service Line.

Projection, population   A calculated figure indicating the size of the population for a particular area or population category for some point in the future.

Promotion   Any activity intended to promote an organization, service or product. Promotion is considered an important component of marketing and can involve public relations, advertising, direct mail and many other types of activities.

Proprietary data   Data gathered by or generated by an organization for exclusive use internal by that organization.

Provider   An individual or organization that is licensed to provide health services, products or equipment.

Provider network   A group of providers that have been formally contracted to provide services to enrollees in a particular health plan; in many plans, enrollees are restricted to providers that belong to the network.

Psychographics   Subjective information reported by people regarding their beliefs, feelings, attitudes and behavior patterns; also referred to as lifestyles and utilized as a basis for predicting health behavior.

Public health   The set of activities designated for public health agencies that include disease surveillance, health status monitoring, air and water monitoring, food inspection, the registration of vital events, and the control of infectious conditions.

Public relations   The maintaining of communication and relationships with the general public, various constituents, and consumer groups. As a dimension of marketing, public relations involves press releases, public speaking, "infomercials", and other means of communicating with those outside the organization.

Purchaser (of health services)   Any organization or individual that pays for health services that are provided. In common usage, purchaser has come to refer to "group purchasers" such as large employers and business coalitions that represent large numbers of covered lives and can negotiate with providers due to their purchasing power.

Qualitative research   Inductive, subjective and process-oriented research methods utilized to describe, understand, and interpret research issues.

Quantitative research   Postivistic, deductive and objective research methods primarily designed to identify relationships between variables.

Rate   The level of occurrence of a phenomenon per a specified number of persons—e.g., per 100, 1,000, 10,000 or 100,000.

Ratio   The proportion of a characteristic in relation to another characteristic. E.g., a sex ratio of 95 means there are 95 males per 100 females.

Region, geographic   Generally a geographic area the extends beyond any one political jurisdiction to create an internally consistent region of some type (e.g., Appalachia). Also, refers to officially designated regions into which the United States is divided by the federal government.

Registry   The systematic recording and reporting of events or situations characterizing a population—e.g., a registry containing all reported cases of cancer within a specified area or all licensed physicians within a particular state.

Research design   A blueprint or framework that is followed in conducting research.

Research question   A specific statement concerning components of a business problem or opportunity that drive the research process; research questions are referred to as hypotheses in more formalized research circumstances.

Respondent   A person or other unit (e.g., household) that takes part in a survey research project.

Return on investment (ROI)   The expected percentage profit hat can be expected measured against the amount of resources that are invested in a project.

Risk   The exposure that individuals or population groups experience with regard to various health problems. The risk of contracting AIDS, for example, varies with the types of behaviors in which an individual participates.

Risk analysis   An actuarial process in which the anticipated utilization and resultant healthcare costs for a particular population or enrollee group are determined.

Rural area   An area designated by the Census Bureau for data collection purposes that does not meet the minimum standards for an urban area. I.e., the population is limited in size and contains no population concentrations of any significance.

Sample   A subset of the population selected for inclusion in a survey.

Sample size   The number of individuals or other units selected for inclusion in a survey based on specified rules for determining the number.

Sample survey   A survey in which a subset of the population has been selected for participation in a study. The intent is to draw conclusions concerning the total population based on the sample of respondents that have been interviewed.

Sampling frame   The list of the target population from which the sample will be drawn—e.g., all addresses in a particular community.

Satisfaction survey   A survey that attempts to measure the level of satisfaction with regard to health services or health plans on the part of patients, family members, plan enrollees, or other categories of customers.

Scenario   The hypothetical presentation of a situation that reflects the possible effects of a variety of factors on an existing situation.

Secondary care   A level of health services that involves moderate intensity care and a moderate level of resources and skill levels. Secondary care is more complex than routine care but less intensive than specialized tertiary services.

Secondary data   Data collected for some other purpose (such as routine administrative records) but used for some other research application. E.g., census data collected for federal statistical purposes might be used for market research.

Segmentation, benefit   The grouping of people based on the benefits (such as convenience or value) sought from a product or service.

Segmentation, demographic   The grouping of individuals into market segments based on such demographic characteristics as age, sex, income, and race.

Segmentation, geographic   The grouping of individuals into market segments based on location of residence or work.

Segmentation, psychographic   The grouping of individuals into market segments based on lifestyle and attitudinal characteristics.

Segmentation, usage   The grouping of individuals into market segments based on their level of utilization of a product or service. Segments may initially be identified as user and non-users, with the users broken down into subcategories based on their level of usage.

Self-administered questionnaire   Survey forms that are completed by the respondents with little or no input from survey administrators.

Service area   The geographic area from which a health care organization draws the majority of its customers; often used interchangeably with "market area".

Service line   A business development approach that involves the identification of a vertical set of services (e.g., cardiac care) and the subsequent operation and marketing of the set of services as a business line.

Sex ratio   An indicator of the relative proportions of males and females within a population. Typically calculated in terms of the number of males per 100 females.

Significance, statistical   The determination that a research finding reflects a statistical association and not simply a chance correlation.

Socioeconomic status   An indicator of an individual or group's position in the social structure based on such measures as income, occupation and education.

Spatial analysis   An analytical technique that involves the study of the spatial relationships between various phenomena—e.g., the analysis of the geographic distribution of physician offices.

Stakeholder   Any individual, organization or constituency that has a stake in the operation of an organization or a healthcare system. Formal stakeholders may be stockholders or other investors, while informal ones may include medical staffs, suppliers, consumers groups, and so forth.

Standardization   A process through which dissimilar populations are statistically adjusted to allow for meaningful comparisons.

Strategy   A generalized approach to positioning an organization relative to the market and its competitors in that market. The strategy provides one parameter in the development of a strategic plan.

Surrogate data   Data used as a substitute for data that cannot be readily obtained.

Survey instrument   Questionnaires used in survey research re sometimes called survey instruments.

SWOT analysis   An analytical technique that involves the evaluation of a community's or an organization's strengths, weaknesses, opportunities and threats.

Syndicated research   A form of contract survey research in which a professional research firm conducts a survey and sells the results to interested parties in the area or, alternatively, the research firm enlists the front-end participation of area healthcare organizations in the development of the survey.

Synthetic data   Population estimates and projections that are generated using statistical techniques and models. Synthetic data are distinguished from actual data collected by means of censuses and surveys.

Tactics   The actions that are initiated in order to pursue a strategy within the context of a strategic plan.

Target marketing   A marketing technique that focuses on specific market segments rather than the mass market.

Tertiary care   Specialized health services for the treatment of serious health conditions that require specialized clinicians, sophisticated equipment and facilities, and substantial support services.

Third-party payer (payor)   Any agency or organization that is responsible for reimbursing the cost of health services provided on the part of an insured individual.

The provider delivers the service to the patient, with the insurer being the "third party" that pays for the care.

Trend analysis The longitudinal analysis of data for the purpose of identifying the presence or absence of consistency over time; a form of time series analysis.

Uncompensated care Health services provided to medically indigent populations that have no ability to pay for care. Uncompensated care is sometimes informally used to refer to any shortfall between charges and reimbursement for services.

Underinsured Individuals or groups in a population who are technically covered under some insurance plan but have such limited benefits or unfavorable copay or deductible provisions that they do not have adequate coverage.

Uninsured Individuals or groups in a population who are not covered under any insurance plan.

Universal coverage Situation in which an entire population is covered by a standard form of medical insurance.

Urbanized area A Census Bureau designation for a geographic area that meets specific requirements for being considered "urban". An urbanized area may or may not be incorporated, since designation is a function of the size and characteristics of the population.

Utilization (of health services) The number and type of health services actually used by a particular population, as opposed to the demand for services.

Utilization management Theoretically, the process of assuring that a patient receives the appropriate care at the appropriate time in the appropriate setting. In actual practice, utilization management is often seen as a means of restricting utilization in order to reduce costs.

Variable A concept of interest in a research study, operationalized in a manner that will allow for statistical analysis.

Vendor, commercial data A private sector corporation that generates and disseminates data and/or software for data manipulation.

Vital statistics Data collected by government agencies related to "vital events"— e.g., births, deaths, marriages, divorces, and abortions.

Vulnerable population Any population segment within a population that is placed at inordinate risk of health problems due to health status, environmental factors, lack of insurance, marginality, and any number of other factors.

What-if analysis The creation of hypothetical situations in which the relevant variables can be manipulated to determine the effects of chances in the model being utilized.

Years of potential life lost A measure of disability and premature death that is calculated in terms of the number of years that an individual would have expected to live (or to have quality of life) had it not been for disability or death. This is sometimes transformed into "productive" years of life lost.

ZIP code An administrative district created by the U.S. Postal Service for the efficient delivery of mail. Although not originally intended as units for data collection and dissemination, ZIP codes are often used as a basis for planning), and marketing studies.

Appendixes

───────── IA ─────────

A Statewide Planning Initiative

OVERVIEW

The materials that follow offer a realistic example, albeit hypothetical, of a community-wide planning process. The state of Columbia (the newly added 51st state) was embarking upon its initial statewide health plan. Since the state had no previous experience with health planning, the process had to be established from the ground up. The initiative was to be spearheaded by the newly-formed Office of Health Planning and Development (OHPD) within the state Department of Health.

PLANNING FOR PLANNING

The first step in the planning process was to establish the mission for this component of the Department's activities. In this case, the mission was established by the state Department of Health in consultation with the governor's office and other relevant state agencies. The mission as formulated was: The Office of Health Planning and Development will establish a comprehensive plan for the coordination of all public and private healthcare organizations in the State with the intent of providing accessible, high quality care to all of the State's citizens.

The next step involved establishing a planning team for carrying out the mission. A process was established by OHPD for soliciting recommendations for planning team participants. Guidelines were provided to assure that representatives of all stakeholders were included. Membership was to include not only health professionals but also adequate representation by consumer groups and patient advocates. It also called for the inclusion of "neutral" individuals who possessed technical expertise in the areas of healthcare administration, information management, clinical areas, and public health, among others. The staff of OHPD was to provide technical support for the project.

An outline of the planning process was developed that indicated the procedures that would be followed, the roles of the various participants, and a time frame for completing the plan. This outline would serve as the basis for the project plan that would ultimately be developed.

INITIAL INFORMATION GATHERING

The information gathering process began with the compilation of existing materials on healthcare in the state. Since this was the first planning initiative, little planning-specific material was expected to be available. However, the Department of Health had begun reporting vital statistics, collecting utilization data from hospitals, and compiling inventories of various health professionals. This information served as a starting point for data collection and as a basis for identifying data gaps that would be filled during the intensive research phase.

The next step was to conduct interviews with a wide range of key informants who held a perspective on various aspects of the system. A general outline for information gathering was established, with the intent of identifying the key issues and the most pressing health-related needs. Representatives of the various government agencies that were involved in any way with healthcare were included. In addition to Department of Health staff, these informants included representatives of the state mental health agency, the alcohol and drug bureau, the traffic safety bureau, the environmental protection office, the Department of Children's Services, the insurance regulation office, and the Medicaid office. The information from these informants was supplemented by representatives of local health departments.

Additional interviews were conducted with representatives of private sector healthcare organizations. These included representatives of the major general and specialty hospitals, allied health personnel, and alternative therapists. Professional organizations were represented by spokespersons for the statewide hospital association, nursing home association, home health association, medical society, and dental society. Interviews were conducted with representatives of the two medical schools in the state, as well as officials with selected nursing schools.

Interviews were conducted with representatives of voluntary associations and consumer groups. Either the statewide office or the most active of the chapters of the Cancer Society, Heart Association, and other voluntary organizations were tapped for information. Consumer groups representing the mentally ill, the disabled, the elderly, and other relevant groups were interviewed.

Interviews were also conducted with representatives of the business community, including the Chamber of Commerce, major employers, and local business coalitions.

Once these interviews were completed and the information compiled, it was possible to begin identifying the issues and considering the direction that the planning initiative would take. The issue that appeared to be the most pervasive centered on the lack of access to basic primary care services, particularly for residents of rural areas and impoverished urban areas, although most of the population was at some disadvantage in this regard. Within this context, the specific issues that were identified included: teenage and out-of-wedlock pregnancies, the unmet needs of the severely mentally ill, and chronic disease management for the growing elderly population. Many additional issues were identified and all would be further explored during the research process.

STATING ASSUMPTIONS

As the planning team began to compile information, it formulated the assumptions that would drive the planning process. Since this was a new initiative, there were no explicit assumptions in place. The following assumptions were initially stated, with the notion that they would be revised as appropriate as the process progressed.

1. There are no preconceived notions concerning the goals of the plan or the form that any solution should take.
2. It will be possible to obtain cross-agency cooperation from the various agencies of relevance for the planning process.
3. Private sector organizations will gladly offer input but may be less willing to effect radical changes.
4. The business community is behind the process and is willing to provide a wide range of support services.
5. A lack of adequate information management capabilities is likely to be a major barrier to data collection and processing.
6. Any successful plan implementation will require the support of certain powerful consumer advocacy groups.

BASELINE DATA COLLECTION

The first step in the formal data collection process involved an environmental assessment. Although the focus was to be restricted to the District of Columbia for planning purposes, it was still important to consider national trends that might have implications for developments at the state level.

Broad societal trends were analyzed and their implications for the local environment considered. These societal trends included demographic trends, economic considerations, and lifestyle and consumer attitude trends. The same type of analysis was applied to healthcare industry trends to identify any developments that are likely to affect the local community. These included trends in healthcare financing, changing organizational structures within the delivery system, and the introduction of new treatment modalities.

Regulatory, political, and legal developments were reviewed for their implications for the community and affected organizations. At the state level itself, a number of initiatives were being considered by various agencies and by the state legislature that would have implications for the issues being addressed in the planning process.

Developments in the area of technology were reviewed, including medical and surgical treatment modalities, pharmaceuticals, biomedical equipment, and information management.

National trends in reimbursement were reviewed and the implications for the state considered. Of particular importance were trends in managed care and in government-sponsored insurance programs. The emergence of managed care within the state had already influenced both practice patterns and provider relationships. Potential changes in either the Medicare or Medicaid programs needed to be considered for their impact on the provision of healthcare within the state.

This review of the social, political, economic, and technological trends affecting the environment provided a starting point for subsequent background research and a context in which additional knowledge could be framed.

Profiling the State's Population

In profiling the population to be affected by the plan, it was initially assumed that the state's boundaries appropriately delineated the geographic unit for planning purposes. While this was generally the case, it was found that three health service areas in the state actually crossed state lines. These "irregularities" had to be taken into consideration for planning purposes.

The characteristics of the state and its resident population were determined through the environmental assessment. The main categories of data that were collected are listed below.

✓ *Demographic Characteristics*
    Age distribution
    Sex distribution
    Racial/ethnic distribution
✓ *Sociocultural Characteristics*
    Marital status
    Household characteristics
    Income distribution
    Educational level

Occupational characteristics
Industry characteristics
✓ *Psychographic Characteristics*
✓ *Insurance Coverage*
✓ *Attitudes*
Perceptions
Preferences
Expectations

The data necessary for environmental assessment were obtained from various state agencies, from secondary sources like the Census Bureau, and from commercial data vendors that offer population estimates and projections and psychographic profiles. A general profile of insurance coverage was pieced together using data from various sources. Ultimately, however, primary research had to be conducted to develop better data on insurance coverage and consumer attitudes.

Determining Health Status

The next step in establishing a baseline involved an examination of the health status of the community and the target populations identified. Information was collected on fertility patterns within the community, the target population's morbidity characteristics, and its patterns of mortality. Some data on all three of these categories were available from county health departments, and this information was supplemented by data from the state health department. Fertility and mortality data were relatively easy to acquire since these data are officially compiled by the health department.

Morbidity data, on the other hand, was more difficult to obtain. Except for the collection of data on certain notifiable diseases by the health department, there was no systematic source of data on morbidity. This data gap was approached from a couple of different angles. The first involved the collection of data from those organizations that were most heavily involved in serving the state's population. Data that indicated the types of diagnoses characterizing their patient populations and the types of procedures performed on their clients were obtained from the public hospital and the health department. Information was also available from some of the community-based clinics and mental health centers that serve this population. These steps provided some actual data from which to begin to understand the morbidity profile.

A second approach involved obtaining data from the National Center for Health Statistics that indicated, based on national survey data, the types of health conditions that would characterize populations with various attributes. This survey data could be used to estimate the morbidity profile of the target population. By looking at prevalence rates for the population with certain racial, income, and age characteristics, it was possible to develop a "proxy" profile of the population's morbidity status. Selective information was also available on indicators of morbidity at the state level from various national sources. Indicators of obesity and cholesterol levels, for example, were available from various federally-sponsored surveys.

Health status indicators were subsequently developed that allowed comparisons with various standards. For example, the infant mortality rate was compared to that for other comparable states, to the national average, and to the standards set out in the Healthy People 2010 initiative. The same process was followed for such other relevant indicators as mortality rates, premature and low birth weight births, and teenage pregnancy.

A critical step here was to convert indicators of health status into health service needs. The prevalence of certain conditions could be directly converted into some measure of need; in other cases, the conversion was more indirect. Ultimately, however, the planning team was required to estimate the types and characteristics of the health services required by the state's population.

Health Behavior

The next step in the process involved determining the level of activity for a broad range of health behavior. The following types of formal health behavior were reviewed as part of the research.

✓ *Inpatient Admissions*
  Hospital admissions
  Nursing home admissions
  Residential treatment center admissions
  Mental health facility admissions
✓ *Outpatient Visits*
  Hospital outpatient visits
  Hospital emergency room visits
  Physician office visits
  Other clinician office visits
  Urgent care visits
  Diagnostic center visits
  Surgicenter visits
  Mental health center visits
✓ *Other Service Utilization*
  Home health visits
  Physical therapy treatments
  Alternative therapy visits
✓ *Procedures Performed*
✓ *Prescriptions Written*

Informal types of health behavior were also reviewed, although there was considerably less "hard" data on these activities. Some state-level data were available from national sources on a number of factors such as seat belt use, dietary patterns, and patterns of smoking and alcohol use. Certain other data were available from state records, including information on the use of prenatal care and the level of childhood immunization.

This information was supplemented by primary research that involved a sample survey of the state's population. This survey collected data on health status characteristics and health behavior. In addition, it obtained data on the attitudes, perceptions, and expectations of the state's population.

Community Resources Inventory

For a statewide comprehensive planning effort such as this, a wide range of resources needed to be identified and inventoried. These included, at a minimum, healthcare facilities and equipment, healthcare programs and services, health personnel, and financing options. Examples of the components of each category that were identified include the following.

✓ *Healthcare Facilities*
   Hospitals
   Nursing homes
   Physician offices
   Community clinics
   Nonphysician clinical offices
   Residential treatment centers
   Assisted living facilities (and other residential units for seniors)
   Mental health facilities
   Home health agencies/hospices
   Urgent care centers
   Freestanding diagnostic centers
   Freestanding surgery centers
   Specialty treatment centers (e.g., pain management)
✓ *Healthcare Equipment*
   Biomedical equipment
   Information technology
   Emergency services equipment
✓ *Health Personnel*
   Physicians
   Nurses
   Nurse clinicians, physician's assistants, and other physician extenders
   Dentists
   Optometrists
   Podiatrists
   Chiropractors

Mental health professionals
Rehabilitation therapists (e.g., physical therapists, speech therapists)
Clinical support personnel (e.g., radiology technologists)
Administrative support personnel (e.g., medical records technicians)
Alternative therapists
✓ *Programs and Services*
Inpatient programs/services
Hospital outpatient programs/services
Ambulatory care programs/services
Long-term care services
Community-based services
Home health services
✓ *Funding Sources*
Commercial insurance (including managed care)
Medicare (including Medicare HMOs)
Medicaid
Other federally funded programs (e.g., Veterans Administration)
State funding sources (e.g., mental health services)
Local funding sources (e.g., public hospital subsidy)
✓ *Networks and Relationships*
Formal hospital alliances
Integrated delivery systems
Provider networks
Chain-operated facilities (e.g., hospitals, nursing homes)
Contractual relationships

This process resulted in the establishment of the first inventory of health-care resources in the state, thereby serving an important purpose in its own right. This information was incorporated into a computerized database that would allow for ongoing updating and enhancement as the planning process continued. This inventory was invaluable for the next step in the process, the assessment of the healthcare situation across the state.

ASSESSING HEALTH STATUS AND HEALTHCARE RESOURCES

At this point, a gap analysis was conducted to determine the extent of the mismatch between identified health problems and the resources available. The healthcare needs of the population identified were compared to the types, levels, and characteristics of the resources available across the state. Thus, the number of hospital beds required for the population was compared to the number of beds in operation.

The number of physicians needed in various specialty categories was compared to the existing physician pool. The level of behavioral health needs was compared to the behavioral health resources available, and so on for each category of need.

It was important to not only examine the existing relationship between needs and resources, but also to project this relationship into the future. If the need for a certain service was decreasing, the future availability of that service should be considered. More important, if the need for a service was increasing, the extent to which the services available was also increasing became an issue. In this case, it was found, for example, that the need for services related to the AIDS population and the Alzheimer's population was increasing rapidly, with every indication that these needs would continue to grow in the future. In contrast, there had been only limited expansion in the resources available to meet these needs, and this shortfall had to be considered in the planning process.

SUMMARIZING THE PRELIMINARY ANALYSIS

Enough information was now available to present a state-of-the-state report to the various stakeholders. This report included a comprehensive description of the community environment, a status report on key organizations, and a report assessing the overall status of the community or market area. This status report also included the strengths, weaknesses, opportunities and threats identified during the analysis.

The major conclusions derived from the analysis to this point included the following

✓ The health status of the state's population could be considered "normal" overall.
✓ On the other hand, there were a number of indicators for which the state deviated negatively from national averages.
✓ A number of subgroups could be identified that were well below accepted standards for health status.
✓ A number of issues existed that required immediate attention.
✓ Private sector healthcare resources were highly developed (to the point of experiencing overcapacity).
✓ The public sector was poorly developed statewide; in fact, the "safety net" appeared to be deteriorating.

These generalized conclusions were supported by specific details for each category of healthcare issues. These conclusions became the basis on which subsequent plan development was founded.

DEVELOPING THE PLAN

The effort up to this point provided the foundation for the actual development of the plan. If the initial work was properly carried out, the planning process should flow smoothly, at least from a technical perspective.

A mission statement that had been developed at the outset was reviewed. This step represented an opportunity to clarify the mission of the organization before moving forward with the planning process.

Setting the Goal(s)

Since planning was being conducted for the entire state, a number of goals were identified by the planning team. Separate goals were developed for each of the following areas.

✓ Primary care access
✓ Reproductive health
✓ Chronic disease management
✓ Behavioral healthcare
✓ Lifestyle education
✓ Elder care
✓ HIV/AIDS management

A number of additional goals were considered, and it was determined that this first effort at a state plan should focus on those issues considered the most pressing.

Each of the goals was clearly stated. As an example, the goal related to reproductive issues was stated as: To create an environment that fosters quality reproductive health for all segments of the state's population.

Setting Objectives

For every goal a number of objectives was specified. The objectives for the goal for reproductive issues just stated included the following.

✓ To reduce the infant mortality rate from a state average of 12/1,000 live births to 9/1,000 within five years
✓ To reduce the proportion of births that are premature from 18% to 12% within three years
✓ To reduce the proportion of births that occur to adolescents from 13% to 9% within three years
✓ To reduce the proportion of births that occur out-of-wedlock from 32% to 20% within three years.

For each of these objectives, any barriers to accomplishing the stated objectives were considered. In this case, it was found, for example, that a lack of educational programs on sexual activities available to junior high and high school students would be a significant barrier to reducing teen pregnancies. This was considered a barrier that could be addressed, so the objective was retained.

Prioritizing Objectives

Since it was not possible to achieve all of the identified objectives within a reasonable time period, the prioritization of objectives became necessary. A set of criteria were agreed upon to help determine the order of priority. Among the selected criteria were the following.

> ✓ What are the most urgent issues—issues that will bring about dire consequences if they are not resolved?
> ✓ What are the pivotal issues—issues that contribute most directly to the mission and goals?
> ✓ Which objectives will provide the greatest return for the planning "investment"?
> ✓ Which objectives can be achieved quicker, easier, and less expensively than others?
> ✓ Which objectives will result in the most visible and most tangible results?
> ✓ Which objectives will have the most lasting impact and/or can maintain themselves over time?
> ✓ Which objectives will involve multiple benefits if they are achieved?

With these criteria in mind, it was possible to review the numerous objectives and prioritize them for treatment in the implementation plan. The unanticipated consequences of meeting the various objectives were discussed, and any potentially negative consequences were addressed. Few negative implications were identified but, in the case of reproductive health, there was some concern raised with regard to aggressive efforts at birth control within certain minority populations.

Specifying Actions

Once the objectives were identified, the next step was to specify the actions necessary for carrying out the objectives. For each objective a number of action steps was identified. For the objective of reducing infant mortality, for example, the actions that were identified included the following.

> ✓ Develop a promotional campaign encouraging good health practices during pregnancy.
> ✓ Develop school-based programs that teach healthy lifestyles before, during, and after pregnancy.

✓ Develop materials to be distributed to organizations, clubs, and other groups that interface with high-risk women.

✓ Develop financial incentives and disincentives that discourage additional births to unmarried women.

✓ Develop a monitoring system to assure that all pregnant women obtain adequate nutrition during pregnancy.

IMPLEMENTING THE PLAN

As is often the case, plan implementation turned out to be a greater challenge than plan development. Although the OHPD had the authority to carry out certain actions and to influence the actions of some other entities, it did not have much leverage with most private sector healthcare organizations. Thus, in developing the implementation plan, the focus was on those activities over which OHPD was likely to have the most control.

The first step in plan implementation involved the development of a project plan. The project plan originally developed for the planning process was extended to include the implementation phase. It indicated the sequence of events that must occur and established the critical path for the achievement of each objective.

Further, an implementation matrix was developed using a spreadsheet that laid out who was to do what and when they were to do it. The matrix listed every action called for by the plan, breaking each action down into tasks. For each action or task the responsible party was identified, along with any secondary parties that should be involved in this activity. The matrix indicated resource requirements (in terms of staff time, money, and other requirements) and the start and end dates for each activity. Finally, benchmarks were established that allowed the planning team to determine when the activity had been completed.

Means of Implementation

Two important considerations in preparing for plan implementation dealt with the need for more effective internal communications and the need to present a coordinated effort to address issues in the statewide healthcare environment. A major component of implementation involved the development of internal communication mechanisms among various state agencies. This included agencies directly involved with health issues and those that had some indirect involvement (e.g., traffic safety, drug abuse). The intent here was to assure that all parties had adequate information on needs and resources and that information flowed freely from one component of state government to the next.

This implementation plan relied heavily on the information systems within state government. It came as no surprise, however, that the current information management system could not adequately support this initiative. This led to the initiation of a feasibility study on cross-departmental information systems that would serve a number of purposes besides communicating on healthcare issues.

The other implementation initiative involved developing more formal relationships with agencies outside of state government, including private sector providers. This was to begin with a period of general discussions or a "get to know you" phase, followed by more formal attempts at data sharing and coordination of activities. The ultimate goal was to develop a statewide system of public/private care that assured that no gaps existed in the provision of services to any segment of the population.

THE EVALUATION PLAN

During the early stages of the planning process, an evaluation plan was outlined that involved both process and outcome evaluation. The project's technical support staff constantly monitored the activities that were occurring and submitted regular reports on the extent to which the process was on schedule and the various processional benchmarks were being met.

The objectives that were established during plan development were used as the ultimate outcome criteria, and the extent to which these objectives were met would be the final measure of success. However, since most objectives called for a three- to five-year time frame, it was important that the team's success in meeting intermediate targets be assessed. Thus, the technical staff used the project plan and the implementation matrix as the basis for evaluating interim progress. This ongoing evaluation not only provided a regular source of information for those involved in planning but it also encouraged those charged with carrying out the various steps to act in an expeditious manner.

REVISION AND REPLANNING

It is unlikely that a health plan will be completed without being modified in one way or another. This type of "on-the-fly" revision is inevitable in a rapidly changing environment. There will always be developments that occur subsequently to the initiation of planning that will affect the plan or its implementation. Additional information may become available during the course of the plan. Various parties may take actions in anticipation of the plan that have implicatioins for the process and plan implementation. Developments may occur that affect resource requirements.

Ideally, each component of the planning process should be revisited with these concerns in mind. All assumptions should be reviewed along with the mission statement. Baseline data should be updated to account for the time lapse since the planning process was initiated. The strategy chosen should be reviewed to determine if it is still the best approach in view of possible changes in the environment. For example, has the collaborative strategy selected failed due to unanticipated turnover on the part of key officials? The goals and objectives should be revisited to assure that they are still appropriate in the light of any changes in either the internal or external environment.

The process should have the flexibility to adapt to developments that occur during the course of plan development and implementation. Planners must remain open to these developments and realize that planning is an iterative process that will be constantly reshaped by a wide range of factors.

1B

Community Health Planning Initiative

OVERVIEW

Metro County Government has established a Department of Health Policy (DHP) that is charged with coordinating the provision of primary care to the medically indigent population within the county. In order to carry out its mission, a plan of action was required. DHP staff initiated a process that would allow for the development of a comprehensive approach to meeting the healthcare needs of the community's medically indigent. Since "medically indigent" was defined in the DHP mission statement as those enrolled in the Medicaid program, those without any form of health insurance, and those whose insurance does not provide an adequate level of coverage, these populations were the target for the planning initiative.

PLANNING FOR PLANNING

The first step in planning for planning was to identify the various public sector agencies that were involved in the provision of health services to the medically indigent. Key individuals involved with these organizations were identified and tapped for participation. Any organizations within the private sector that were providing health services to the medically indigent were also identified. These

345

included hospitals that provided a significant level of charity care, community-based health clinics, and the major community mental health centers, among others. Community physicians who serve a primarily indigent population were identified as well.

DHP established a planning task force that involved representatives of the above groups. Two DHP staff persons were assigned to provide technical support to the task force. An expert on health services research in the community was identified and engaged as a consultant to provide external oversight to the project. The task force reviewed the DHP mission statement, established an outline of the process to be followed during the planning initiative, made initial assignments to subcommittees, and laid out a tentative timetable for the planning process.

INITIAL INFORMATION GATHERING

Although some preliminary information had been collected prior to establishing the task force, another phase of information gathering was initiated once the task force was in place. The task force itself was a good place to start, since it represented the key stakeholders with regard to the medically indigent. Interviews with task force members identified many of the key issues and provided the foundation for developing an outline to be used in interviewing other members of the community.

It was discovered in this initial round of interviews that (1) certain key public officials had not been included, (2) there was more private sector involvement in dealing with this population than originally thought, and (3) several of the truly vulnerable populations were not represented on the task force. Steps were taken to obtain input from representatives from each of these categories in order to round out the task force's understanding of the issues.

The initial data gathering process also involved a review of existing reports, studies, and previously prepared technical papers. The public hospital and the health department had both utilized consultants at various times in the past, and these reports were obtained. Financial audits had been performed on most of the key organizations at one time or another, and this information was obtained as well. The health department had applied for numerous grants, and the data included in these applications was very useful. Information was obtained from several certificate-of-need applications that the public hospital had filed with the state. The local university had, through its healthcare administration program, carried out a number of studies on this population that also provided useful background information.

At the same time, efforts were made to identify any existing databases on the local health system in general and on the medically indigent population in particular. The availability of data from the public hospital, the county health department, the publicly-operated nursing homes, and other local healthcare organizations was determined. Any data resources maintained by local universities were identified, along with data available from community-based clinics and mental health centers. The local offices of the Medicaid program, the Food Stamp program, the state welfare agency, and the state nutritional program were contacted for information. Statewide agencies such as the Department of Health, the Department of Children's Services, the environmental monitoring agencies, and other relevant agencies were contacted to determine the types of data they could make available. Data from these sources were collated, processed, and analyzed by the task force's technical staff.

Numerous conclusions were drawn from this initial round of information gathering. It was determined that the task force did not adequately represent the various stakeholders in the process, and it was subsequently expanded. It was determined that the process was going to be seriously hampered by a lack of solid data on the target population, and additional resources were allocated for primary research. It was also determined that there were between three and five organizations that accounted for the management of most of the medically indigent, and that these organizations should be the focus of the planning initiative.

It was also possible to state some basic assumptions at this point, some of which were derived from the preliminary conclusions above.

✓ There appear to be adequate resources available to meet the basic needs of the medically indigent, but these resources are not efficiently employed.
✓ Information management capabilities must be put into place for the process to be effective.
✓ Private sector organizations are not likely to play a meaningful role in planning for the needs of the medically indigent.
✓ State and federal regulations and actions that are beyond the control of the local community will be a major factor in the ability to plan for this population.
✓ The most effective course of action will be to focus on the key organizations that serve the target population.

These assumptions would, of course, be revisited throughout the process, but they allowed some initial parameters to guide the planning initiative to be set. The task force was now in a position to initiate more formal data collection activities.

BASELINE DATA COLLECTION

The first step in the formal data collection process involved an environmental assessment. Since this was a local initiative, conditions and developments at the national and state level were less important than they might be for other types of planning. Nevertheless, the task force required knowledge of various trends at the national and state levels.

Broad societal trends were reviewed and their implications for the local environment considered. These included demographic trends, economic considerations, lifestyle trends, and consumer attitude trends. Health industry trends were analyzed to identify any developments that were likely to affect the local community. These included trends in reimbursement and changing approaches to public sector delivery systems.

Regulatory, political, and legal developments were of particular importance, since the majority of the citizens for whom planning was taking place were Medicaid enrollees. At the federal and state levels, likely regulatory developments had to be considered. Of particular importance were reimbursement trends for Medicaid services. It was also important to identify any trends in federal or state funding for targeted populations (e.g., the homeless, the working poor) that might have implications for the local planning initiative.

This review of the social, political, economic, and technological trends affecting the environment provided a starting point for subsequent background research and a context in which additional knowledge could be framed.

Profiling the Service Area and Its Population

The characteristics of the community had to be determined as part of the environmental assessment. The analysis initially focused on the total community and then targeted the medically indigent. The categories of data that were collected are listed below.

✓ *Demographic Characteristics*
 Age distribution
 Sex distribution
 Racial/ethnic distribution
✓ *Sociocultural Characteristics*
 Marital status
 Household characteristics
 Income distribution
 Educational level
 Occupational characteristics
 Industry characteristics
✓ *Psychographic Characteristics*
✓ *Financing Characteristics*
 Payor categories
 Insurance coverage
✓ *Attitudes*
 Perceptions
 Preferences
 Expectations

Most of this information was obtained from secondary sources of data. Census Bureau data were used to develop a demographic and sociocultural profile of the community in general and the affected population in particular, supplemented by data generated by commercial data vendors. Data on the payor mix of the resident population was pieced together from a variety of sources to provide a general picture of the population's distribution among the commercial insurance, government insurance, and uninsured categories. This same process was repeated for the areas of the city that were characterized by concentrations of the medically indigent. As this process unfolded, the planners realized that there were significant gaps in existing knowledge with regard to the characteristics of the medically indigent.

Even at this early stage, some conclusions could be drawn relevant for the planning process. First, the location of the medically indigent population was found to be changing; it was becoming less concentrated and more spread among the "normal" population. Second, it was found that the medically indigent did not have the stereotypical characteristics historically associated with this population; they were much more like the general population than had been thought. Third, it was found that the extent of medical indigence was much more widespread than originally thought, particularly when it came to the working poor who had neither private insurance nor Medicaid.

Determining Health Status

The next step in establishing a baseline of knowledge was to examine the health status of the community and the target population. Information was collected on fertility patterns within the community, its morbidity characteristics, and level of mortality. Some data relevant to all three of these categories were available from the county health department, and this was supplemented with data from the state health department. Fertility and mortality data were relatively easy to acquire since these data are officially compiled by the health department.

Morbidity data, on the other hand, were more difficult to acquire. Except for the collection of data on certain notifiable diseases by the health department, there was no systematic source of data on morbidity. This situation was approached from a number of different angles. The first involved the collection of data from those organizations that were most heavily involved with this population. Data were obtained from the public hospital and the health department that indicated the types of diagnoses characterizing their patient populations and the types of procedures performed on their clients. Information was also available from some of the community-based clinics and mental health centers that serve this population. This provided some actual data from which to begin to understand the mortality profile.

A second approach involved obtaining data from the National Center for Health Statistics that indicated, based on national survey data, the types of health conditions that would characterize populations with various attributes. This survey data could be used to estimate the morbidity profile of the target population. By looking at prevalence rates for a population with certain racial, income, and age characteristics, it was possible to develop a "proxy" profile of the population's morbidity status.

A third approach involved the administration of a sample survey within the target population. Respondents from over 500 households were interviewed in an attempt to gain a more "grassroots" understanding of the health problems faced by this population. This primary research understandably slowed down the planning process but turned out to provide invaluable data for the project.

Some other approaches were attempted but with limited success. Mortality data was reviewed to determine if the cause of death might be a useful indicator of morbidity in the population, but this turned out to be unfruitful. An attempt was made to obtain data from the state Medicaid files on the encounters reported for the target population. This turned out to be such a complex process that it was abandoned.

The data collection process on health status offered some additional conclusions to help guide the planning process. First, the target population was not nearly as outside the mainstream of medicine as conventional wisdom held. Most of the medically indigent did have access to basic medical care. The working poor without insurance or Medicaid were the exception; they seemed to have limited access to care. Second, the type of problems characterizing this population were little different from those of the general population. Third, it was reconfirmed that many of the health problems that exist reflect the presence of nonhealth factors in the environment. Health problems stemming from housing conditions, nutritional factors, crime, violence, and drug abuse were much more significant within this population.

Health Behavior

While general patterns of health behavior were identified, the research focused on those indicators of health behavior most relevant for the target population. The following types of health behavior were considered in the research process.

✓ *Inpatient Admissions*
  Hospital admissions
  Nursing home admissions
  Residential treatment center admissions
  Mental health facility admissions
✓ *Outpatient Visits*
  Hospital outpatient visits
  Hospital emergency room visits
  Physician office visits
  Other clinician office visits
  Urgent care visits

    Diagnostic center visits
    Surgicenter visits
    Mental health center visits
✓ *Other service Utilization*
    Home health visits
    Physical therapy treatments
    Alternative therapy visits
✓ *Procedures Performed*

The same sources of data were employed as for health status. Data on utilization were obtained from the public hospital, the health department, and the community-based clinics that maintained good records. In this case, data were also obtained from private sector providers, particularly hospitals, to determine the health behavior patterns of the medically indigent within the context of the overall community. The data collected through the sample survey were invaluable in this regard, since they revealed a great deal about the services that the medically indigent utilize and why they use them. Again, proxy data was applied based on NCHS surveys in order to round out the profile of service utilization.

One of the major findings from this research was that the medically indigent were more like the general public in their utilization patterns than was originally believed. Most preferred to use private physicians when they could, and there appeared to be declining dependence on strictly public sources of healthcare. The differences that were found in health behavior (e.g., the higher use of emergency rooms) reflected access issues more than preferences. A second finding from the primary research confirmed the contention that this population was much less focused on prevention than the general population. While their aspirations were similar to those of the general population, their concern with personal health behavior appeared to lag behind.

Community Resources Inventory

A number of categories of community resources needed to be identified and inventoried. These included healthcare facilities and equipment, healthcare programs and services, health personnel, and financing options, among others. Examples of the components of each category that were identified included the following.

✓ *Healthcare Facilities*
    Hospitals
    Nursing homes
    Physician offices
    Community clinics
    Nonphysician clinical offices
    Residential treatment centers
    Assisted living facilities (and other residential units for seniors)

Mental health facilities
Home health agencies/hospices
Urgent care centers
Freestanding diagnostic centers
Freestanding surgery centers
Specialty treatment centers (e.g., pain management)
✓ *Healthcare Equipment*
Biomedical equipment
Information technology
Emergency services equipment
✓ *Health Personnel*
Physicians
Nurses
Nurse clinicians, physician's assistants, and other physician extenders
Dentists
Optometrists
Podiatrists
Chiropractors
Mental health professionals
Rehabilitation therapists (e.g., physical therapists, speech therapists)
Clinical support personnel (e.g., radiology technologists)
Administrative support personnel (e.g., medical records technicians)
Alternative therapists
✓ *Programs and Services*
Inpatient programs/services
Hospital outpatient programs/services
Ambulatory care programs/services
Long-term care services
Community-based services
Home health services
✓ *Funding Sources*
Commercial insurance (including managed care)
Medicare (including Medicare HMOs)
Medicaid
Other federally-funded programs (e.g., Veterans Administration)
State funding sources (e.g., mental health services)
Local funding sources (e.g., public hospital subsidy)
✓ *Networks and Relationships*
Formal hospital alliances
Integrated delivery systems
Provider networks
Chain-operated facilities (e.g., hospitals, nursing homes)
Contractual relationships

All of these components were important in one way or another, and almost any one of them could have a substantial impact on the system. In particular, the extent to which they were available to the medically indigent had to be determined.

ASSESSING HEALTH STATUS AND HEALTHCARE RESOURCES

Once the community's needs and resources had been identified and inventoried, they could be evaluated. A number of approaches were considered for performing this assessment, and a gap analysis technique was selected for the initial assessment. The needs of the target population that had been identified were compared to the services available. As a result of this process a number of gaps were identified. These included the following:

- ✓ The number of practitioners required to serve the medically indigent population was much greater than the current supply of providers.
- ✓ The providers primarily serving the medically indigent were poorly located with regard to the current residential distribution of this population.
- ✓ The service complement offered by public sector providers serving this population was not appropriate for the current needs of the population.
- ✓ The traditional models for serving this population (e.g., public health, educational) were no longer in keeping with its needs.
- ✓ Access to care, not the ability to pay for it, was the major impediment.

To further assist in the analysis, a health status index was developed for the entire community. Using a number of different indicators of health status, an index number was developed for each ZIP code and each census tract within the county. The health status index allowed the quantification of the level of unmet needs characterizing various parts of the community. It also served as a basis for determining priorities and, eventually, for evaluating the success of the planning initiative.

SUMMARIZING THE PRELIMINARY ANALYSIS

Enough information was now available to present a state-of-the-community report. This report included a comprehensive description of the community and the medically indigent population. This status report also included a review of the local system's strengths, weaknesses, opportunities, and threats identified during the analysis. It included an "issues statement" based on the results of the analysis to this point.

A number of conclusions could be reached at this point, and they informed subsequent planning activities. These conclusions included the following.

- ✓ The medically indigent population was currently much different than it was in the past.
- ✓ The characteristics of the medically indigent were changing, and the population displayed few of the stereotypical traits generally associated with this group.
- ✓ The location of the medically indigent was changing over time, resulting in a mismatch between the locations of service providers and concentrations of the medically indigent.
- ✓ The medically indigents were becoming more similar to the general population over time in terms of their health-related characteristics.
- ✓ Many of the more serious issues related to the medically indigent involved newly-emerging ethnic populations that were not being integrated into the healthcare system.
- ✓ A lack of access was the major impediment to obtaining adequate care, not finances, transportation, knowledge, or any of the other traditional explanations.
- ✓ While the resources available to this population are not totally adequate, a more coordinated system could stretch existing resources much further.
- ✓ It will be increasingly important to take health services to this population, both in social and geographic terms.

At this point planners considered the importance of developing a strategy that would guide the rest of the planning process. It was decided that an integrated delivery system approach would be utilized in an attempt to create efficiencies in the provision of health services to this population. This would involve the integration of various public health functions under one umbrella and the development of critical linkages with private sector providers. Further, it was determined that a heavy outreach component must be included in order to take health services to the population and, at the same time, identify individuals or groups that are falling through the cracks in the system.

DEVELOPING THE PLAN

The effort up to this point provided the foundation for the actual development of the plan. The original mission statement of DHP was reviewed, and it was felt that the approach being taken was in keeping with that mission.

It was now possible to consider the appropriate goal or goals for the organization. In this case, the goal involved the development of a delivery system that assured that all segments of the medically indigent population had adequate access to basic healthcare.

A number of objectives were established subsidiary to this goal. These objectives included the following.

✓ Establishing an integrated public health delivery system within two years
✓ Affecting a redistribution of existing public sector services to more appropriate locations within two years
✓ Establishing a comprehensive database of the community's medically indigent within one year
✓ Developing a mechanism for implementing an aggressive outreach program to this population within two years
✓ Developing an outreach program targeting specific ethnic populations within one year
✓ Formally incorporating participation by at least one of the major private sector providers within one year

As the planning team established the objectives, barriers to accomplishing the stated objectives were considered. The major barrier in this case related to the challenge of merging existing public health organizations involving very different cultures into an integrated system.

At this point, it became necessary to prioritize the objectives, since all could not be accomplished at the same time. Representative questions asked in setting priorities included the following.

✓ What are the most urgent issues—issues that will bring about dire consequences if they are not resolved?
✓ What are the pivotal issues—issues that contribute most directly to the mission and goal?
✓ Which objectives must be addressed as prerequisites for achieving other objectives?
✓ Which objectives will result in the most visible or most tangible results?
✓ Which objectives face the least barriers?
✓ Which objectives will involve multiple benefits if they are achieved?
✓ To what extent is there likely to be a negative response to the achieving of an objective?

The unanticipated consequences of meeting the various objectives were discussed and any potentially negative consequences were addressed. One major consequence that was considered was the reaction of private sector providers if the public sector became more aggressive in attempting to address health problems. This was recognized as a concern but, given the seriousness of the health problems of the medically indigent, it was considered a risk that must be taken.

Once the objectives were identified, the next step was to specify the actions necessary for carrying out the objectives. For each objective a number of action steps was identified. For the objective of developing a database on the medically indigent, for example, the actions that were identified included the following.

- ✓ Acquire data on clients from the key organizations that are involved in providing services to the medically indigent.
- ✓ Engage an information management consultant to assist in designing the database.
- ✓ Develop a community survey mechanism for identifying medically indigent individuals who might not appear in existing databases.

IMPLEMENTING THE PLAN

DHP had limited authority to implement many of the objectives on its own. It would, instead, have to facilitate these activities through other players. In this case, considerable political manipulation was necessary in order to get implementation started.

The first step in plan implementation involved the development of a project plan. The project plan originally developed for the planning process was extended to include the implementation phase. It indicated the sequence of events that must occur and established the critical path for the achievement of each objective.

Further, an implementation matrix was developed using a spreadsheet that laid out who was to do what and when they were to do it. The matrix listed every action called for by the plan, breaking each action down into tasks. For each action or task the responsible party was identified, along with any secondary parties that should be involved in this activity. The matrix indicated resource requirements (in terms of staff time, money, and other requirements) and the start and end dates for each activity. Benchmarks were established that allowed the planning team to determine when the activity had been completed.

THE EVALUATION PLAN

During the early stages of the planning process, an evaluation plan was outlined that involved both process and outcome evaluation. The project's technical support staff constantly monitored the activities that were occurring and submitted regular reports on the extent to which the process was on schedule and the various processional benchmarks were being met.

The objectives that were established during plan development were used as the ultimate outcome criteria, and the extent to which these objectives were met would be the final measure of success. However, since most objectives called for a three- to five-year time frame, it was important that the team's success in meeting intermediate targets be assessed. Thus, the technical staff used the project plan and the implementation matrix as the basis for evaluating interim progress. This ongoing evaluation not only provided a source of constant information for those involved in planning, but it also encouraged those charged with carrying out the various steps to act in an expeditious manner.

REVISION AND REPLANNING

It is unlikely that a health plan will be completed without being modified in one way or another. This type of "on the fly" revision is inevitable in a rapidly changing environment. There will always be developments that occur subsequently to the initiation of planning that will affect the plan or its implementation. Additional information may become available during the course of the plan. Various parties may take actions in anticipation of the plan that have implications for the process and plan implementation. Developments may occur that affect resource requirements.

Ideally, each component of the planning process should be revisited with these concerns in mind. All assumptions should be reviewed along with the mission statement. Baseline data should be updated to account for the time lapse since the planning process was initiated. The strategy chosen should be reviewed to determine if it is still the best approach in view of possible changes in the environment. For example, has the collaborative strategy selected failed due to unanticipated turnover on the part of key officials? The goals and objectives should be revisited to assure that they are still appropriate in the light of any changes in either the internal or external environment.

The process should have the flexibility to adapt to developments that occur during the course of plan development and implementation. Planners must remain open to these developments and realize that planning is an iterative process that will be constantly reshaped by a wide range of factors.

IIA

A Strategic Planning Case Study

OVERVIEW

Southern NeuroScience Center (SNC) is a major specialty practice in the southeastern United States that includes nine neurologists and neurosurgeons. With 55 employees, SNC represented a major business operation. The organization had been highly successful in the traditional healthcare environment but was concerned about its positioning for the future direction of healthcare. SNC had never developed a strategic plan but was now faced with a number of important issues that required some type of framework for decision making.

Although SNC was the dominant provider of "neuro" services in its market (roughly one-fourth of the state), it faced minor but persistent competition from a few other well-established neuro specialists in the community. Further, it was constantly faced with the prospect of national organizations entering the market. SNC was concerned that it had outgrown its existing market area and would be unable to increase its market share in the future. The organization had also made some decisions in previous years that needed to be revisited in the light of new developments in the environment.

The key decision makers in SNC realized that they would require outside resources in order to develop a strategic plan. They did not have the expertise for such an undertaking in house, and there were a number of competing agendas that needed to be isolated from the planning process. SNC already had a relationship with an organization that had performed a financial analysis for them, and this organization was engaged to prepare the strategic plan.

INITIAL INFORMATION GATHERING

The initial steps in the planning process involved preliminary interviews with the practice manager, the business manager, the managing physician, and a representative from both the neurology and neurosurgery components of the organization. The practice manager was identified as the liaison with the consultant. This stage also involved acquiring and reviewing any information that was available on the organization. This included any materials for public distribution (e.g., promotional materials), annual reports, internal documents such as executive committee minutes, any planning reports or analysis that had been previously performed, and the *vitaes* of all the organization's physicians.

This initial stage of information gathering provided an overview of the organization and its position within the market, an indication of the key players within the organization, and some notion of internal decision making and communications.

This process also served to identify the key issues as seen from the perspective of those interviewed and as suggested by a review of existing materials. Some of the issues that were identified at this stage were: declining physician revenues despite increasing workload; continuous agitation between the neurologists and neurosurgeons; an unsatisfactory compensation formula for physician partners; gaps in certain clinical areas; and unproductive and/or poorly located satellite offices. Additional issues were identified, and all of these were considered for future analysis. Potential internal barriers to the planning process were also identified at this time.

A general outline of the planning process was developed in conjunction with the practice manager, and this was presented to the SNC executive committee. This document served as the starting point for the planning process, with the assumption that it would continue to be modified as the process unfolded.

The organization did not have an official mission statement, beyond its intention to provide quality neurological care to the community. It was agreed that a more definitive mission statement would be formulated in the course of the process.

Initial assumptions were also formulated to create some basic parameters for the process. It was assumed, for example, that a joint neurology/neurosurgery practice was the form the organization should take; current relationships with hospitals and other providers were appropriate; little expansion could take place within the current market area; and there were no effective competitors within the market area. It was further assumed that managed care would continue to grow in significance, and major local employers would play an increasingly active role in the management of their employees' health insurance. All of these assumptions, of course, were open to revision as the planning process proceeded.

BASELINE DATA COLLECTION

With this background, it was possible to begin collecting detailed data on the organization and its environment. This process began with an internal audit of the practice and its operations. In addition to previously acquired documents, the consultants obtained detailed financial statements, medical staff policies, personnel policies, and other documents that might provide insights into the organization.

Another round of interviews was conducted involving all of the SNC physicians, the department heads of each of the six departments, and two other individuals who were thought to be particularly knowledgeable about the organization.

A full-scale internal audit was then performed that included a detailed financial analysis, an organizational analysis, a patient profile, and an employee survey. The audit also examined the services that were being offered, the pricing for these services, and the locations at which these services were being provided. It further determined existing utilization patterns for all services and identified trends in these patterns. The customers for the practice were profiled along a number of different dimensions, and referral relationships were identified and assessed. The characteristics of practice personnel were reviewed, and all internal processes were identified and evaluated. Current marketing activities were inventoried.

The operations analysis component of the internal audit involved a review of patient flow and paper flow. It also reviewed internal processes for managing services and for communications. Information systems were reviewed, as were the processes for billing patients and collecting fees.

The internal audit took approximately three weeks to perform. Each of the items mentioned above included a number of subtopics. The consultants worked closely with business and clinical personnel in order to develop this information.

The initial findings from the internal audit were presented as an interim report to the SNC executive committee. Even at this early stage, there were a number of conclusions that could be drawn from the research. Some examples of the conclusions included the following.

✓ The neurosurgeons felt that the neurologists were not carrying their load but were being compensated as if they were.
✓ There was limited communication among the various clinical components and a number of misperceptions had emerged.

✓ None of the physicians was satisfied with the existing compensation formula.

✓ The existing organizational structure reflected the historical situation but was not appropriate for the new healthcare environment.

✓ While SNC employees were satisfied overall, there were certain important areas of concern that were affecting morale and productivity.

✓ There were certain procedures that were not being performed to the extent they should have been.

✓ There was no internal marketing program in place, resulting in frequent patient complaints and public relations problems.

The external audit began with a review of societal trends that were likely to have implications for the practice and/or its market. Demographic trends were reviewed, particularly as they related to the neuro specialties. Trends in lifestyles and consumer attitudes and expectations were considered. The overall economic outlook was examined, since upturns or downturns in the economy may effect utilization and payment capabilities. These same factors were examined at the state level as well.

This planning initiative took place during the period when the Clinton administration was seriously considering healthcare reform legislation. Attention was paid to the potential impact that the enactment of various reform provisions would have on specific components of healthcare, including neurology and neurosurgery.

Health industry trends were carefully reviewed, again with an eye for their impact on the neuro specialties. Of particular interest were the implications of managed care for the reimbursement of neuroscience services. Trends in rehabilitation care were another area of interest to the practice, as was the controversy over back pain treatment.

An analysis of national trends in reimbursement was also considered crucial. This involved a review of reimbursement trends by commercial insurance carriers and, as noted above, managed care plans. Proposed changes in Medicare coverage and reimbursement was also an important topic. Changes in workers' compensation reimbursement and the provision of rehabilitation services also had to be considered. Although there were few state programs that would significantly impact a neuro practice, any state or local developments along these lines were identified.

Recent and emerging technological developments that would impact the provision of neurology and neurosurgery services were identified and evaluated for their implications for the practice.

A thorough analysis of the practice's market area was subsequently undertaken. Beginning with a review of secondary data sources, a complete demographic profile of the market area was established. Available sources of data were also used to determine the health status of the population and its patterns of health behavior. These characteristics of the general population were compared to the characteristics of the practice's patients.

Despite the availability of a reasonable amount of secondary data, the specialized nature of neurological care meant that somewhat less information was available than might have been for more common specialties. For this reason, this project relied more heavily on primary research than many similar planning initiatives might. There were a number of groups for which surveys were conducted. These included the following:

✓ The practice's patients
✓ Competitors' patients
✓ Referring physicians
✓ Nonreferring physicians
✓ Major employers (especially benefits managers)
✓ Key health plans (including managed care)

Personal interviews were also conducted with selected hospital administrators and other key informants who might have an opinion on SNC or the neurological specialties.

A thorough competitive analysis was undertaken as well. This involved the identification and evaluation of all potential competitors with the practice. In this case, the numbers were few and competitors were easily identified. These competing specialists were profiled in terms of practice characteristics, personal demographics, specialty areas (if any), practice volumes, and case mix.

As a result of the primary research conducted, there was also considerable qualitative information available on competitors within the market area. This turned out to be a valuable exercise and revealed that the potential for serious competition was less salient than originally believed. It was found, for example, that the only competing group of any size was in the process of splitting up, that the major individual competitor was planning to leave the area, and that certain other neurologists and neurosurgeons were being forced to limit their practices because of impairments or personal circumstances. This was useful information for the formulation of the plan.

A final component of the research was a locational analysis. Most of SNC's office-based services were developed at the primary site, and most of the hospital care was administered at the market's largest hospital. The practice had maintained three satellite locations for at least two years, and the appropriateness of these sites needed to be reviewed.

It was ultimately concluded that the location of the main office was appropriate and that the hospital relationship was favorable (although other options were not ruled out). It was further determined that two of the satellite operations were not appropriately sited, while one of them was.

Once the market data had been collected and reviewed, a SWOT analysis was performed. This technique was used to identify the strengths and weaknesses of the practice, the opportunities that existed for the practice in its market area (and beyond), and the threats and potential threats found in the market area or as a result of national trends.

The findings from the internal and external audits were reviewed first with the practice manager and the managing physician and, subsequently, with the executive committee. After a review of the findings with the key participants, a strategic planning retreat was scheduled.

The planning retreat—involving all nine physicians, the practice manager and the business manager—was conducted by the consultants. They presented a review of the research methodology and a summary of the findings. A state-of-the-practice report was provided that summarized "who SNC was and what it was doing." The organization's strengths and weaknesses were outlined, and a report on its position within the market was presented. The major issues, as identified during the data collection process, were reviewed and discussed. Opportunities that existed for the organization were outlined, along with threats that might exist.

DEVELOPING THE PLAN

This information provided the basis for formulating the strategic plan. The process started with the specification of the primary goal for the organization. The goal that emerged from the planning retreat read: To become the premier neuroscience practice in the southern half of the state. Once this goal was established, a strategy was adopted. The proposed strategy called for an aggressive program of expansion that involved the addition of new services and staff and the development of a decentralized network of service outlets.

With this goal and strategy in mind, a number of objectives were established in order to support their achievement. These objectives included the following:

✓ Increase the number of staff physicians from 9 to 15 over a three-year period.
✓ Add sports medicine as a product line within one year.
✓ Open one new satellite office per year over the next three years.
✓ Add unique, state-of-the-art diagnostic technology over the next year.
✓ Immediately restructure the governance of the practice to support the type of aggressive initiative being proposed.
✓ Establish a major presence at a second local hospital within one year.

An additional objective that fell into a different category was identified during the planning retreat. This involved a revision of the compensation arrangements for practice physicians. It was agreed that this issue would be addressed independently of the strategic planning process.

The next step was to review the barriers that might exist with regard to any of the objectives. The only serious barrier that was identified involved the relationship with the second local hospital. Upon additional information gathering, the consultants found that a poor past relationship with the hospital would be a major impediment to closer ties Further, the one group that represented any form of competition for SNC was very much in favor at this hospital. This objective was eliminated from the list.

Similarly, the consequences of meeting the various objectives were considered, both positive and negative, intended and unintended. There were few negatives implications for any of the objectives that could be identified. Admittedly, some toes would be stepped on as the practice expanded into other market areas and added new services. This was to be expected and all parties agreed that, in the current competitive environment, ruffled feathers were inevitable. The bottom line called for an aggressive approach that could not take the narrow interests of competing practices into consideration.

The planning team then addressed the prioritization of the remaining objectives. Based on the agreed upon goal and strategy, the highest priority was given to increasing the size of the physician staff to 15 and to setting up additional practice locations. The remaining objectives became second-tier objectives.

For each objective, a number of actions was specified. For the objective related to staff expansion, for example, the following actions were identified:

✓ Establish a screening committee to review all applicants.
✓ Budget funds for the recruitment process.
✓ Identify the specialties that are to be recruited.
✓ Engage a recruitment firm to begin the search.
✓ Prepare office space for the new physicians.

IMPLEMENTING THE PLAN

Once action steps had been identified for all of the objectives, an implementation matrix was created. For each of the dozens of actions that had been identified, the matrix specified the following.

✓ The primary responsible party
✓ Other responsible parties
✓ The effort in terms of time anticipated
✓ A deadline for completion
✓ The necessary resources
✓ Any prerequisites

This matrix essentially determined who was to do what, at what time, and how they were to do it. This was a critical step in the process, without which it was unlikely that many of the actions would have been carried out in a timely fashion.

The preliminary implementation matrix developed at the planning retreat was carried back to be finalized by the practice manager and the managing physician.

The last step in the process carried out at the planning retreat was the creation of a ten-year future scenario for the practice. Given the plan laid out during the session, participants were asked to contribute to the creation of a vision for the future practice. The scenario should envision who would be involved, where the practice locations would be, the types of services that would be offered, and so forth. In the end, the planning team had essentially "invented" the future for SNC. In carrying out the plan that had been developed, they would be responsible for making this scenario an actuality.

The final step in the planning process involved the evaluation component of the project. Using the implementation matrix as the basis, a mechanism was established for tracking the progress of plan implementation over the three-year time period it covered.

IIB

A Case Study in Marketing Planning

OVERVIEW

SouthCoast Institute, a rehabilitation hospital with a historical focus on inpatient services, desired to expand its outpatient capabilities in response to various developments within the environment. This new direction would require considerable reorientation of the staff towards an outpatient mind-set, as well as the establishment of a number of new services.

Among the options for new services was the development of an aquatherapy program to supplement the services currently provided to rehabilitation patients. An aquatherapy program would expand the capabilities of the existing program and make physical therapy possible for a wider range of patients. Since Medicare and most commercial health plans provided reimbursement for aquatherapy services, the program should be a source of additional revenue. It would further serve to differentiate SouthCoast Institute from other providers of rehabilitation services. While aquatherapy services would be utilized by the Institute's hospitalized rehabilitation patients, the intent was to bolster the fledgling outpatient program and attract other clients who were not involved with the hospital's inpatient rehabilitation program.

The decision to develop and market an aquatherapy program was one result of a major strategic planning initiative that was being carried out by SouthCoast Institute. Many of the organizational issues had been handled within the context of the ongoing strategic plan. A planning team was already in place, and a planning framework had been established. The aquatherapy initiative was incorporated as a component of the overall implementation plan. It remained for the staff to develop and implement a marketing plan to support the development of this new program.

INITIAL INFORMATION GATHERING

The initial steps in the information gathering process involved collecting background data on existing aquatherapy programs. Data were compiled on the types of procedures and services offered by most programs, the types of patients typically served, reimbursement prospects, and so forth. A general notion of what was involved in operating an aquatherapy program was developed.

At the same time, a preliminary internal information gathering process was carried out. This focused on the potential for developing the program within the confines of the existing rehabilitation therapy framework. The analysis examined the availability of personnel to provide aquatherapy services, the potential for training additional staff, existing equipment and additional equipment needs, and, perhaps most important, the attitude of the medical staff with regard to this service.

The internal information gathering process uncovered a certified aquatherapist on staff who could serve as the product line champion. There was also a pool of physical therapy aides who, with minimal additional training, could support the aquatherapy program. Although the hospital did not have a therapy pool, existing plans for renovating the rehabilitation facility included the construction of such a pool, along with a regulation-size exercise pool. Further, the medical staff who were primarily involved in referring patients to the Institute were generally supportive and, in some cases, enthusiastic about the prospects of aquatherapy.

BASELINE DATA COLLECTION

These positive findings set in motion the formal data collection process, starting with data on the market potential for this service within the Institute's market area. The number of potential customers, in fact, turned out to be much greater than anticipated. Potential sources of referral were identified and subsequently interviewed concerning their interest. Local health plans were contacted to determine their willingness to reimburse for this service, and aquatherapy programs in other markets were identified and contacted for their input.

Several secondary target audiences were identified that, while contributing no major revenue streams, would increase utilization of the pools and perhaps contribute to some fixed costs. These included community groups, swim teams, social service programs, and even a "commercial" audience of water aerobics customers who could be expected to pay a fee for use of the facility. Employees of the Institute were also queried with regard to their interest in using these facilities as part of the employee fitness program.

A competitive analysis was conducted, and it was determined that no medically-supported aquatherapy was being offered within the community. Options for interim use of existing area pools were explored, and a suitable temporary site was identified for piloting the program. Preliminary financial statements were prepared to provide an estimate of the potential profitability of the service.

When the potential barriers were examined, few if any were found to exist. The only barrier identified was a lack of knowledge about aquatherapy in the community (even among some medical practitioners). No inherent resistance was identified from any segment of the community.

DEVELOPING THE PLAN

With this background data indicating significant potential for a successful and profitable service, the planning team set a goal of establishing the Institute's program as the premier aquatherapy program in the region. In terms of strategy, the team decided that an approach that emphasized education and relationship-building was appropriate. The intent was to stay away from aggressive advertising and flashy promotions.

In support of this goal, the following objectives were established:

✓ Create and implement a comprehensive internal marketing program for aquatherapy within six months.

✓ Directly contact all potential referrers outside the Institute and its affiliates within six months.

✓ Recruit and train a marketing/liaison person to work with the aquatherapy program on a full-time basis within six months.

✓ Identify and contact within six months all community groups that might potentially benefit from the standard swimming pool and the aquatherapy pool.

✓ Integrate aquatherapy services into the sports medicine and occupational medicine programs within one year.

With these objectives in mind, a number of actions were identified. The following marketing-related actions were included:

✓ Create promotional material for distribution to potential referral agents.
✓ Set up meetings with relevant internal parties (including medical staff) to explain the program.
✓ Identify an appropriate person to train for liaison with the community.
✓ Identify any appropriate external targets for promotional and educational activities.

The fact that the program was new and unique in the area guided the development of the marketing plan. The appropriate message to be delivered was formulated and the means of spreading it were determined.

In keeping with the educational/relationship-building approach, the marketing mix focused on low-key promotional activities and avoided high-profile media techniques. For internal marketing, the plan included a newsletter, internal publications, a flyer in each Institute employee's paycheck, posters, special information sessions for staff and referring physicians, and a videotape to explain the program. For external audiences, the plan called for a newsletter, press releases (and other media coverage as appropriate), print advertising (probably limited to the *Yellow Pages*), limited electronic media (for the grand opening), videotape, exhibits (e.g., schools, health fairs), and public presentations (support groups, medical society, voluntary health associations).

An implementation plan was developed as part of the marketing plan that identified the resources needed, the required financial commitment, the responsible parties for the various tasks, and timelines for all activities. The SouthCoast program director was given primary responsibility for implementing the plan. The physical therapist with the aquatherapy certification would assist the program director.

An evaluation procedure was put into place to assess the progress of the program. Since it was a start-up operation, it would be easy to track the volume of services utilized. The plan also called for a pretest and post-test to be administered to referral agents to determine the extent to which they were made aware of the program. Satisfaction surveys were to be developed for administration to patients and referrers. The extent to which the program generated secondary benefits in the community (e.g., with community groups, schools, swim clubs) would be tracked and periodically reported.

IIC

A Case Study in Business Planning

OVERVIEW

A clinical psychologist had formulated an innovative program for the treatment of certain types of eating disorders. The program represented a unique approach and appeared to have substantial potential in the healthcare marketplace. The program's approach was predicated upon the fact that many cases of eating disorders could be attributed to a history of sexual abuse.

In order to initiate the program, external funding would be required. A business plan was developed as a basis for seeking investors and as a means of guiding project development. The following sections represent an abbreviated version of the business plan, since the full text would be inappropriately long for appendix material.

Eating disorders are an increasingly prevalent health condition in the United States. They were labeled the "disease of the 1980s" but the estimated size of the problem continued to grow through the 1990s. Research now indicates that between 3 percent and 10 percent of the female population in the United States is affected by anorexia or bulimia at any one time and perhaps as many as 40 percent over their lifetimes. It is further estimated that 30 percent of college women suffer from some form of eating disorder and that 10 percent of high school girls are anorexic. The exact prevalence is difficult to determine, however, since many individuals suffering from eating disorders, especially men, are reluctant to admit their condition. However, even at the lowest identified rates, there are an estimated one million women in the United States suffering from an eating disorder at any given time.

Similarly, sexual abuse is also prevalent in the United States. Recent studies have shown that one out of every three women will have been abused by the time she reaches adulthood. As with eating disorders, there may be many more cases of undiagnosed sexual abuse. This is particularly the case with men in our society, among whom both of these conditions are more common than was thought in the past.

It now appears that there is a strong connection between eating disorders and a history of sexual abuse. An estimated one-fourth to one-third of adult females in the United States are thought to have suffered from childhood sexual abuse. Of individuals identified with eating disorders researchers and therapists report from 50 percent to 90 percent have suffered from sexual abuse as children. Despite these startling figures, there are virtually no treatment programs that take the interrelationship between these two conditions into consideration.

THE PROPOSED PROGRAM

This business plan describes a residential program that offers an innovative therapy approach for individuals suffering from eating disorders, sexual abuse symptomatology or, typically, a combination of both. Many individuals may suffer from one or the other of these conditions (eating disorders or sexual abuse) but may not realize the connection with the other. Unless they enter a program such as this, the relationship between the two conditions may not be discovered.

A residential program offers a cost-effective alternative to traditional inpatient programs. Hospitalization for six weeks typically costs $30,000 or more. While some insurance programs will cover a portion of these charges, many do not. Individuals are often left owing large amounts. Not only would a residential program be less expensive than inpatient care, but it also promises to be more effective than existing hospital-based programs.

PROGRAM GOALS

The mission of the proposed project involves the development of a demonstration program for the treatment of individuals with eating disorders that may be related to a history of sexual abuse. The following goals and objectives have been identified:

Short-Term Goals

Goal 1: To establish the innovative treatment program as a therapeutically and financially viable operation

Goal 2: To publicize this form of treatment in order to gain attention and support for the program

Long-Term Goals

Goal 1: To establish a residential therapy center dedicated to the effective treatment of individuals suffering from eating disorders and sexual abuse using an approach that is sensitive to the relationship between these two conditions

Goal 2: To refine our understanding of the linkage between eating disorders and sexual abuse and subsequently improve the therapeutic techniques available

Goal 3: To develop a foundation for promoting the concepts and techniques of this form of eating disorder therapy on a national basis and expanding the program on a franchise basis

Examples of objectives developed pursuant to the short-term goal of establishing the treatment program as a therapeutically and financially viable operation include the following:

✓ Acquire and adapt a suitable facility for initial services within six months.

✓ Identify and negotiate with potential staff to complement existing personnel within three months.

✓ Acquire all licenses, permits and certificates within three months.

✓ Negotiate and finalize the contract for program management services within three months.

✓ Identify and contact the major sources of referrals to the program within four months.

THE POTENTIAL MARKET

For planning purposes, it is assumed that the county in which the treatment center will be located is the primary market area. The surrounding medical trade area will be considered the secondary service area. The primary market area includes around 870,000 inhabitants. The metropolitan area (five counties) includes a million residents, and along with the remainder of the surrounding medical service area contains a resident population of approximately two million.

Since there is no consensus on the exact prevalence of either eating disorders or sexual abuse and even less precise prevalence figures on the two combined, it is difficult to generate precise market estimates. However, based on national figures for sexual abuse alone, it is estimated that in the primary market area there are over 38,000 females between the ages of 21 and 39 who have experienced sexual abuse as children. If one considers the population that is believed to be afflicted with eating disorders, another 5,200 college-aged females fall into this category, along with nearly 5,000 high school-aged residents. Thus, if only females in certain age groups who have experienced childhood sexual abuse and females in certain age groups who are thought to have eating disorders are counted, the potential market in the primary market area alone amounts to approximately 50,000 individuals. Viewed another way, if 20 percent of the female population aged 15 to 39 years had either an eating disorder or a history of sexual abuse, the potential market would equal 34,000 individuals. Based on a reasonable ratio of male to female prevalence, an additional 8,000 to 10,000 males could be added to this number.

These approximations of the local market should be adjusted to reflect certain characteristics of the local population. Because of the expense of treatment for eating disorders, few people without health insurance or the ability to pay for treatment out of pocket can be expected to participate in the typical program. Further, nonwhites historically have not been attracted to this type of program. To be very conservative, one might adjust the potential market to reflect the importance of low-income and/or nonwhite populations within the primary service area. In addition, the program may want to restrict its clients to certain age ranges and, for the residential program, to women. After adjustment, there should still be a market in the range of 25,000 to 30,000 patients.

It would not be unreasonable to add an additional potential patient population of 10,000 individuals (unadjusted for demographic characteristics) in the remainder of the metropolitan area and another 10,000 unadjusted potential patients from the medical service area outside of the primary market area. Thus, even if these figures turn out to be overstated, it is clear that an adequate market for this type of program exists in the market area.

EXISTING TREATMENT APPROACHES

Many professionals are beginning to realize that each eating disorder, as well as each patient, should be treated as a unique case. Outpatient treatment generally entails individual psychotherapy but may also involve the family, especially in the case of the younger patient. It is important that the underlying patterns of interaction are recognized and that the family accept help in changing them.

Hospitalization is usually required when weight loss has reached a danger level—about 25 percent or more below normal weight. In most cases, weight can be restored by a combination of psychotherapy and learning new eating behavior patterns. Weight gain alone will not solve the problem. The underlying issues must be dealt with; otherwise, quite often people with eating disorders comply with the hospital rules until they gain enough weight to be released and then immediately return to serious dieting and weight loss.

Although a number of weight management programs have been developed and marketed nationally, no nationwide effort exists with regard to eating disorders in general and the eating disorder/sexual abuse syndrome in particular. There are a few programs in the market area that purport to deal with eating disorders. However, eating disorder treatment is not highly developed, and no existing program emphasizes treatment that takes past sexual abuse into consideration. While a variety of programs offer treatment for sexual abuse, eating disorder syndromes are typically not targeted by these programs.

Currently, no inpatient program is operating within the market area, nor are there any residential treatment programs for these types of problems. The only inpatient program to be offered in the area was discontinued in the 1980s due to poor reimbursement for inpatient care. None of the existing outpatient programs appear to have captured a significant share of the market. It is difficult to assess the quality, acceptance, or success rate for the existing programs because they have operated sporadically with little follow-up on their patients.

EXISTING FINANCING MECHANISMS

Historically, eating disorders have not been widely covered by insurers. Typically only the larger insurance carriers (e.g., Prudential, Equitable, and Metropolitan) have provided this sort of coverage and, when provided, it is almost exclusively through employer-sponsored plans. A review of existing practices has indicated very limited reimbursement locally for the treatment of eating disorders. Coverage for treatment of past sexual abuse is sometimes available, but reimbursement is often difficult to justify. Neither eating disorder treatment nor sexual abuse treatment is routinely covered under most health plans.

Hospital-based programs have had difficulty admitting patients for treatment of eating disorders because of the paucity of coverage. One approach has been to obtain a diagnosis of depression and use this as a basis for admission. Even so, it is unlikely that many health plans will cover inpatient care for these conditions in the future.

The reimbursement situation suggests that out-of-pocket payments will be the primary source of revenue for a program such as this. The financial analysis assumes that 80 percent of the program's revenues will come directly from patients and their families. This is fairly typical for programs of this nature and, considering the socioeconomic status of many of the affected, it is not unreasonable to anticipate an adequate market willing to pay out of pocket.

Discussions have been held with the major health insurance carriers in the market area, and there does appear to be general support for a cost-effective and efficacious program that would address eating disorders and their underlying causes. As it stands, insurers are often reimbursing enrollees for expensive stomach stapling surgery and/or other resource-intensive attempts at weight control. It appears that any evidence of success may open the doors to a greater willingness to provide insurance benefits for the program. The state Workers' Compensation program also appears to be another possible source of reimbursement, given the cost to employers of workers who suffer from these problems. This has been a source of coverage in other states, and the possibility is being explored with regard to this project.

EXISTING REFERRAL SOURCES

Individuals follow a variety of routes in entering eating disorder treatment programs. The most common referral patterns involve primary care physicians who immediately recognize an eating disorder and/or sexual abuse problem and make a referral to an appropriate program (if they can find one). Often, primary care physicians attempt to treat such patients and, after limited success, refer them to a more appropriate resource. Mental health providers are another source of referrals. Many of them are not prepared to treat either eating disorders or sexual abuse and are willing to refer their patients to experts in these areas.

Many other referrals can be expected from counselors, social workers and other professionals who come into contact with individuals experiencing these problems but who do not have the resources to manage the patients. Another large group of patients is expected to be self-referred. Many of these patients will have obtained treatment for their condition without any measurable improvement. These conditions are such that affected individuals will go to great lengths to obtain any treatment that holds promise.

The program director is well positioned to capitalize on the major sources of referrals. She is well known within the behavioral health community and has extensive contacts among both private and public providers of mental health services. She is also well connected within the physician community, not only through family members but through previous services she has provided for referring physicians.

PROGRAM STRUCTURE

The proposed program would treat patients in a residential setting, rather than the traditional hospital setting. In the residential program, participants will stay for a period of three months followed up by three months of aftercare. Participants will be encouraged to receive ongoing support through Overeaters Anonymous meetings and/or incest survivor groups when appropriate. During the three-month period of residence, patients will be encouraged to begin part-time work or attend school as they become ready.

Treatment includes individual counseling, group therapy, education seminars, behavior modification, meditation, family group therapy, exercise physiology, nutritional counseling, body image exercises, and psychodrama. All patients will be treated as unique individuals, each going through his or her own process of recovery. Because this treatment program has an emphasis on sexual abuse, it is important that this issue is handled properly.

PROGRAM PERSONNEL

The residential program will be under the direction of a program director as well as a medical director. Clients entering the program will be assigned to a treatment team. The team will consist of a physician, a social worker, a psychologist, a nutritionist, and a nursing staff member. The treatment team will be responsible for developing a written treatment plan for each client.

Most of the initial staff are already involved with the program director at one level or another. The program could begin immediately with limited need to hire additional staff. However, potential staff members will be identified and held in reserve until their employment becomes necessary.

MARKETING PLAN

Much of the work on the initial marketing plan for the program has already been completed. This work includes: refining the understanding of local, regional, and national demand; adjusting these figures for various modifying factors to arrive at the effective demand; identifying and evaluating existing potentially competing programs; determining the share of the market that could potentially be captured and relating that to the eating disorders program threshold for success; and collecting the additional data required to clearly delineate the market and the manner in which it is being served. This would certainly include a study of existing attitudes and perceptions of patients and potential patients with regard to existing programs and treatment approaches.

In recruiting clients, the priority would be placed on individuals who have insurance coverage for eating disorders. Secondarily, those with the ability to pay out of pocket for these services will be targeted. However, this emphasis is primarily to ensure the financial viability of the program and does not seek to exclude any individual in need of these services. As cash flow warrants, individuals with less ability to pay will be targeted by the program, with their expenses being subsidized by better paying patients or, alternatively, subsidized by outside funds.

A separate marketing plan component will be developed for each of the target populations, since the respective target markets require different approaches. The discussion of marketing mix will describe the different types of marketing appropriate for the various targets.

During the planning process decisions must be made with regard to the promotional mix that will be utilized. The use of a variety of approaches is envisioned, and the list of options must be refined and prioritized. The budget available for promotions will probably be a factor in the promotional mix and vice versa. The options currently being considered include the following.

✓ *Establishing Referral Relationships*
Medical/social services
Employers/employer alliances
Insurers
✓ *Community Outreach*
Public service announcements
Community presentations
Health fairs
✓ *Professional Participation*
Presentations at conferences
Displays at conferences
✓ *Direct mail*
Potential referrers
Individuals
✓ *Media Advertising*
Traditional print media
Radio
Television
Yellow Pages
✓ *Newsletter Production*
✓ *Video/audiotape Production*

Regardless of the eventual promotional mix, a variety of promotional materials must be prepared. At a minimum, tasteful brochures must be developed. There should probably be at least two different brochures, one for potential referrers and one for individuals. This will entail some creative input and technical production expenses. A logo should be developed and thought given to stylistic factors that will be interwoven throughout the material.

The use of a marketing consultant will be necessary, at least in the early stages of program development, in order to contribute to marketing planning. A marketing consultant who specializes in healthcare has been identified to provide this support. It is also possible that the affiliated hospital will be able to provide some marketing support once the program is underway.

RESOURCE REQUIREMENTS

The appendix (not included) provides a detailed listing of the resource requirements necessary for startup and operations. This section covers information on facilities requirements, furnishings and equipment, personnel, materials and supplies, overhead costs, and marketing resources.

LEGAL CONSIDERATIONS

A number of legal issues must be dealt with in establishing and operating the residential treatment center. Although a state certificate-of-need is not required, a number of licenses and certificates are required by the state and local authorities. Further, issues related to patient confidentiality, malpractice, and liability considerations must be addressed.

An attorney with extensive background in this type of project has been involved from the idea's inception. He will continue to provide ongoing input in his areas of expertise as the project progresses.

FINANCIAL ANALYSIS

Detailed financial statements are provided in the appendix (not included), including five-year pro forma statements. These documents detail sources of revenue and expenses for start-up and the first five years of operations. As indicated from this supplementary material, minimal market penetration could generate significant program volume. Even with pricing well below traditional inpatient fees, this represents a significant business opportunity.

DEVELOPMENT SCHEDULE

The appendix (not included) also includes a detailed project plan that outlines start-up requirements and carries the program through the first five years of operation. The project plan includes detail on responsibilities, resource requirements, task sequencing, and benchmarks that will be used to measure progress.

APPENDIX MATERIALS

The following sections are included in the appendix (but not reproduced here).

- ✓ Description of proposed facility (including floor plans)
- ✓ Resumes and qualifications of program director and other key personnel
- ✓ Qualifications of the management consultant
- ✓ Financial statements
- ✓ Project plan
- ✓ Detailed marketing plan

Index

Health Services Planning
Second Edition